T0324991

Paternal Influences on Human Reproductive Success

Paternal Influences on Human Reproductive Success

Douglas T. Carrell, PhD
Department of Obstetrics and Gynecology, Department of Human Genetics, and the
Andrology and IVF Laboratories at University of Utah School of Medicine,
Salt Lake City, Utah, USA

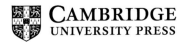

CAMBRIDGE
UNIVERSITY PRESS

University Printing House, Cambridge CB2 8BS, United Kingdom

One Liberty Plaza, 20th Floor, New York, NY 10006, USA

477 Williamstown Road, Port Melbourne, VIC 3207, Australia

314-321, 3rd Floor, Plot 3, Splendor Forum, Jasola District Centre, New Delhi - 110025, India

79 Anson Road, #06-04/06, Singapore 079906

Cambridge University Press is part of the University of Cambridge.

It furthers the University's mission by disseminating knowledge in the pursuit of
education, learning and research at the highest international levels of excellence.

www.cambridge.org
Information on this title: www.cambridge.org/9781107024489

First published 2013

A catalogue record for this publication is available from the British Library

Library of Congress Cataloging in Publication data
Paternal influences on human reproductive success / [edited by] Douglas T. Carrell, Ph.D., Andrology and IVF Laboratories,
Department of Surgery (Urology), Department of Obstetrics and Gynecology, Department of Human Genetics, University
of Utah School of Medicine, Salt Lake City, Utah, USA.
   pages   cm
Includes bibliographical references and index.
ISBN 978-1-107-02448-9
1. Infertility, Male – Social aspects.   I. Carrell, Douglas T.
RC889.P32   2013
616.6´921–dc23

2012038443

ISBN 978-1-107-02448-9 Hardback

....

This book is dedicated to my family, who is always supportive of my small efforts to expand our understanding of infertility and assisted reproduction and improve our therapies for infertile couples.

Contents

Color plates are to be found between pp. 116 and 117.

Contributors

Naif Al-Hathal MD
McGill University, Royal Victoria Hospital,
Department of Surgery, Division of Urology,
Montreal, Quebec, Canada.

Kenneth I. Aston PhD, HCLD
University of Utah School of Medicine,
Department of Surgery, Division of Urology,
Andrology & IVF Laboratories, Salt Lake City,
Utah, USA.

Marc A. Beal BSc, MSc
University of Regina, Department of Biology, Regina,
Saskatchewan, Canada.

Lars Björndahl MD, PhD
Karolinska University Hospital, Centre
for Andrology and Sexual Medicine,
Andrology Laboratory, Huddinge,
Stockholm.

Jens Peter Bonde MD, PhD
Copenhagen University, Bispebjerg Hospital,
Department of Occupational and Environmental
Medicine, Copenhagen, Denmark.

William O. Brant MD, FACS
University of Utah School of Medicine, Department
of Surgery, Division of Urology
Salt Lake City, Utah, USA.

Douglas T. Carrell PhD, HCLD
University of Utah School of Medicine, Department of
Surgery, Andrology and IVF Laboratories,
Department of Obstetrics and Gynecology,
Department of Human Genetics, Salt Lake City,
Utah, USA.

Chiara Chianese MS
University of Florence, Department of Clinical
Physiopathology, Sexual Medicine and Andrology
Unit, Florence, Italy.

Donald F. Conrad PhD
Washington University School of Medicine,
Department of Genetics, Department of Pathology &
Immunology, St. Louis, Missouri, USA.

Simon L. Conti MD
Stanford University School of Medicine, Department
of Urology, Stanford, California, USA.

Jessie Dorais MD
University of Utah School of Medicine, Department of
Obstetrics and Gynecology, Salt Lake City, Utah, USA.

Michael L. Eisenberg MD
Stanford University School of Medicine, Department
of Urology, Male Reproductive Medicine and Surgery,
Department of Obstetrics and Gynecology, Stanford,
California, USA.

Harry Fisch MD
New York Presbyterian Hospital, Weill Cornell
Medical College, Urology and Reproductive Medicine,
New York, New York, USA.

John R. Gannon MD
University of Utah School of Medicine, Department
of Surgery, Division of Urology, Salt Lake City,
Utah, USA.

Aleksander Giwercman MD, PhD
Lund University, Skåne University Hospial Malmö,
Reproductive Medicine Centre, Malmö, Sweden.

Ahmad O. Hammoud MD, MPH
University of Utah School of Medicine, Department
of Obstetrics and Gynecology, Division of
Reproductive Endocrinology and Infertility, Salt Lake
City, Utah, USA.

David Iles BSc, PhD
University of Leeds, Faculty of Biological Sciences,
Institute for Integrative and Comparative Biology,
West Yorkshire, Leeds UK.

Csilla Krausz MD, PhD
University of Florence, Department of Clinical
Physiopathology, Sexual Medicine and Andrology
Unit, Florence, Italy.

Oumar Kuzbari MD
University of Utah School of Medicine, Department of
Obstetrics and Gynecology, Division of Reproductive
Endocrinology and Infertility, Salt Lake City,
Utah, USA.

Cristina Joana Marques PhD
University of Porto (FMUP), Faculty of Medicine,
Department of Genetics, Portugal.

David Miller BSc, PhD
University of Leeds, Faculty of Medicine and Health,
Leeds Institute for Genetics, Health and Therapeutics,
Division of Reproduction and Early Development,
West Yorkshire, Leeds, UK.

Jeremy B. Myers MD
University of Utah School of Medicine, Department of
Surgery, Division of Urology, Salt Lake City, Utah, USA.

Queenie V. Neri BSc
The Ronald O. Perelman and Claudia Cohen Center
for Reproductive Medicine, Weill Cornell Medical
College, New York, New York, USA.

Gianpiero D. Palermo MD, PhD
The Ronald O. Perelman and Claudia Cohen Center
for Reproductive Medicine, Weill Cornell Medical
College, New York, New York, USA.

Zev Rosenwaks MD
The Ronald O. Perelman and Claudia Cohen Center
for Reproductive Medicine, Weill Cornell Medical
College, New York, New York, USA.

Denny Sakkas PhD
Boston IVF Inc., Waltham, Massachusetts, USA.

Heide Schatten MD
University of Missouri-Columbia, Department
of Veterinary Pathobiology, Columbia, Missouri,
USA.

Christopher M. Somers BSc, MSc, PhD
University of Regina, Department of Biology, Regina,
Saskatchewan, Canada.

Mário Sousa MD, PhD
University of Porto and Centre for Reproductive
Genetics Alberto Barros, UMIB, Institute of
Biomedical Sciences Abel Salazar (ICBAS), Lab of Cell
Biology, Porto, Portugal.

Qing-Yuan Sun PhD
Chinese Academy of Sciences, Institute of Zoology,
State Key Laboratory of Reproductive Biology, Beijing,
China.

Armand Zini MD
McGill University and St. Mary's Hospital, Royal
Victoria Hospital, Department of Surgery, Division of
Urology, Montreal, Quebec, Canada.

Preface

One theme that draws abundant attention from the world's press is the theory of the imminent demise of human males. Whether it be due to reports of a "degenerating Y chromosome," advances in cloning technologies, the theory of an "ultimate revenge of women," or some combination of the three scenarios, the public seems to relish a sensational account of the impending extinction or irrelevance of the male. This book is not such an account. Indeed, the objective of this book is to summarize and explore the recently growing emphasis on the paternal role in reproductive fitness.

It is interesting that a book emphasizing the role of the male gamete in reproduction is necessary. While the necessity of sperm for normal reproduction has been known since the studies of Spallanzani, the role that the sperm play in forming a normal embryo has not been clear, and in fact is evolving rapidly. Our understanding of the male contribution evolved from the "spermist theory" promoted by Hartsoeker in the late seventeenth century that postulated a fully formed "homunculus" within a sperm cell, then shifted with the "epigenesis" theory, supported by Harvey and others, which held that both the oocyte and sperm were necessary for embryogenesis. Epigenesis was firmly established with the identification of chromosomes as the heritable component, however, the contribution of the sperm has largely been considered to only consist of a haploid set of chromosomes, while the oocyte has been looked upon as the controlling force for embryogenesis and the provider of the necessary factors for early embryogenesis. Ironically, the recent explosion of research into "epigenetics," a term related to the early developmental theory of epigenesis, has changed the paradigm of the possible importance of the male contribution to embryogenesis and reproductive fitness.

This book explores the current understanding of the role of sperm in reproductive success. Areas of interest include genetic factors, including DNA integrity, aneuploidy, structural variations, and mutations within the germline, as well as epigenetic factors and mechanisms, including epigenetic influences in normal embryogenesis, the role of sperm epigenetic abnormalities in infertility, and the effects of environmental factors on the epigenome. Since it is becoming increasingly common for men to father children later in life, the role of aging is carefully considered in several chapters, not only from a clinical perspective, but also with an eye towards the basic science of changes in spermatogenesis in the older male. Lastly, since fertilization and early embryogenesis are increasingly performed in the laboratory through assisted reproduction techniques, emerging laboratory concepts are also discussed.

I thank all who have assisted in the preparation of this book, particularly the chapter authors. This distinguished group of scientists and clinicians are the cutting edge of the field of male factors involved in reproductive success. I also thank my assistant, Lori Barnard, for her consistent energy and expertise in helping to move this book forward. Lastly, I thank my colleagues, especially those from my own clinic and laboratories, for their stimulating work and discussions that have helped to move the field forward, aid patients in need, and assist me in endeavors such as this book.

Chapter

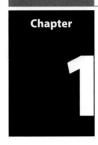

The reproductive fitness of the human male gamete

Douglas T. Carrell

Introduction

Our understanding of the contribution of the male gamete to reproductive success has a long and intriguing history. It has been known since ancient times that the male provides a vital force that is essential for embryogenesis, however, the functions and relative contributions of the male and female contributions have been debated. For example, Aristotle wrote of the necessity of the male "fluids" (semen) in terms of "that which generates," in contrast to the female fluids, which he described as "that out of which it generates." In other words, components of both the male and female "fluids" were necessary and contributory to development of the offspring, but semen was the controlling force while female "fluids" provided the resources necessary for embryogenesis [1].

The first reports of the visualization of sperm within semen were made separately by Anton Leeuwenhoek, Nicolaas Hartsoeker, and Christian Huygens, beginning in 1677 [2]. The visualization of the small "animal-cues" which we now know as spermatozoa was made at a time of philosophical debate over two competing theories of reproduction: "epigenesist," whose proponents held that development (embryogenesis) resulted from a systematic progression of development from the components provided by the male and female fluids according to laws or principles, versus the theory of "preformation," which held that either the sperm or ova contained a fully formed individual that was stimulated to grow under the influence of the mixture of the two fluids [3, 4]. The "preformist theory" of development was partially influenced by religious doctrine, and comprised two competing camps, the "ovists," who

believed that the preformed individual was contained within the ovum, and the "spermists," who held that the sperm contained the preformed person. The "spermist theory" is often represented by a drawing made by Hartsoeker in his publication *Dioptrique* in 1694 in which a homunculus is seen within the sperm cell (Figure 1.1) [5]. Interestingly, Hartsoeker did not claim to have seen a person within a sperm cell, although others later would make such claims, rather he was suggesting what the possible appearance of such a "homunculus" may reflect [5, 6]. Nevertheless, the "preformist" era, and specifically the "spermist" view, was the pinnacle of emphasis of the role of the contribution of the sperm to embryogenesis.

Although the "preformist theory" of reproduction was subsequently disproved through classical descriptive and experimental studies, the relative contribution of the sperm versus the oocyte to embryogenesis has continued to be debated. Clearly, the oocyte contributes the environment and most support organelles, enzymes, energy sources, and other molecules for the first few cleavage cycles, which perhaps has in some ways minimized the view of the contribution of the sperm to the embryo as simply a static haploid set of chromosomes (and in the human a centrosome) that are controlled and regulated entirely by the oocyte. This view is reflected in the paucity of studies from the "early days" of human in vitro fertilization (IVF) in regards to the effects of sperm on embryo morphology and fitness as compared with the much greater focus on the effects of the oocyte or of embryo culture conditions on embryo quality [7]. Whether this bias is due simply to the progress of technological advances that promoted

Paternal Influences on Human Reproductive Success, ed. Douglas T. Carrell. Published by Cambridge University Press.
© Cambridge University Press 2013.

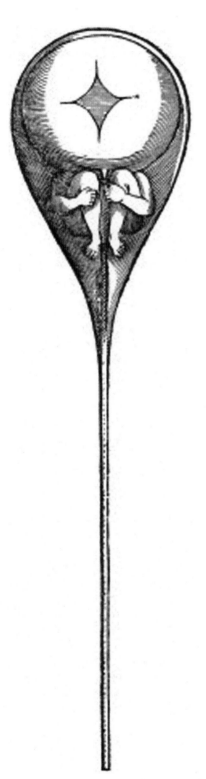

studies on culture conditions and oocyte development or underlying biases in scientific thought, or a combination of the two factors, can be debated. However, it is clear that the general trend of sperm biology research moved towards a focus on fertilization, first with a focus on biological events such as capacitation, zona binding and oocyte fertilization events, and later, based on technological advances, to assisted fertilization techniques, such as partial zona dissection (PZD), sub-zona injection (SUZI), and intracytoplasmic sperm injection (ICSI) [8].

Recent studies have demonstrated that the role of the male gamete in embryogenesis is significant in ways not previously understood [9]. Advances in our understanding of the biology of the sperm have highlighted genetic and epigenetic mechanisms that can preclude normal cleavage of the embryo, often observed as fragmented embryos that undergo cleavage arrest, or can result in serious health concerns for the offspring (Figure 1.2) [10–12]. These advances in understanding the biology of the gamete have also facilitated an increased appreciation of the potential influence of environmental influences on the gametes and resulting embryo, including such influences as aging, obesity, air quality, and drugs. This brief chapter will highlight some of these advances and concerns, which are discussed in detail in the remaining chapters.

Sperm biology

Recent studies have clearly demonstrated genetic mechanisms and defects contributing to subfertility. Clearly, diminished sperm DNA integrity, as defined by an increase of single- and double-strand DNA breaks, has been shown to be associated with embryo quality and IVF outcome [13, 14]. Since sperm lack the ability to self-repair DNA strand breaks, an accumulation of damage may overwhelm and affect the repair processes that occur during embryogenesis [15]. The emergence of sperm DNA damage as a potential cause of poor embryo development is important and relevant in its own right, but has also been beneficial in focusing more attention on sperm factors in general, as well as focusing the need for improved sperm preparation and selection techniques to be used prior to assisted reproduction technologies (ART) [16].

Structural alterations to sperm DNA have been shown to alter the reproductive potential of an individual. Such alterations may include defects ranging from whole chromosome losses or gains to sub-microscopic

Figure 1.1. This drawing by Hartsoeker is an extreme postulation of the contribution of the sperm to embryo development, proposing that the sperm provides a "homunculus", which is a preformed person with fully differentiated physical features.

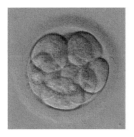
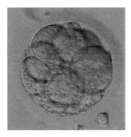
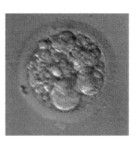

Figure 1.2. Examples of normal embryotic cleavage at the 8 cell stage (level 1), moderately abnormal cleavage with some blastomere fragmentation (level 2), and poor cleavage with extreme fragmentation (level 3). This figure is presented in color in the color plate section.

Level 1 Embryo   **Level 2 Embryo**   **Level 3 Embryo**

variations, and even individual base mutations. Large structural alterations, such as chromosome aneuploidies, often preclude normal embryogenesis and result in miscarriage [17]. While oocytes have long been known to be the major contributor to embryo aneuploidy, recent studies have highlighted the contribution of sperm to embryonic aneuploidy as well [18, 19]. While chromosome aneuploidy is seen in 2–3% of men evaluated for infertility, the percentage increases dramatically in men with oligozoospermia or azoospermia [20, 21]. Meiotic errors are increasingly frequent in aging women, however, clear evidence of such an effect has not been demonstrated in men [22]. Smaller, sub-microscopic variations to the genome, typically termed "structural variants," have recently been reported to be related to male infertility and are becoming a focus of research by several laboratories [23–25].

While the effects of structural variations and point mutations on embryogenesis have not been demonstrated in humans, it is interesting to note that a recent study on the effects of mutation accumulation in *Drosophila melanogaster* demonstrated that an increased "mutation accumulation" results in a decrease in post-fertilization embryo potential [26]. This is intriguing in light of the observation that the incidence of rare polymorphisms is elevated in severely infertile men [27]. The observations of increased levels of rae polymorphisms and structural variations may indicate that some subfertile men carry a form of genetic instability, which may have profound implications for the embryo and offspring [28].

Gametes of oligozoospermic men have been reported to contain errors of imprinting, an observation that is emphasized by reports that there is a small, but very significant increase in the rate of imprinting disorders in offspring conceived by IVF [29–31]. A larger, programmatic epigenetic role has also been proposed for sperm [10, 29]. Recent studies have demonstrated that the sperm epigenome is uniquely marked at genes involved in embryogenesis,

and that severe abnormalities are observed in the epigenetic marks at many development-related genes in the sperm of some men who consistently contribute to very poor embryogenesis when undergoing IVF [32–34]. These observations need to be studied in more depth, but they may suggest a major mechanism whereby sperm influence early embryogenesis. Importantly, these studies have also highlighted a major mechanism by which the environment and lifestyle factors may alter sperm epigenetics and reproductive potential [35].

Two other emerging areas of sperm biology are explored in this book, the role of the sperm centrosome and the possible function of non-coding RNAs carried by the sperm. In humans, the sperm provides the functional centrosome, of which the proximal centriole and the centrosomal proteins are functional from the first embryonic cleavage onwards [36]. While our understanding of centrosomal function is in its infancy, defects of centrosome function have been described, while other studies have focused on identifying models to evaluate and better understand the role of centrosomal proteins in normal embryogenesis [37–39]. Similarly, recent studies have begun to identify differences in the RNA transcripts present in sperm, both in coding and non-coding RNAs [40, 41]. While mRNAs may be more reflective of the status of spermatogenesis (a historical record of spermatogenesis), it is thought that small non-coding RNAs may be functional in embryogenesis [10, 42]. These two areas highlight the growing scope of sperm factors potentially affecting embryogenesis.

What is the role of the male gamete in embryogenesis?

The advances in our understanding of sperm biology, briefly highlighted above and discussed in detail in the following chapters, open the door to better answering questions relevant to the contribution of the male to reproductive success. The following are some of the questions that are considered and are explored in the remaining chapters:

1. Do genetic factors, including structural variations and polymorphisms, affect embryogenesis, and if so, what is the mechanism?
2. Is the sperm epigenome programmed to influence or support early embryogenesis?
3. How might environmental factors, including diet and stress, affect the programmatic epigenome?
4. Is the epigenome responsible for transmission of an increased risk in late-onset diseases such as diabetes or heart disease?
5. How is the epigenome altered as a male ages?
6. Does aging affect genetic features of male reproductive fitness?
7. Is there an increased risk of late-onset diseases in children conceived by older men?
8. Is altered sperm centrosome function responsible for poor embryogenesis in some couples?
9. Do RNA transcripts carried by sperm have a function in embryogenesis?
10. Can DNA integrity of sperm be improved?
11. How do medications and supplements affect sperm integrity, especially in the aging male?
12. Does obesity affect sperm function?
13. What evidence is there of transmission of diseases through epigenetic mechanisms?
14. How does the variability of semen production affect interpretation of clinical data?
15. Is ICSI safe?
16. What medical and surgical therapies can improve sexual function in the older man?
17. How can safety of ART techniques be better monitored and assessed?
18. Can sperm selection techniques select sperm with increased fitness?

Conclusions

As noted above, our increased understanding of sperm biology has highlighted the potential of the male gamete to affect embryogenesis and reproductive success. Many important questions are being investigated, and some important answers are emerging. Naturally, the advances we are making are also stimulating new and profound questions. As discussed in the following chapters, the ramifications of our growing knowledge are profound.

References

1. Aristotle. *Generation of animals*, translated by A. L. Peck. Cambridge, MA: Harvard University Press; 1979.
2. Needham DM, Williams JM. Some properties of uterus acomyosin and myofilaments. *Biochem J.* 1959;**73**:171–81.
3. Bowler PJ. The changing meaning of "evolution". *J Hist Ideas.* 1975;**36**(1):95–114.
4. Maienschein J. Epigenesis and preformationism. In Zalta EN, editor. *The Stanford Encyclopedia of Philosophy*; 2012.
5. Pinto-Correia C. Homunculus: Historiographic misunderstandings of preformationist terminology. In Gilbert SF, editor. *Devbio: A Companion to Developmental Biology*. 9th edn. Sunderland, CN: Sinauer Associates; 2006.
6. Hill KA. Hartsoeker's homonculus: a corrective note. *J Hist Behav Sci.* 1985;**21**(2):178–9.
7. Templeton A, Morris JK, Parslow W. Factors that affect outcome of in-vitro fertilisation treatment. *Lancet.* 1996;**348**(9039):1402–6.
8. Palermo GD, Cohen J, Alikani M *et al.* Development and implementation of intracytoplasmic sperm injection (ICSI). *Reprod Fertil Dev.* 1995;**7**(2):211–17; discussion 7–8.
9. Carrell DT. Epigenetics of the male gamete. *Fertil Steril.* 2012;**97**(2):267–74.
10. Jenkins TG, Carrell DT. The sperm epigenome and potential implications for the developing embryo. *Reproduction.* 2012;**143**(6):727–34.
11. Le Bouc Y, Rossignol S, Azzi S *et al.* Epigenetics, genomic imprinting and assisted reproductive technology. *Ann Endocrinol (Paris).* 2010 May;**71**(3):237–8.
12. Leidenfrost S, Boelhauve M, Reichenbach M *et al.* Cell arrest and cell death in mammalian preimplantation development: Lessons from the bovine model. *PLoS One.* 2011;**6**(7):e22121.
13. Simon L, Lutton D, McManus J *et al.* Sperm DNA damage measured by the alkaline comet assay as an independent predictor of male infertility and in vitro fertilization success. *Fertil Steril.* 2011;**95**(2):652–7.
14. Zini A. Are sperm chromatin and DNA defects relevant in the clinic? *Syst Biol Reprod Med.* 2011;57 (1–2):78–85.
15. Grenier L, Robaire B, Hales BF. The activation of DNA damage detection and repair responses in cleavage-stage rat embryos by a damaged paternal genome. *Toxicol Sci.* 2012;**127**(2):555–66.
16. Henkel R. Sperm preparation: State-of-the-art – physiological aspects and application of advanced

sperm preparation methods. *Asian J Androl.* 2012;**14**(2):260–9.

17. Brown S. Miscarriage and its associations. *Semin Reprod Med.* 2008;**26**(5):391–400.

18. Tempest HG. Meiotic recombination errors, the origin of sperm aneuploidy and clinical recommendations. *Syst Biol Reprod Med.* 2011;**57**(1–2):93–101.

19. Zhou D, Xia Y, Li Y et al. Higher proportion of haploid round spermatids and spermatogenic disomy rate in relation to idiopathic male infertility. *Urology.* 2011;**77**(1):77–82.

20. Chandley AC, Edmond P, Christie S et al. Cytogenetics and infertility in man. I. Karyotype and seminal analysis: results of a five-year survey of men attending a subfertility clinic. *Ann Hum Genet.* 1975;**39**(2):231–54.

21. Carrell DT. The clinical implementation of sperm chromosome aneuploidy testing: pitfalls and promises. *J Androl.* 2008;**29**(2):124–33.

22. Fonseka KG, Griffin DK. Is there a paternal age effect for aneuploidy? *Cytogenet Genome Res.* 2011;**133**(2–4):280–91.

23. Tuttelmann F, Simoni M, Kliesch S et al. Copy number variants in patients with severe oligozoospermia and sertoli-cell-only syndrome. *PLoS One.* 2011;**6**(4): e19426.

24. Giachini C, Nuti F, Turner DJ et al. Tspy1 copy number variation influences spermatogenesis and shows differences among y lineages. *J Clin Endocrinol Metab.* 2009;**94**(10):4016–22.

25. Noordam MJ, Westerveld GH, Hovingh SE et al. Gene copy number reduction in the azoospermia factor c (azfc) region and its effect on total motile sperm count. *Hum Mol Genet.* 2011;**20**(12):2457–63.

26. Mallet MA, Kimber CM, Chippindale AK. Susceptibility of the male fitness phenotype to spontaneous mutation. *Biol Lett.* 2012;**8**(3):426–9.

27. Aston KI, Carrell DT. Genome-wide study of single-nucleotide polymorphisms associated with azoospermia and severe oligozoospermia. *J Androl.* 2009;**30**(6):711–25.

28. Aston KI, Carrell DT. Emerging evidence for the role of genomic instability in male factor infertility. *Syst Biol Reprod Med.* 2012;**58**(2):71–80.

29. van Montfoort AP, Hanssen LL, de Sutter P et al. Assisted reproduction treatment and epigenetic inheritance. *Hum Reprod Update.* 2012;**18**(2):171–97.

30. Eroglu A, Layman LC. Role of ART in imprinting disorders. *Semin Reprod Med.* 2012;**30**(2):92–104.

31. Hiura H, Okae H, Miyauchi N et al. Characterization of DNA methylation errors in patients with imprinting disorders conceived by assisted reproduction technologies. *Hum Reprod.* 2012;**27**(8):2541–8.

32. Hammoud SS, Nix DA, Hammoud AO et al. Genome-wide analysis identifies changes in histone retention and epigenetic modifications at developmental and imprinted gene loci in the sperm of infertile men. *Hum Reprod.* 2011;**26**(9):2558–69.

33. Miller D, Brinkworth M, Iles D. Paternal DNA packaging in spermatozoa: More than the sum of its parts? DNA, histones, protamines and epigenetics. *Reproduction.* 2010;**139**(2):287–301.

34. Hammoud SS, Nix DA, Zhang H et al. Distinctive chromatin in human sperm packages genes for embryo development. *Nature.* 2009;**460**(7254):473–8.

35. Hamatani T. Human spermatozoal RNAs. *Fertil Steril.* 2012;**97**(2):275–81.

36. Schatten H. The mammalian centrosome and its functional significance. *Histochem Cell Biol.* 2008;**129**(6):667–86.

37. Navara CS, First NL, Schatten G. Phenotypic variations among paternal centrosomes expressed within the zygote as disparate microtubule lengths and sperm aster organization: correlations between centrosome activity and developmental success. *Proc Natl Acad Sci USA.* 1996;**93**(11):5384–8.

38. Hinduja I, Baliga NB, Zaveri K. Correlation of human sperm centrosomal proteins with fertility. *J Hum Reprod Sci.* 2010;**3**(2):95–101.

39. Tachibana M, Terada Y, Ogonuki N et al. Functional assessment of centrosomes of spermatozoa and spermatids microinjected into rabbit oocytes. *Mol Reprod Dev.* 2009;**76**(3):270–7.

40. Lee TL, Xiao A, Rennert OM. Identification of novel long noncoding RNA transcripts in male germ cells. *Methods Mol Biol.* 2012;**825**:105–14.

41. Krawetz SA, Kruger A, Lalancette C et al. A survey of small RNAs in human sperm. *Hum Reprod.* 2011;**26**(12):3401–12.

42. Ostermeier GC, Goodrich RJ, Diamond MP et al. Toward using stable spermatozoal rnas for prognostic assessment of male factor fertility. *Fertil Steril.* 2005;**83**(6):1687–94.

The sperm genome: effect of aneuploidies, structural variations, single nucleotide changes, and DNA damage on embryogenesis and development

Kenneth I. Aston and Donald F. Conrad

Introduction

A principal role of the sperm is to serve as a vessel for the delivery of paternal genetic material to the oocyte. Following penetration of the cumulus complex and zona pellucida by the sperm, the sperm membrane binds to and fuses with the oolemma triggering oocyte activation, which results in the resumption of meiosis, extrusion of a second polar body, and formation of male and female pronuclei. Subsequently male and female pronuclei migrate together and fuse to form a single, diploid pronucleus that will undergo replication and undergo multiple rounds of mitosis to form an embryo that will, under ideal circumstances, result in a healthy offspring. Successful sexual reproduction depends on, among other factors, a normal sperm genome. Aberrations in the sperm genome including DNA damage, aneuploidies, gene mutations, and structural variations can result in failed fertilization, arrested or abnormal embryo development, early or late miscarriage, or in rare cases the birth of genetically abnormal offspring. This chapter will discuss the known sperm genetic abnormalities that can impact embryogenesis, pregnancy, or offspring health.

Spermatogenesis

A brief review of the events required for successful spermatogenesis and fertilization is important in understanding how the complete sperm genome arises and how insults at different stages in development can lead to genetic anomalies that can be transmitted to the embryo.

Prenatal germ cell development

The initiation of germ cell development occurs in the early stages of embryogenesis with primordial germ cell (PGC) precursors arising in the yolk sac during gastrulation [1]. Primordial germ cells migrate from the epithelium of the yolk sac to the gonadal ridges in an amoeboid fashion during which time the cells continue to divide by mitosis [2]. Primordial germ cells are guided in their migration to the gonadal ridge by chemotactic molecules CXCR4, expressed on PGC surface and SDF1, secreted by gonadal ridge cells [3].

Upon reaching the gonadal ridge, PGCs colonize the region and begin sex-specific differentiation to form gonocytes [4]. While the timing of PGC development in the human is not well established, the cells are readily detectable in the developing embryo by 3 weeks gestation [5], and they have begun to colonize the gonadal ridge by the fifth week [4]. The gonads remain undifferentiated in terms of gender until week seven, at which time differentiation of the gonadal cortex and sexual differentiation begins [4].

Upon initiation of sexual differentiation seminiferous cords, precursors to seminiferous tubules begin to form and encompass PGCs and mesodermal cord cells in the medullary region of the gonads. The PGCs will eventually give rise to spermatozoa, while the mesodermal cord cells will give rise to Sertoli cells. Interstitial stromal tissue becomes vascularized, and precursors to Leydig cells develop [6]. Sexual differentiation continues, driven in part by the endocrine activities of Sertoli and Leydig cells. The number of fetal gonocytes doubles every 6 days between week 6 and week 9, increasing from about 3,000 to about 30,000 [7]. Between weeks 13–15 of development fetal gonocytes begin to differentiate into prospermatogonia triggered by the downregulation of a

Paternal Influences on Human Reproductive Success, ed. Douglas T. Carrell. Published by Cambridge University Press.
© Cambridge University Press 2013.

number of genes including KIT, OCT4, NANOG, and TFPA2C [8]. As fetal development continues, testes continue to develop and begin their descent from the lumbar region near the kidneys, over the pubic bone, and through the abdominal canal to finally reach the scrotum by 35–40 weeks gestation.

Postnatal development

The differentiation of fetal gonocytes to prospermatogonia continues throughout fetal development and is finally completed in infancy [8]. Sertoli and Leydig cells increase in number in infants during the first 3 months after birth accompanied by a rise in testosterone and inhibin B levels [8]. The testes grow slowly prior to puberty, and germ cell development remains relatively quiescent.

Puberty is a process wherein secondary sexual characteristics are developed in a gradual and stepwise manner and culminates in reproductive competence [9]. Associated with puberty is a sudden increase in testicular size resulting from the formation of seminiferous tubules from the solid seminiferous cords, increase in size and activity of Sertoli cells, and the resumption of mitotic activity by the germ cells as spermatogenesis initiates. In addition, endocrine secretion activity by Leydig cells increases, which drives many of the morphologic changes that occur at puberty [9]. These events mark the onset of sexual maturity, the resumption of spermatogenesis, and the concomitant acquisition of fertility, which will continue throughout a man's life.

At puberty, spermatogenesis is initiated and proceeds in three main phases. First, prospermatogonial stem cells enter mitosis to produce large numbers of spermatogonial stem cells in the mitotic proliferation phase. As these stem cells replicate morphologically distinct cells called A1 spermatogonia emerge marking the start of spermatogenesis.

Type A1 spermatogonia undergo several rounds of mitosis to form subsequent generations of type A spermatogonia, eventually giving rise to intermediate spermatogonia then type B spermatogonia, which undergo a final round of mitosis to form resting primary spermatocytes. The cells derived from a single A1 spermatogonium remain linked by thin cytoplasmic bridges, which persist until residual cytoplasm is shed just prior to the release of sperm into the lumen [10].

Following the proliferative stage, which occurs just inside the basement membrane within seminiferous tubules, primary spermatocytes undergo a round of DNA replication without cell division, they pass through Sertoli cell junctions toward the tubule lumen, and meiotic division begins. During the first meiotic prophase, crossing over and the exchange of genetic material between homologous chromosomes at recombination foci occurs. The event of homologous recombination is the basis for new combinations of alleles in each gamete, mixing genetic material from both paternal and maternal genomes. A minimum of one recombination site per chromosome is required for proper chromosomal segregation, and errors in meiotic recombination are a primary cause of aneuploidy in gametes [11]. As homologous chromosomes separate, cytokinesis results in two secondary spermatocytes to complete the first round of meiosis. Following the first meiotic division, sister chromatids separate followed by a second cytokinesis event resulting in haploid early round spermatids, which remain linked by cytoplasmic bridges.

The completion of meiosis is followed by dramatic nuclear and cytoplasmic remodeling events during the process of spermiogenesis. At the nuclear level, gene transcription ceases and DNA becomes more tightly compacted as the majority of nuclear histones are replaced first by transition proteins and finally by protamines. Also during this phase, each cell elongates, the tail and midpiece form, enzymes are packaged to form the acrosome, residual cytoplasm is shed and phagocytized by the Sertoli cell, cytoplasmic bridges dissolve, and mature spermatozoa are released into the lumen through the process of spermiation.

Following the completion of spermatogenesis and spermiation, spermatozoa move through the seminiferous tubules to the rete testis, through the vasa efferentia and into the epididymus where sperm are concentrated and undergo a process of maturation that renders spermatozoa motile and capable of fertilization.

Fertilization

Following the long process of male germ cell development which began just a few weeks after conception with the migration of primordial germ cells to the gonadal ridge and culminates with spermiation and epidydimal maturation of spermatozoa, the final step in the transmission of the male germline to the next generation involves the process of fertilization. Through copulation, semen, composed of seminal plasma and spermatozoa is deposited in the female reproductive tract. The seminal plasma serves a role in buffering the acidic vaginal pH as well as providing an energy source (fructose and sorbitol) for the sperm as well as antioxidants such as ascorbic acid and hypotaurine to guard against oxidative damage to sperm.

A small fraction of the spermatozoa deposited in the vagina will enter the cervix, and in the absence of progesterone, coincident with ovulation a few sperm will be allowed to penetrate the cervical mucus to eventually reach the uterus. In the female reproductive tract, sperm undergo a process of capacitation in which sperm surface glycoproteins are removed resulting in a change in the membrane properties of the sperm and the transition to a state of hyperactive motility and the ability to undergo the acrosome reaction [12]. Finally a few hours after coitus a few sperm (tens to hundreds) will reach the ampullary region of the oviduct where spermatozoa come in contact with a recently ovulated oocyte surrounded by a mass of cumulus cells [13].

As sperm penetrate the loosely packed cumulus cells they reach the zona pellucida, the proteoglycan structure surrounding the oocyte. Interaction of the spermatozoan with the zona pellucida protein ZP3 initiates the acrosome reaction, and by vesiculation of the acrosomal membranes enzymes are released enabling penetration of the zona pellucida by the sperm [14]. Following zona pellucida penetration, the sperm membrane fuses with the oolemma, and in addition to introducing a haploid genetic complement to the oocyte also triggers oocyte activation, characterized by a series of intracellular calcium spikes that initiate the cortical reaction which is critical for the prevention of polyspermia [15].

In addition, activation of the oocyte results in the resumption of meiosis in the oocyte, which precedes male and female pronuclear formation. Oocyte meiosis concludes with the extrusion of a second polar body, yielding a diploid zygote. As the sperm nucleus is introduced to the oocyte cytoplasm, the nuclear membrane breaks down, and chromatin decondensation occurs relatively rapidly as protamines are removed and replaced by maternally derived histones. At this point both maternal and paternal sets of chromosomes acquire a membrane and form pronuclei. Male and female pronuclei migrate toward the center of the zygote, and at the same time DNA replication of each haploid set of chromosomes occurs. As DNA replication is completed and the pronuclei come in close proximity, the membranes break down, and syngamy occurs marking the final event of fertilization and the initiation of embryonic cell division [16].

The role of the sperm genome in embryogenesis

The paternal genome contributes half of the genetic material to the offspring, and therefore, the genetic state of the spermatozoon can have profound impacts on the viability and health of the early embryo, the fetus, and finally the offspring. As the process of spermatogenesis is very complex, and the entire sperm population arises from a single sperm and egg and subsequently from a small number of primordial germ cells, subtle defects in the originating gametes or early in the process of gametogenesis can have profound impacts on the spermatozoa population and ultimately on the next generation. Genetic defects in sperm such as aneuploidies and *de novo* mutations or structural variations will be directly transmitted to the early embryo, and these effects have been well documented. Another potential source for a disruptive genetic state in offspring is elevated DNA fragmentation in the sperm, a relatively common feature in infertile men.

Single nucleotide polymorphisms and point mutations in sperm

In terms of size, single nucleotide polymorphisms (SNPs) and point mutations represent the smallest type of genetic variation, however their impact can be significant. These single-base changes are the most abundant source of DNA sequence variation in the human genome. Recent whole genome sequencing studies have revealed approximately 3.3 million single nucleotide differences within a given individual [17]. Single nucleotide polymorphisms are often, albeit arbitrarily, defined as polymorphisms whose minor allele is present in > 1% of the population; by contrast, point mutations are rare or *de novo* changes in DNA sequence. Recently, using whole-genome sequencing of two parent–offspring trios, the rate of *de novo* point mutation was directly estimated to be on the order of 1×10^{-8} per base per generation. This translates to an average of 30 *de novo* mutations per gamete [18].

Both SNPs and mutations in coding regions can be silent, with no effect on amino acid sequence; or they can be missense, resulting in the change of an amino acid; or nonsense, introducing a premature stop codon in a coding region. Alternatively they can be located outside of coding regions of genes and can have no effect, or can alter gene regulation by affecting gene regulatory elements such as promoters, enhancers, or microRNAs.

Since by definition each individual SNP occurs in a significant proportion of the population there are few such common variants that are individually causal of disease, but they can confer increased risk for disease propensity. There are numerous examples of SNPs that confer risk for diverse diseases, and the number of SNPs identified as being associated with various complex diseases has grown rapidly in the past decade with the significant discovery power of genomic tools including SNP microarrays and whole genome sequencing. The maternal and paternal contributions of SNPs to offspring will be approximately equal because half of the DNA is derived from each parent. While numerous studies have evaluated the involvement of SNPs in male factor infertility, none has evaluated the effect of SNPs on embryogenesis and early development. We recently reported a small but significant increase in the frequency of minor alleles in somatic DNA from azoospermic men compared with controls based on a pilot genome-wide SNP association study [19]. The implications of these findings are currently unclear and warrant further research.

Because spermatogenic progenitors undergo a significantly greater number of cell divisions than germ cell progenitors in the female germline, it was predicted in the mid-1900s that the male germline would be more mutagenic than the female germline [20], and in fact whole-genome sequence analysis of human and chimpanzee indicates a six-fold higher mutation rate in the male germline [21]. While this male-driven mutation process has been observed across several million years of evolution, mutation rates and the source of mutations within a single generation can vary greatly [18]. The implication of a general increase in mutation rates in male versus female gametes is that on average, the majority of *de novo* mutations in offspring will be derived from the sperm.

As with SNPs, the studies to identify sperm-derived mutations that affect embryogenesis or early development have not been performed, however there have been numerous genes identified by mouse knock-out studies that result in embryonic lethality, so clearly functional mutations in sperm in any number of genes or regulatory elements could be responsible for disorders in embryo development, miscarriage, or developmental problems. The huge number of genes required for normal development and the diversity of phenotypes associated with reproductive complications make the identification of causal *de novo* mutations a daunting task.

Advanced paternal age is a reported risk factor for over a dozen Mendelian diseases, as well as a small number of complex developmental disorders such as autism [22]. One straightforward interpretation of this observation is that mutations are distributed stochastically across the genome, and sperm from older fathers are more likely to harbor random *de novo* mutations in Mendelian disease loci. However, a fascinating mechanism for the paternal age effect has been recently uncovered in the study of Apert syndrome, achondroplasia, and Costello syndrome [23]. These diseases are caused by *de novo* gain-of-function mutations in the genes FGFR2, FGFR3, and HRAS, which cause clonal expansion of the spermatogonia in which they occur. This mechanism, which is reminiscent of oncogenesis, is mediated through the growth factor receptor-RAS signaling pathways and is likely to occur in all men. Over the lifetime of a human male, their frequency is reported to reach as high as 1/10,000 spermatogonia within the testis despite their inception in one or a few spermatogonia. It remains to be seen to what extent selfish germline mutations such as these contribute to the pathogenesis of common human disease, and whether their existence can be detected by deep sequencing of germ cells or individuals. Because growth factor receptor-RAS signaling is used extensively throughout the body to control cell proliferation, it seems inevitable that mutations that confer selective advantages to spermatogonia will also perturb embryogenesis.

Genomic structural variations in sperm

Structural variations include insertions, deletions, duplications, and inversions in the genome. The term "structural variant" (SV) typically refers to sub-microscopic changes in DNA, while larger events are termed cytogenetic or chromosomal abnormalities, which will be discussed in the following section. Early definitions described SVs as events > 1 kb in length [24], however this definition was primarily based on technical limitations in the ability to detect smaller events. The coming of age of routine whole-genome sequencing has resulted in the expansion of the definition of SVs to include much smaller events – down to 50 bp in size [25]. Structural variants can be

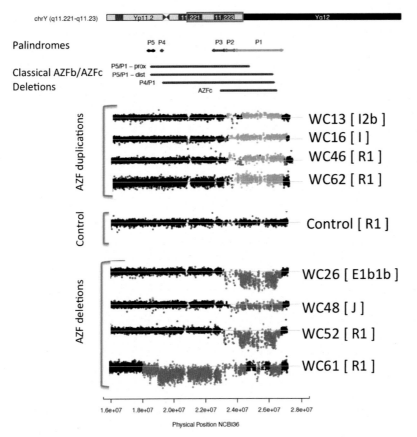

Figure 2.1. Copy number variation on the Y chromosome in men with azoospermia. We used the Affymetrix 6.0 oligonucleotide array to screen a small group of azoospermic individuals ascertained at a tertiary care clinic, and identified a number of classical AZF deletions, as well as duplications of AZFc. Next to each CNV is listed the sample ID and Y haplogroup of the sample. These data demonstrate that existing array platforms can cleanly identify Y chromosome rearrangements involving both gain and loss of sequence, and will facilitate investigation of the full spectrum of Y chromosome variation in future studies of male infertility. In both panels, for each individual, deviations of probe $\log_2$ ratios from 0 are depicted by gray lines or black dots, and probes spanning CNV calls are colored as either red (losses) or green (gains). The location of the region plotted is highlighted by a red box on the Y karyogram at top, followed by horizontal lines depicting the location of DNA sequence features that facilitate the formation of recurrent CNVs in the region ("palindromes"), and the location of the "classical" AZFb/c deletions described in the literature. This figure is presented in color in the color plate section.

identified using genomic microarray analysis or whole genome sequencing. Figure 2.1 illustrates deletions and duplications of the Y-chromosome identified by SNP microarray analysis.

While SVs can arise by a variety of mechanisms, a predominant source for *de novo* SVs occurs during meiotic recombination of meiotic prophase I. Low copy repeat regions serve as a substrate for the genesis of SVs through non-allelic homologous recombination (NAHR) [26]. Because both male and female gametes only undergo meiosis once during gametogenesis, the rate of SV formation via NAHR is likely to be equal between males and females for most genomic locations. While several groups have evaluated the role of SVs in spermatogenic impairment [27–30], the role of sperm-derived SVs on fertilization and embryo development is unclear at present.

The best-characterized SVs that affect male fertility are the deletions of the azoospermia factor (AZF) regions of the Y chromosome, present in a significant proportion of azoospermic and severe oligozoospermic men [31], and first identified as distal Yq deletions in a subset of azoospermic men through karyotypic analysis [32]. While sperm retrieval is often possible in men with specific AZF deletions (e.g. AZFc), and embryo development and pregnancy rates following ICSI in AZFc-deleted men are similar to rates in men without deletions, the deletion will be transmitted to all male offspring, who will likewise be infertile.

Many of the structural variations contributed by the sperm to the early embryo will have little or no effect on embryo development, however larger SVs, particularly those that impact genes or regulatory elements may have profound effects on embryo and fetal development, or may increase disease susceptibility in offspring [33]. Numerous groups are working to characterize the extent of SV throughout the genome and to understand the impact that specific SVs have on phenotype. A more thorough assessment of the incidence of SVs in the sperm of infertile men compared with fertile controls will be necessary to better predict potential long-term risks of assisted reproductive technology to offspring health.

Chromosomal abnormalities in sperm

The best-studied genetic defects that impact embryogenesis, pregnancy rates, and offspring health are aneuploidies (monosomies and trisomies). The size of these cytogenetic abnormalities makes them readily detectable with standard karyotypic analysis, and therefore it has been recognized for many years that chromosomal abnormalities are a frequent cause of early pregnancy loss. In fact, chromosomal abnormalities in the early conceptus are the single largest contributor to early pregnancy loss, accounting for approximately half of first trimester miscarriages [34]. Recent data from preimplantation genetic screening of cells biopsied from IVF blastocysts indicates that about half of IVF blastocysts are aneuploid, indicating most selection against embryonic aneuploidy likely occurs following implantation [35].

Embryonic aneuploidy typically arises from aneuploidy in one or both of the gametes. Like the majority of SVs, most aneuploidies are the result of meiotic errors during gametogenesis, with chromosomal non-disjunction resulting in monosomic and trisomic gametes [11]. Maternally derived aneuploidies are the source for the great majority of embryonic aneuploidies (about 90%), with advanced maternal age being a significant risk factor for increased aneuploidy rates [11].

Though the majority of embryonic aneuploidy is derived maternally, about 10% of cases are of paternal origin [36]. Interestingly, about half of XXY pregnancies arise due to paternal non-disjunction [36], and X monosomies are also generally paternally derived [37]. Additionally, 5–10% of trisomies 13, 14, 15, 21, and 22 are of paternal origin, with the remaining autosomal aneuploidies almost always originating from the oocyte [36]. While the impact of paternal age on chromosome abnormalities is much less than the age effect seen in women, it does appear that advanced paternal age is a slight risk factor for increased sperm chromosomal anomalies [34, 38].

Importantly, the incidence of constitutional aneuploidies as well as balanced and unbalanced translocations is significantly higher in infertile men than in the general population. In 1599 unselected men attending a subfertility clinic, 2.2% displayed some form of chromosomal abnormality, a rate five times higher than the rate in the general population [39]. In more severe cases of male infertility the rate is higher still, with 5.1% of oligozoospermic and 14.1% of azoospermic men displaying somatic chromosome abnormalities [40].

An aneuploid and a euploid spermatozoon identified by chromosome fluorescence *in situ* hybridization (FISH) are depicted in Figure 2.2.

A small body of data indicates that carriers of somatic chromosomal abnormalities also exhibit higher rates of sperm aneuploidy [41, 42], and increased rates of sperm aneuploidy have in fact been observed in infertile men [38, 43, 44]. In addition, increases in chromosomally abnormal embryos have been observed following IVF with sperm exhibiting increased sperm chromosome abnormalities [45]. Importantly, Y chromosome microdeletions appear to be a risk factor for increased sperm aneuploidy rates, particularly for the sex chromosomes [46–48].

While the majority of embryonic aneuploidies result in early pregnancy loss, some aneuploidies are compatible with development to term. Approximately 0.3% of newborns are aneuploid, with trisomy 21 and sex chromosome trisomies (XXX, XXY, and XYY) and XO monosomy being the most common [36]. Additionally trisomies 13 and 18 are compatible with live birth on rare occasion.

Though the majority of embryonic aneuploidies are of maternal origin, clearly, the sperm genome plays a significant role in the chromosomal constitution of the early embryo, and chromosomal status affects implantation and delivery rates as well as the health of offspring. Further, in cases of male factor infertility or advanced paternal age, the risk of transmission of an aneuploid paternal genome to the oocyte is increased.

Sperm DNA damage

In addition to the genetic contribution of sperm to the early embryo in terms of DNA sequence and ploidy, fragmentation of the sperm genome can also affect embryogenesis. Sperm DNA damage can arise through a number of different mechanisms and at various stages of the spermatogenic process. Sperm DNA fragmentation can occur: (a) through leaky apoptotic mechanisms during spermatogenesis, (b) from persistent strand breaks that are necessarily induced during the chromatin remodeling stage of spermiogenesis, (c) in post-testicular sperm as a result of reactive oxygen species in the epididymis or vas deferens, (d) through the actions of oxygen-radical-induced endogenous caspases and endonucleases, and (e) by extrinsic factors such as radiation, chemotherapy, or environmental exposures [49]. Sperm DNA damage can be assessed by a variety of

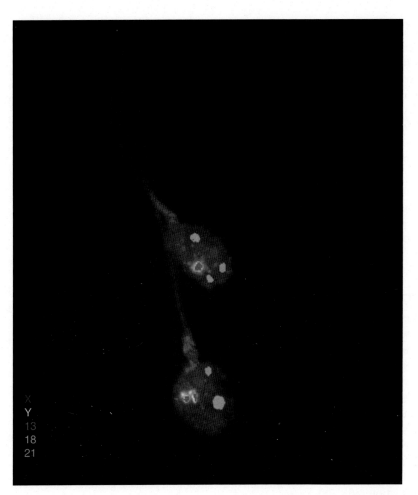

Figure 2.2. A chromosomally normal sperm (upper) and aneuploid sperm aneuploid for chromosome 13 (lower) identified by 5-color chromosome FISH. Sperm were probed for chromosomes X, Y, 13, 18, and 21 (photo courtesy of Benjamin Emery, University of Utah Andrology and IVF Laboratories). This figure is presented in color in the color plate section.

methodologies including terminal deoxynucleotidyl transferase-mediated dUDP nick-end labeling (TUNEL), Comet assay, and sperm chromatin structure assay (SCSA). Figure 2.3 illustrates a spermatozoon displaying minimal DNA damage (top panel) and a spermatozoon with excessive DNA damage (bottom panel) as assessed by the Comet assay.

Sperm DNA damage is significant because sperm lack the machinery to efficiently repair damage once it has occurred. While it has been demonstrated in the mouse that oocytes have the capacity to repair sperm DNA fragmentation following fertilization [50], there are certainly limits to the oocyte's capacity for repair. Improper or incomplete repair may lead to developmental problems in the early embryo, and that capacity likely decreases with increasing female age [49], while the risk of sperm DNA fragmentation may increase with age [51, 52].

The impact of sperm DNA damage on the embryo is not completely characterized, however it has been demonstrated that increased sperm DNA damage is associated with reduced embryo quality [53], reduced implantation rates [54], and increased miscarriage rates [55–58]. The impact of sperm DNA damage on embryogenesis is further demonstrated by observations of improved ART outcomes in couples with repeated pregnancy failures using testicular sperm, where DNA damage is normally significantly lower than in ejaculated sperm [59, 60].

In addition to the negative impact of increased sperm DNA fragmentation on fertilization, embryogenesis, and pregnancy rates, of particular concern is the potential long-term impact of sperm DNA fragmentation on offspring health. Mice produced by ICSI using sperm with induced DNA fragmentation exhibited significantly increased incidence of solid

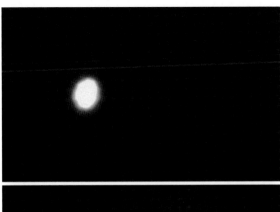
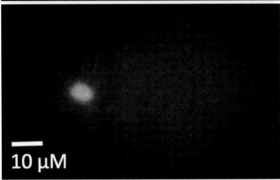

Figure 2.3. Photomicrographs of spermatozoa analyzed for DNA damage using the Comet assay. The top panel displays a cell with minimal DNA damage, and the bottom panel displays a cell with extensive DNA fragmentation, resulting in a pronounced comet-like tail (photos courtesy of Luke Simon, University of Utah Andrology and IVF Laboratories). This figure is presented in color in the color plate section.

tumor formation, more frequent death by 5 months of age, and generally shorter lifespan [61]. The data in humans are sparse, but it is certainly feasible that extensive sperm DNA fragmentation could lead to increased mutation rates and *de novo* SVs in the early embryo which could have significant long-term consequences to offspring health [62].

Conclusions

The paternal genome delivered to the oocyte at fertilization can have profound impacts on embryogenesis, pregnancy, and offspring health. Failures in early embryogenesis, implantation, and early pregnancy can be the result of abnormal sperm chromatin constitution, mutations or larger SVs in any number of genes or regulatory elements, or increased sperm DNA fragmentation. In other cases, these genomic features may be compatible with normal birth, but they may affect childhood health or have long-term

health consequences. Given the importance of the paternal genomic contribution to embryogenesis, pregnancy outcomes, and even offspring health, additional research to evaluate the incidence of sperm aneuploidy, DNA fragmentation, and potentially genomic instability in infertile men, and the development of improved techniques for selecting the most "normal" sperm for ART are clearly warranted.

References

1. Ginsburg M, Snow MH, McLaren A. Primordial germ cells in the mouse embryo during gastrulation. *Development*. 1990;**110**(2):521–8.

2. Tam PP, Snow MH. Proliferation and migration of primordial germ cells during compensatory growth in mouse embryos. *J Embryol Exp Morphol*. 1981;**64**:133–47.

3. Richardson BE, Lehmann R. Mechanisms guiding primordial germ cell migration: strategies from different organisms. *Nat Rev Mol Cell Biol*. 2010;**11**(1):37–49.

4. Pereda J, Zorn T, Soto-Suazo M. Migration of human and mouse primordial germ cells and colonization of the developing ovary: an ultrastructural and cytochemical study. *Microsc Res Tech*. 2006;**69**(6):386–95.

5. De Felici M, Scaldaferri ML, Lobascio M *et al.* Experimental approaches to the study of primordial germ cell lineage and proliferation. *Hum Reprod Update*. 2004;**10**(3):197–206.

6. Wu X, Wan S, Lee MM. Key factors in the regulation of fetal and postnatal Leydig cell development. *J Cell Physiol*. 2007;**213**(2):429–33.

7. Bendsen E, Byskov AG, Laursen SB *et al.* Number of germ cells and somatic cells in human fetal testes during the first weeks after sex differentiation. *Hum Reprod*. 2003;**18**(1):13–18.

8. Virtanen HE, Cortes D, Rajpert-De Meyts E *et al.* Development and descent of the testis in relation to cryptorchidism. *Acta Paediatr*. 2007;**96**(5):622–7.

9. Traggiai C, Stanhope R. Delayed puberty. *Best Pract Res Clin Endocrinol Metab*. 2002;**16**(1):139–51.

10. Alberts B, Johnson A, Lewis J *et al. Molecular Biology of the Cell*. New York, NY: Garland Science; 2002.

11. Hassold T, Hunt P. To err (meiotically) is human: the genesis of human aneuploidy. *Nat Rev Genet*. 2001;**2**(4):280–91.

12. Bedford JM. Significance of the need for sperm capacitation before fertilization in eutherian mammals. *Biol Reprod*. 1983;**28**(1):108–20.

13. Suarez SS, Pacey AA. Sperm transport in the female reproductive tract. *Hum Reprod. Update.* 2006;**12** (1):23–37.

14. Brewis IA, Wong CH. Gamete recognition: sperm proteins that interact with the egg zona pellucida. *Rev Reprod.* 1999;**4**(3):135–42.

15. Ducibella T. The cortical reaction and development of activation competence in mammalian oocytes. *Hum Reprod. Update.* 1996;**2**(1):29–42.

16. Perreault SD. Chromatin remodeling in mammalian zygotes. *Mutat Res.* 1992;**296**(1–2):43–55.

17. Wheeler DA, Srinivasan M, Egholm M *et al.* The complete genome of an individual by massively parallel DNA sequencing. *Nature.* 2008;**452**(7189):872–6.

18. Conrad DF, Keebler JE, DePristo MA *et al.* Variation in genome-wide mutation rates within and between human families. *Nat Genet.* 2011;**43**(7):712–14.

19. Aston KI, Carrell DT. Genome-wide study of single-nucleotide polymorphisms associated with azoospermia and severe oligozoospermia. *J Androl.* 2009;**30**(6):711–25.

20. Haldane JB. The mutation rate of the gene for haemophilia, and its segregation ratios in males and females. *Ann Eugen.* 1947;**13**(4):262–71.

21. Taylor J, Tyekucheva S, Zody M *et al.* Strong and weak male mutation bias at different sites in the primate genomes: insights from the human-chimpanzee comparison. *Mol Biol Evol.* 2006;**23**(3):565–73.

22. Tarin JJ, Brines J, Cano A. Long-term effects of delayed parenthood. *Hum Reprod.* 1998;**13**(9):2371–6.

23. Goriely A, Wilkie AO. Paternal age effect mutations and selfish spermatogonial selection: causes and consequences for human disease. *Am J Hum Genet.* 2012;**90**(2):175–200.

24. Feuk L, Carson AR, Scherer SW. Structural variation in the human genome. *Nat Rev Genet.* 2006;**7**(2):85–97.

25. Alkan C, Coe BP, Eichler EE. Genome structural variation discovery and genotyping. *Nat Rev Genet.* 2011;**12**(5):363–76.

26. Molina O, Anton E, Vidal F *et al.* Sperm rates of 7q11.23, 15q11q13 and 22q11.2 deletions and duplications: a FISH approach. *Hum Genet.* 2011;**129** (1):35–44.

27. Tuttelmann F, Simoni M, Kliesch S *et al.* Copy number variants in patients with severe oligozoospermia and Sertoli-cell-only syndrome. *PLoS One.* 2011;**6**(4):e19426.

28. Hansen S, Eichler EE, Fullerton SM *et al.* Spanx gene variation in fertile and infertile males. *Syst Biol Reprod Med.* 2010;**55**:18–26.

29. Giachini C, Nuti F, Turner DJ *et al.* Tspy1 copy number variation influences spermatogenesis and shows differences among y lineages. *J Clin Endocrinol Metab.* 2009;**94**(10):4016–22.

30. Noordam MJ, Westerveld GH, Hovingh SE *et al.* Gene copy number reduction in the azoospermia factor c (AZFc) region and its effect on total motile sperm count. *Hum Mol Genet.* 2011;**20**(12):2457–63.

31. Reijo R, Lee TY, Salo P *et al.* Diverse spermatogenic defects in humans caused by Y chromosome deletions encompassing a novel RNA-binding protein gene. *Nat Genet.* 1995;**10**(4):383–93.

32. Tiepolo L, Zuffardi O. Localization of factors controlling spermatogenesis in the nonfluorescent portion of the human Y chromosome long arm. *Hum Genet.* 1976;**34**(2):119–24.

33. Stankiewicz P, Lupski JR. Structural variation in the human genome and its role in disease. *Annu Rev Med.* 2010;**61**:437–55.

34. Brown S. Miscarriage and its associations. *Semin Reprod Med.* 2008;**26**(5):391–400.

35. Fragouli E, Wells D. Aneuploidy in the human blastocyst. *Cytogenet Genome Res.* 2011;**133** (2–4):149–59.

36. Hassold T, Abruzzo M, Adkins K *et al.* Human aneuploidy: incidence, origin, and etiology. *Environ Mol Mutagen.* 1996;**28**(3):167–75.

37. Hassold T, Pettay D, Robinson A *et al.* Molecular studies of parental origin and mosaicism in 45, X conceptuses. *Hum Genet.* 1992;**89**(6):647–52.

38. Martin RH. Meiotic errors in human oogenesis and spermatogenesis. *Reprod Biomed Online.* 2008;**16** (4):523–31.

39. Chandley AC, Edmond P, Christie S *et al.* Cytogenetics and infertility in man. I. Karyotype and seminal analysis: results of a five-year survey of men attending a subfertility clinic. *Ann Hum Genet.* 1975;**39**(2):231–54.

40. Retief AE, Van Zyl JA, Menkveld R *et al.* Chromosome studies in 496 infertile males with a sperm count below 10 million/ml. *Hum Genet.* 1984;**66**(2–3):162–4.

41. Perrin A, Basinko A, Douet-Guilbert N *et al.* Aneuploidy and DNA fragmentation in sperm of carriers of a constitutional chromosomal abnormality. *Cytogenet Genome Res.* 2011;**133**(2–4):100–6.

42. Wong EC, Ferguson KA, Chow V *et al.* Sperm aneuploidy and meiotic sex chromosome configurations in an infertile XYY male. *Hum Reprod.* 2008;**23**(2):374–8.

43. Tempest HG. Meiotic recombination errors, the origin of sperm aneuploidy and clinical recommendations. *Syst Biol Reprod Med.* 2011;**57**(1–2):93–101.

44. Zhou D, Xia Y, Li Y *et al.* Higher proportion of haploid round spermatids and spermatogenic disomy rate in

relation to idiopathic male infertility. *Urology*. 2011;**77** (1):77–82.

45. Rodrigo L, Peinado V, Mateu E *et al*. Impact of different patterns of sperm chromosomal abnormalities on the chromosomal constitution of preimplantation embryos. *Fertil Steril*. 2010;**94**(4):1380–6.

46. Ferlin A, Arredi B, Speltra E *et al*. Molecular and clinical characterization of Y chromosome microdeletions in infertile men: a 10-year experience in Italy. *J Clin Endocrinol Metab*. 2007;**92**(3):762–70.

47. Siffroi JP, Le Bourhis C, Krausz C *et al*. Sex chromosome mosaicism in males carrying Y chromosome long arm deletions. *Hum Reprod*. 2000;**15**(12):2559–62.

48. Mateu E, Rodrigo L, Martinez MC *et al*. Aneuploidies in embryos and spermatozoa from patients with Y chromosome microdeletions. *Fertil Steril*. 2010;**94** (7):2874–7.

49. Sakkas D, Alvarez JG. Sperm DNA fragmentation: mechanisms of origin, impact on reproductive outcome, and analysis. *Fertil Steril*. 2010;**93**(4):1027–36.

50. Brandriff B, Pedersen RA. Repair of the ultraviolet-irradiated male genome in fertilized mouse eggs. *Science*. 1981;**211**(4489):1431–3.

51. Hammiche F, Laven JS, Boxmeer JC *et al*. Sperm quality decline among men below 60 years of age undergoing IVF or ICSI treatment. *J Andrology*. 2011;**32**(1):70–6.

52. Belloc S, Benkhalifa M, Junca AM *et al*. Paternal age and sperm DNA decay: discrepancy between chromomycin and aniline blue staining. *Reprod Biomed Online*. 2009;**19**(2):264–9.

53. Simon L, Lutton D, McManus J *et al*. Sperm DNA damage measured by the alkaline comet assay as an independent predictor of male infertility and in vitro fertilization success. *Fertil Steril*. 2011;**95**(2):652–7.

54. Benchaib M, Braun V, Lornage J *et al*. Sperm DNA fragmentation decreases the pregnancy rate in an assisted reproductive technique. *Hum Reprod*. 2003;**18** (5):1023–8.

55. Lewis SE, Simon L. Clinical implications of sperm DNA damage. *Hum Fertil (Camb)*. 2010;**13**(4):201–7.

56. Zini A. Are sperm chromatin and DNA defects relevant in the clinic? *Systems Biol Reprod Med*. 2011;**57** (1–2):78–85.

57. Borini A, Tarozzi N, Bizzaro D *et al*. Sperm DNA fragmentation: paternal effect on early post-implantation embryo development in Art. *Hum Reprod*. 2006;**21**(11):2876–81.

58. Carrell DT, Liu L, Peterson C M *et al*. Sperm DNA fragmentation is increased in couples with unexplained recurrent pregnancy loss. *Arch Androl*. 2003;**49** (1):49–55.

59. Weissman A, Horowitz E, Ravhon A *et al*. Pregnancies and live births following ICSI with testicular spermatozoa after repeated implantation failure using ejaculated spermatozoa. *Reprod Biomed Online*. 2008;**17**(5):605–9.

60. Greco E, Scarselli F, Iacobelli M *et al*. Efficient treatment of infertility due to sperm DNA damage by ICSI with testicular spermatozoa. *Hum Reprod*. 2005;**20** (1):226–30.

61. Fernandez-Gonzalez R, Moreira PN, Perez-Crespo M *et al*. Long-term effects of mouse intracytoplasmic sperm injection with DNA-fragmented sperm on health and behavior of adult offspring. *Biol Reprod*. 2008;**78** (4):761–72.

62. Aitken RJ, De Iuliis GN, McLachlan RI. Biological and clinical significance of DNA damage in the male germ line. *Int J Androl*. 2009;**32**(1):46–56.

Chapter 3

The sperm epigenome: a role in embryogenesis and fetal health?

Douglas T. Carrell and Jessie Dorais

Introduction

It is interesting and instructive to note that the underlying foundations in our studies of fertilization and early embryogenesis are evolving. Until recently, the mechanisms and foci of research regarding events in the fertilization continuum have been largely based on sperm physiology (i.e. sperm motility, hyperactivation, capacitation, the acrosome reaction, zona binding, sperm chromatin decondensation, etc.), whereas post-fertilization embryogenesis events have been investigated almost exclusively from the perspective of the oocyte's contribution to embryo competence and the transition of control in early embryogenesis to the embryo itself. However, it has become apparent that the sperm cell provides more than a "neutral" set of chromosomes to the oocyte [1]. Furthermore, it has been shown that in a subset of infertile couples undergoing in vitro fertilization (IVF), the sperm may be responsible for altered embryogenesis [2–4]. Several mechanisms exist by which sperm may affect embryogenesis, including DNA damage in the form of single- and double-strand breaks, chromosome aneuploidy, altered sperm-derived centrosome function, and sperm DNA packaging abnormalities through both "classical epigenetic" and "non-classical epigenetic" mechanisms.

"Epigenetics" is defined as "the study of mitotically and/or meiotically heritable changes in gene function that can not be explained by changes in DNA sequence" [5]. A key component of this "classical" definition of epigenetics is the issue of heritability. While many sperm factors may ultimately affect gene transcription (i.e. DNA strand breaks or protamine packaging defects), such factors are usually not heritable. The two "classical" forms of epigenetic marks are DNA methylation and various chemical modifications on histone tails. Either of these epigenetic marks is sufficient to regulate gene activation independently, or in concert with each other.

In many somatic cell types, the effects of epigenetic marks on the functions of cellular homeostasis, differentiation, and pathologies are relatively well characterized. Epigenetic modifications have been shown to not only affect normal cellular function, but also to be involved in aging, cancer, and as a mechanism whereby environmental influence may affect cell function [6, 7]. Therefore, one may easily envision the profound potential that epigenetic modifications play in normal embryogenesis, and the potential negative impact that abnormal epigenetic programming in the germline could have on the highly choreographed and intricate interplays of differentiation present during normal development.

Embryogenesis is the result of the activation of an oocyte, including its maternal set of chromosomes, by the delivery of a paternal set of chromosomes from the fertilizing sperm cell. Oocytes and sperm, both terminally differentiated cells, are vastly different in their function, morphology, and individual contribution to the embryo. Thus, it is to be expected that their epigenetic marks on their respective haploid sets of DNA would also likely be vastly different. For example, DNA packaging varies greatly between the mature sperm and egg. In mature sperm, DNA packaging is largely due to packaging by protamines, specialized nuclear proteins not used in any other cell type. Therefore, it is likely that embryogenesis depends on the normalcy of epigenetics of the sperm, the oocyte, and post-fertilization epigenetic modifications in the embryo.

Ultimately, our understanding of the epigenetics of embryogenesis and development will depend on

---

Paternal Influences on Human Reproductive Success, ed. Douglas T. Carrell. Published by Cambridge University Press.
© Cambridge University Press 2013.

advancements in our understanding of the epigenetics of the sperm, oocyte, and embryo, and we are beginning to gain greater insight into each of these areas. However, for both practical and ethical reasons, the sperm cell has been the most extensively studied and recent reports have better defined the mechanisms by which human sperm may influence normal embryogenesis [8–12]. This chapter will focus on the epigenetic landscape of the sperm and highlight the data regarding the altered epigenetics of sperm in a subset of infertile men. Past and future research on the epigenetic landscape of the sperm and egg will likely have a profound impact on current understanding of normal embryogenesis and provide clinical ramifications in the fields of infertility, recurrent pregnancy loss, imprinting disorders, and other inherited disease states.

Protamination of the sperm chromatin

Sperm function includes complex and diverse processes. Initially, sperm are required to traverse the female reproductive tract to reach the oocyte, penetrate the cumulus oophorus, bind to and penetrate the zona pellucida, fuse to the oolemma, penetrate the oocyte, and undergo numerous post-penetration events [13]. In order to accomplish these functions, the sperm cell has an extremely specialized architecture and physiology, including dramatic modifications to the chromatin structure, largely facilitated by replacement of most (90–95%) histones with protamines [14]. Protamination of sperm chromatin facilitates the nuclear compaction necessary for sperm motility, protects the sperm genome from oxidization and other harmful molecules within the female reproductive tract, and results in a transcriptionally quiescent sperm genome [14].

During protamination, canonical histones in sperm are largely replaced by protamines in a multistep process. First, select histones are replaced by histones variants that are expressed during spermatogenesis, including testis-specific histone 2B (TH2B) which is the most abundant histone variant found in mature sperm [15]. Testis-specific histone 2B has long been of particular interest in sperm chromatin packaging due to both its unique expression pattern and because it has been shown through immunohistological studies to locate in the telomeres of sperm chromosomes [16]. Simultaneously, other histones

undergo hyperacetylation of the histone tail, triggering a cascade of events that ultimately results in protamine replacement [17]. Histone acetylation is regulated by the simultaneous interplay of both acetylases and deacetylases and results in a "relaxed" chromatin structure that may be important in facilitating topoisomerase-induced strand breaks and removal of histones, followed by their transient replacement with transition proteins 1 and 2 (TP1 and TP2), and ultimately protamines [18, 19]. The transition proteins are important for the normal histone to protamine transition and double knock-out studies of these genes results in infertility [20, 21]. Isolated T1 or T2 gene knock-out studies have demonstrated a compensatory benefit from whichever transition protein remains, but the resulting sperm appear to undergo increased DNA damage during epididymal transport [22]. Hence, although the expression of the transition proteins is temporally short and redundancy exists, proper expression of both proteins appears necessary for the normal completion of protamination.

Humans express two protamines, protamine 1 and protamine 2 (P1, P2), which are expressed in roughly equal quantities, and are usually reported clinically as a ratio of the expression of each protein (P1/P2 ratio) [23]. Protamines undergo unique translational regulation, most notably extensive phosphorylation, that is essential for normal protamine function leading to chromatin condensation [24]. Improper temporal regulation of the P1 and P2 transcripts not only leads to altered expression of the mature proteins, but also leads to infertility. In fact, the retention of protamine precursors and/or an altered P1/P2 ratio are both associated with male infertility [14, 25–27].

Protamination results in dramatic compaction of the DNA in the sperm nucleus. This compaction happens as the result of the formation of disulfide bonds between the protamines, which ultimately results in a super-compacted structure of repeating toroidal chromatin structures (Figure 3.1) [28]. Each toroid packages approximately 50 kilobases (kb) of DNA [29]. One current hypothesis is that each toroid is equivalent to one loop domain of DNA with linker regions of histone-bound DNA associated with matrix attachment regions (Figure 3.1) [30, 31]. This model would potentially result in increased protection of protamine-bound DNA from damage by the toroidal compaction and subsequent stacking of toroids, and concurrently predict increased susceptibility of the

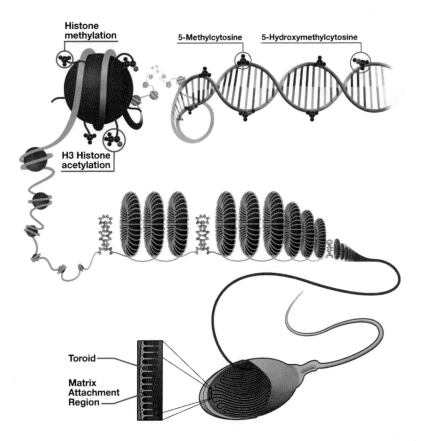

Figure 3.1. Chromatin and epigenetic modifications to sperm. Epigenetic modifications consist of DNA methylation of 5 position of cytosine, including 5-methylcytosine and 5-hydroxymethylcytosine. Histone tail modifications confer structural and spatial confirmations that influence the binding of transcription factors and enzymes to the chromatin. Chromatin modifications result from the extensive, but not complete, removal of most histones and replacement with protamines. Protamines facilitate a higher order of chromatin packaging consisting of toroidal units with interspersed histone regions. This figure is presented in color in the color plate section.

linker regions and histone-bound regions to DNA degradation and strand breaks by endonucleases [32]. As noted above, several studies evaluating abnormal protamination have reported elevated DNA damage in the form of strand breaks [33–35].

Altered protamine expression has been associated with a broad range of sperm anomalies, including diminished sperm counts, decreased sperm function, and diminished embryo quality during in vitro fertilization [34, 36–38]. Furthermore, abnormal protamination is relatively common in the sperm of infertile men, but relatively rare in men with known fertility and normal semen quality [26, 39]. While protamine replacement is generally measured and reported as a mean value for the entire ejaculate, it is important to note that there is a broad range of protamine replacement between individual sperm of an ejaculate, thus sperm isolation/selection techniques may potentially be of use for improving clinical outcome in patients with abnormal protamine replacement [40–42]. The precise relationship between protamination and the diverse and temporally separated events of spermatogenesis is not clearly understood at this time [38].

The role of retained histones

In fertile men, 5–15% of the genome remains bound to histones after protamination. The question of why any histones are retained in fertile, normospermic men is intriguing. It seems illogical from an evolutionary perspective that protamination would be "leaky" or inefficient, and more plausible that retained histones serve a biological function. One could hypothesize that if the retention of histones was the result of inefficient replacement that the retained histones would be randomly distributed throughout the genome, whereas if the retention served a biological function, one may expect to see the histones retained in an orderly and conserved fashion that implies a function. Recent studies indicate the latter scenario. Retained histones are not randomly distributed throughout the genome but rather are retained in a consistent manner that implies a function, and secondly, unique histone modifications that help regulate genome activation and silencing also appear to be programmatically distributed in the sperm genome in the same manner [11, 43, 44]. These observations imply that sperm chromatin may transmit epigenetic regulatory mechanisms that affect post-fertilization transcriptional regulation [44].

Nucleosomes are octomers typically composed of two dimers of histones H3-H4 and two dimers of histones H2A-H2B, with each nucleosome linked by histone H1 [45]. Chemical modifications to the tail of a histone can confer dramatically different functions to the histone specific to their binding affinity to DNA and the accessibility of other regulatory factors to the DNA, which together affect gene activation or silencing for that specific region or gene [46]. The chemical modifications primarily consist of modifications of lysine and serine residues on the histone tail by phosphorylation, methylation, acetylation, and ubiquitination [47, 48]. Histones conferring a generally "active" transcription state include acetylation of H3 and H4, which as discussed above generally facilitates an open chromatin structure and binding of transcription factors [49]. Deacetylation, conversely, is associated with an "inactive" transcriptional status, and generally correlates with DNA methylation [50]. Histone lysine methylation is another key regulator of activation, with H3K9 and H3K27 histones generally associated with "inactive" status [51]. Table 3.1 lists the key histone modifications found in sperm and their activation status.

Arpanahi et al. have utilized endonuclease digestion of human and mouse sperm chromatin to identify endonuclease-sensitive regions, and found that endonuclease-sensitive regions were more likely to be histone-bound regions that were largely associated with regulatory regions of the genome, including gene promoters [52]. Hammoud et al. used repeated digestion of the sperm genome of fertile men to isolate histone-bound DNA from protamine-bound DNA, followed by deep sequencing of the histone-bound and protamine-bound DNA fractions. This study, mapped at base pair resolution, showed a clear, consistent, and highly significant pattern of histone retention at the promoters of gene families involved in development, micro RNAs, and imprinted genes. Conversely, protamines were not enriched at any gene family [11].

Since sperm protamines are rapidly replaced by oocyte-derived histones in the zygote, the same group also repeated the study using an additional step in which antibodies were used to isolate DNA bound to histones with certain tail modifications [53]. It was hypothesized that if an epigenetic role were associated with the retained histones, the conserved localization of specific histone variants or modifications would be necessary and programmatic in the embryo. Indeed, the subsequent studies clearly demonstrated a pattern in which key developmental genes were bivalently marked with H3K4me3, an activating mark, and H3K27me3, a silencing mark, similar to the bivalently marked developmental gene promoters of embryonic stem cells [11, 54].

Interestingly, TH2B represents 40–50% of the retained histones in sperm, and is enriched in the promoters of genes for ion channels and other spermatogenesis genes, but was not enriched at developmental gene promoters. Thus, TH2B retention may be a "historical" epigenetic record of spermatogenesis. Histone variant H2AZ, which has been implicated in poising in certain cell types, is enriched in the pericentromeric heterochromatin regions of sperm, as had previously been reported in immunostaining studies

Table 3.1 A partial list of activating and silencing modifications to histones retained in sperm.

Modification	Activating	Silencing	Bivalency
Acetylation of H3	X		
Acetylation of H4	X		
Ubiquitination of H2B	X		
H3K4me2	X		
H3K4me3	X		
Ubiquitination of H2A		X	
H3K9me		X	
H3K27me3		X	
H3K4me3 and H3K27me3			X

[2, 55]. Regions enriched with isolated H3K4me3 in the absence of H3K27me3, localize to spermatogenesis-related genes, while H3K4me2 is enriched at developmental genes. These patterns are consistent in normospermic, fertile men and seem to reflect a historical record of spermatogenesis and a future program for developmental processes [2].

The data obtained from humans and the theory that sperm chromatin epigenetic marks include both a historical record and a future embryonic program have been supported by data from the zebrafish, which do not employ protamination. Wu *et al.* reported that the zebrafish sperm genome was similar to the human genome in that activating modifications were seen at genes involved in spermatogenesis and bivalency was seen at developmental gene promoters, and were also able to demonstrate a relationship in the temporal expression of developmental genes in the embryo with associated multi-valent activation marks at those loci [56, 57].

Sperm DNA methylation

DNA methylation is the most potent epigenetic mark that promotes gene silencing. Methylation occurs primarily at the 5-carbon position of cytosine-phosphate-guanine dinucleotides (CpGs) through the action of the DNMT family of proteins, which are responsible for both the initiation of methylation and subsequent maintenance of methylation marks [58]. Methylation of cytosines is not only relevant for the regulation of transcription, but also is used for allele-specific imprinting of mono-allelically expressed genes and X chromosome inactivation [59, 60]. CpGs found in high concentrations near gene promoters are termed "CpG islands" and are potent inhibitors of transcription when methylated [61]. The silencing of transcription by CpG methylation is accomplished largely by inhibiting the recruitment and/or binding of other factors directly involved in transcription [62, 63].

Hammoud *et al.* concurrently analyzed DNA methylation and histone modifications in human sperm and showed that the bivalently poised promoters of developmental genes were also associated with hypomethylation, consistent with the "poised" state of bivalently marked genes of embryonic stem cells [11]. Molaro *et al.* have recently sequenced the human sperm methylome and confirmed the generally hypomethylated state of developmental gene promoters [64]. These findings lend strong support to the hypothesis that the sperm

genome delivers an epigenetically "poised" set of developmental genes that may have profound influence in the proper growth and development of the embryo.

Post-fertilization epigenetic changes

It is important to consider the role of epigenetic modifications in the haploid genomes of the sperm and oocyte post-fertilization. In order to re-set imprinted genes and coordinate the events necessary for embryogenesis, significant and broad epigenetic changes occur to the sperm genome (now a portion of the zygotic genome), beginning almost immediately following sperm fertilization (Figure 3.2) [65–67]. Perhaps the most striking change is the "global" DNA methylation erasure that occurs in the paternal pronucleus, which removes most methylation marks from the paternal genome (Figure 3.2) [68]. However, the term global is often misused in describing this event, as there are distinct regions in the paternal genome that escape demethylation, including imprinted genes and retrotransposons [68, 69]. The demethylation of the sperm genome is thought to remove gamete-specific regulatory marks that are the historical records of gametogenesis, and to establish embryogenesis-specific marks [67, 70].

Unlike the maternal pronucleus, demethylation of the paternal pronucleus is active [71–73]. Additionally, protamines are replaced with maternally derived histones (Figure 3.3). Unfortunately, the mechanisms and key enzymes of active demethylation of the paternal pronucleus are not well understood [65]. Due to significant differences in animal models, the timing of demethylation is also not well understood, although it is clear that the re-setting occurs prior to the first cleavage stage [68, 74, 75].

The epigenetic landscape of sperm and the extent to which post-fertilization changes occur to re-set the paternal genome have not yet been established. Clearly, detailed studies in this area are lacking and future studies that characterize this process will more fully elucidate the role of sperm epigenetics in maturation and fertilization and how this landscape changes during embryogenesis.

Investigation of chromatin modifications in sperm of infertile men

The study of the methylation status of imprinted genes in the sperm of severely infertile men has been

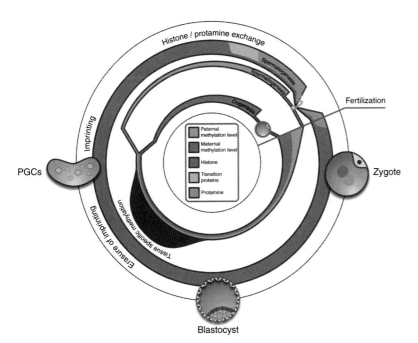

Figure 3.2. Summary of critical chromatin and concurrent DNA methylation modifications in sperm, embryos, and primordial germ cells. Key events include the protamination of sperm during spermiogenesis, followed by replacement of protamines with histones at the pronuclear stage of embryogenesis. After fertilization, sperm-derived DNA is actively demethylated in contrast with passive demethylation of maternally derived DNA. Resetting of imprinting occurs in the primordial germ cells and tissue-specific methylation changes occur throughout development. This figure is presented in color in the color plate section.

accelerated by several epidemiologic studies that show a small, but significantly increased risk of generating offspring with imprinting disorders in couples undergoing IVF and intracytoplasmic sperm injection (ICSI) [76, 77]. Subsequent studies have generally shown altered methylation in the imprinted genes of oligozoospermic men compared with controls [78–80]. It is again important to note the heterogeneous nature of sperm, and the fact that the methylation defects were not universal or consistent within the sperm of an individual, but rather that elevated percentages of sperm with altered methylation were noted. Elevated methylation defects of imprinted genes has also been observed in other pathologies, including men with obstructive azoospermia undergoing testicular aspiration of sperm, men with known defects of protamination, and patients with idiopathic infertility [81–83].

Interestingly, altered methylation in sperm is seen at many-fold higher rates than the rates of altered methylation in the offspring, suggesting the potential corrective ability of the embryo to "re-set" the methylation profile. Additionally, it may be that the sperm actually used for ICSI are not affected at the same level as the sperm analyzed from the ejaculate, since sperm used for ICSI are usually "selected" because they are viable, motile, and the most morphologically normal.

Our laboratory has been interested in studying the methylation status of non-imprinted genes, particularly development-related genes and micro RNAs, and recently reported that gross methylation defects were not seen in the promoters of OCT4, SOX2, NANOG, HOCC11, miR-17 in sperm from men with known abnormalities of protamination, a population previously shown to have elevated risk of defects of methylation of imprinted genes [83, 84]. However, defects were observed in the CREM gene (also known as the cAMP response element modulator gene), which may be a reflection and/or a cause of abnormal spermatogenesis [84, 85]. Recently, we have evaluated the genome-wide methylation status of sperm in two populations of infertile patients, men with abnormal protamination and men with unexplained poor embryogenesis during IVF therapy. Profound methylation abnormalities of numerous CpGs were observed in the sperm of 3/28 of the men analyzed, and subtle differences in others [86]. These studies clearly demonstrate the early current stage of translational research in this area and the difficulties in interpreting subtle variations in methylation patterns.

In the only study of its kind thus far, we have recently evaluated histone localization and modifications genome-wide in the sperm of men with either abnormal protamination or men with unexplained

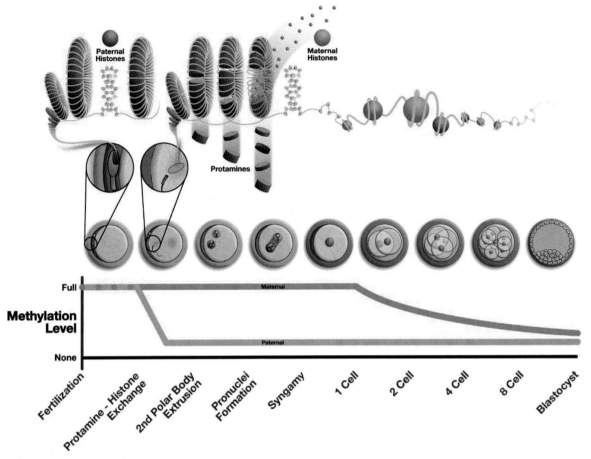

Figure 3.3. Alterations to the epigenome post-fertilization. This figure demonstrates the removal of protamines and their replacement with maternal histones during the very early stages post-fertilization, as well as DNA methylation changes to the paternal and maternal DNA throughout embryogenesis. This figure is presented in color in the color plate section.

poor embryogenesis during IVF [87]. By necessity, all studied men had normal sperm counts. This study clearly demonstrated abnormalities in some of the men of both classifications, both in regards to general histone localization and in regards to the location of specific histone modifications. Methylation of developmental genes was altered in some cases, but was more subtle in most cases [87]. These limited studies of infertile men seem to support the hypothesis that sperm epigenetic marks are programmatic, at least in part, and imply a function during embryogenesis. The observation of abnormalities in IVF patients with unexplained poor embryogenesis is interesting, but must be confirmed in larger populations of such highly characterized patients. While the current studies focus on the effect these defects may have on

fertility, future studies also need to ascertain if such epigenetic changes seen in the gametes of some infertile men actually translate to any heritable risks to the offspring. Such studies are ongoing, but only speculative at this point.

The transmission of environmental effects through sperm epigenetic changes

The understanding of epigenetic mechanisms is particularly important and exciting since epigenetic mechanisms may help explain the link between environmental influences and disease. Additionally, since epigenetic effects can be heritable, abnormalities observed in gametes may not only result in diminished fertility, but also may portend health risks to offspring. Recent studies highlight the phenomenon of paternally, epigenetically driven changes to offspring [88]. For example, it has been demonstrated that when mated with a normal female, male mice fed a low protein diet sire offspring with altered expression of many genes important in metabolism and cholesterol synthesis [88]. Similarly, metabolic alterations, specifically changes in insulin sensitivity, were noted in the female offspring of male rats fed high fat diets [89]. Lastly, utilizing data collected during and following massive crop failures in Sweden in the late 1800s and early 1900s, investigators were able to perform large retrospective studies in human populations observing similar effects. The data from these studies suggest that an alteration in paternal diet may independently affect offspring health and metabolic activity [90, 91]. These studies highlight the need for further studies evaluating the potential influence of epigenetic changes in sperm to health risks in the offspring, including risks that may not be observed until late in life.

Our laboratory has presented preliminary evidence of epigenetic changes in male gametes with age [92]. Briefly, differences in the global levels of DNA methylation were found to increase as the individual aged. It is not known if these changes translate to clinical relevance, however, given the possible link of advanced paternal age to neuropsychiatric disease, cancer, and other diseases (as discussed in detail in Chapter 10, this volume), further studies on age-associated changes in the epigenetic signature of gametes are necessary [93–95]. In addition to diet and aging, numerous other environmental influences will need to be studied in regards to their potential effects on gamete epigenetics, including but not limited to, medications, cancer, smoking, exercise, and stress.

Conclusions

It is apparent that sperm have a unique epigenetic status, including the purposeful replacement of most histones with protamines, the enrichment of retained histones at the promoters of genes associated with development, dual chemical modifications on the retained histones at developmental genes that are consistent with a stem cell-like "bivalency" that may poise the genes for activation during embryogenesis, and DNA demethylation at sites that facilitate transcriptional activation. Furthermore, it appears that abnormalities of these epigenetic marks are more common

and more pronounced in infertile men compared with fertile controls, including men with histories of unexplained poor embryogenesis when going through IVF. These data imply that the sperm epigenome likely serves a functional role in normal embryogenesis. Whether such a role is a significant factor in infertility or recurrent miscarriage remains to be proven.

It is known that there is a small, but significant increased risk of offspring with imprinting abnormalities from IVF patients with severe male infertility, and that abnormal methylation in the sperm of these patients is observed compared with fertile controls. Furthermore, data are beginning to accumulate for heritable epigenetic effects in offspring transmitted through the male germline. This fascinating and clinically important area of sperm epigenetics is in its infancy and upcoming research would likely shed light in the near future on some of these unanswered questions.

References

1. Carrell DT. Epigenetics of the male gamete. *Fertil Steril.* 2012;**97**(2):267–74.

2. Carrell DT, Hammoud SS. The human sperm epigenome and its potential role in embryonic development. *Mol Hum Reprod.* 2010;**16**(1):37–47.

3. Garrido N, Remohi J, Martinez-Conejero JA et al. Contribution of sperm molecular features to embryo quality and assisted reproduction success. *Reprod Biomed Online.* 2008;**17**(6):855–65.

4. Knez K, Zorn B, Tomazevic T et al. The IMSI procedure improves poor embryo development in the same infertile couples with poor semen quality: a comparative prospective randomized study. *Reprod Biol Endocrinol.* 2011;**9**:123.

5. Riggs AD, Martinssen RA, Russo VEA. *Epigenetic Mechanisms of Gene Regulation.* Cold Spring Harbor, NY: Cold Spring Harbor Press; 1996.

6. Herceg Z, Vaissiere T. Epigenetic mechanisms and cancer: an interface between the environment and the genome. *Epigenetics.* 2011;**6**(7):804–19.

7. Liu L, Rando TA. Manifestations and mechanisms of stem cell aging. *J Cell Biol.* 2011;**193**(2):257–66.

8. Puri D, Dhawan J, Mishra RK. The paternal hidden agenda: epigenetic inheritance through sperm chromatin. *Epigenetics.* 2010;**5**(5):386–91.

9. Biermann K, Steger K. Epigenetics in male germ cells. *J Androl.* 2007;**28**(4):466–80.

10. Jenkins TG, Carrell DT. The paternal epigenome and embryogenesis: poising mechanisms for development. *Asian J Androl.* 2010;**13**(1):76–80.

11. Hammoud SS, Nix DA, Zhang H *et al.* Distinctive chromatin in human sperm packages genes for embryo development. *Nature.* 2009;**460**(7254):473–8.

12. Navarro-Costa P, Nogueira P, Carvalho M *et al.* Incorrect DNA methylation of the dazl promoter cpg island associates with defective human sperm. *Hum Reprod.* 2010;**25**(10):2647–54.

13. Yanagimachi R. Male gamete contributions to the embryo. *Ann N Y Acad Sci.* 2005;**1061**:203–7.

14. Oliva R. Protamines and male infertility. *Hum Reprod Update.* 2006;**12**(4):417–35.

15. van Roijen HJ, Ooms MP, Spaargaren MC *et al.* Immunoexpression of testis-specific histone 2b in human spermatozoa and testis tissue. *Hum Reprod.* 1998;**13**(6):1559–66.

16. Churikov D, Siino J, Svetlova M *et al.* Novel human testis-specific histone h2b encoded by the interrupted gene on the x chromosome. *Genomics.* 2004;**84**(4):745–56.

17. Rousseaux S, Gaucher J, Thevenon J *et al.* Spermiogenesis: histone acetylation triggers male genome reprogramming. *Gynecol Obstet Fertil.* 2009;**37**(6):519–22.

18. Rousseaux S, Boussouar F, Gaucher J *et al.* Molecular models for post-meiotic male genome reprogramming. *Syst Biol Reprod Med.* 2011;**57**(1–2):50–3.

19. Song N, Liu J, An S *et al.* Immunohistochemical analysis of histone H3 modifications in germ cells during mouse spermatogenesis. *Acta Histochem Cytochem.* 2011;**44**(4):183–90.

20. Meistrich ML, Mohapatra B, Shirley CR *et al.* Roles of transition nuclear proteins in spermiogenesis. *Chromosoma.* 2003;**111**(8):483–8.

21. Shirley CR, Hayashi S, Mounsey S *et al.* Abnormalities and reduced reproductive potential of sperm from TNP1- and TNP2-null double mutant mice. *Biol Reprod.* 2004;**71**(4):1220–9.

22. Suganuma R, Yanagimachi R, Meistrich ML. Decline in fertility of mouse sperm with abnormal chromatin during epididymal passage as revealed by ICSI. *Hum Reprod.* 2005;**20**(11):3101–8.

23. Corzett M, Mazrimas J, Balhorn R. Protamine 1: protamine 2 stoichiometry in the sperm of eutherian mammals. *Mol Reprod Dev.* 2002;**61**(4):519–27.

24. Aoki VW, Carrell DT. Human protamines and the developing spermatid: their structure, function, expression and relationship with male infertility. *Asian J Androl.* 2003;**5**(4):315–24.

25. de Mateo S, Ramos L, de Boer P *et al.* Protamine 2 precursors and processing. *Protein Pept Lett.* 2011;**18**(8):778–85.

26. Carrell DT, Liu L. Altered protamine 2 expression is uncommon in donors of known fertility, but common among men with poor fertilizing capacity, and may reflect other abnormalities of spermiogenesis. *J Androl.* 2001;**22**(4):604–10.

27. Aoki VW, Liu L, Jones KP *et al.* Sperm protamine 1/protamine 2 ratios are related to in vitro fertilization pregnancy rates and predictive of fertilization ability. *Fertil Steril.* 2006;**86**(5):1408–15.

28. Cree LH, Balhorn R, Brewer LR. Single molecule studies of DNA–protamine interactions. *Protein Pept Lett.* 2011;**18**(8):802–10.

29. Balhorn R. A model for the structure of chromatin in mammalian sperm. *J Cell Biol.* 1982;**93**(2):298–305.

30. Ward WS. Function of sperm chromatin structural elements in fertilization and development. *Mol Hum Reprod.* 2010;**16**(1):30–6.

31. Yamauchi Y, Shaman JA, Ward WS. Non-genetic contributions of the sperm nucleus to embryonic development. *Asian J Androl.* 2011;**13**(1):31–5.

32. Dominguez K, Arca CDR, Ward WS. The relationship between chromatin structure and DNA damage in mammalian spermatozoa. In Zini A, Agarwal A, editors. *Sperm Chromatin: Biological and Clinical Applications in Male Infertility and Assisted Reproduction.* New York, NY: Springer; 2011, pp. 61–8.

33. Garcia-Peiro A, Martinez-Heredia J, Oliver-Bonet M *et al.* Protamine 1 to protamine 2 ratio correlates with dynamic aspects of DNA fragmentation in human sperm. *Fertil Steril.* 2011;**95**(1):105–9.

34. Torregrosa N, Dominguez-Fandos D, Camejo MI *et al.* Protamine 2 precursors, protamine 1/protamine 2 ratio, DNA integrity and other sperm parameters in infertile patients. *Hum Reprod.* 2006;**21**(8):2084–9.

35. Aoki VW, Moskovtsev SI, Willis J *et al.* DNA integrity is compromised in protamine-deficient human sperm. *J Androl.* 2005;**26**(6):741–8.

36. de Mateo S, Gazquez C, Guimera M *et al.* Protamine 2 precursors (pre-P2), protamine 1 to protamine 2 ratio (P1/P2), and assisted reproduction outcome. *Fertil Steril.* 2009;**91**(3):715–22.

37. Simon L, Castillo J, Oliva R *et al.* Relationships between human sperm protamines, DNA damage and assisted reproduction outcomes. *Reprod Biomed Online.* 2011;**23**(6):724–34..

38. Carrell DT, Emery BR, Hammoud S. Altered protamine expression and diminished spermatogenesis: what is the link? *Hum Reprod Update.* 2007;**13**(3):313–27.

39. Nanassy L, Liu L, Griffin J *et al.* The clinical utility of the protamine 1/protamine 2 ratio in sperm. *Protein Pept Lett.* 2011;**18**(8):772–7.

40. Huser T, Orme CA, Hollars CW et al. Raman spectroscopy of DNA packaging in individual human sperm cells distinguishes normal from abnormal cells. *J Biophotonics*. 2009;2(5):322–32.

41. Aoki VW, Emery BR, Liu L et al. Protamine levels vary between individual sperm cells of infertile human males and correlate with viability and DNA integrity. *J Androl*. 2006;27(6):890–8.

42. Hammoud S, Liu L, Carrell DT. Protamine ratio and the level of histone retention in sperm selected from a density gradient preparation. *Andrologia*. 2009;41(2):88–94.

43. Li Y, Lalancette C, Miller D et al. Characterization of nucleohistone and nucleoprotamine components in the mature human sperm nucleus. *Asian J Androl*. 2008;10(4):535–41.

44. Miller D, Brinkworth M, Iles D. Paternal DNA packaging in spermatozoa: More than the sum of its parts? DNA, histones, protamines and epigenetics. *Reproduction*. 2010;139(2):287–301.

45. Campos EI, Reinberg D. Histones: annotating chromatin. *Annu Rev Genet*. 2009;43:559–99.

46. Cairns BR. The logic of chromatin architecture and remodelling at promoters. *Nature*. 2009;461(7261):193–8.

47. Kouzarides T. Chromatin modifications and their function. *Cell*. 2007;128(4):693–705.

48. Handy DE, Castro R, Loscalzo J. Epigenetic modifications: basic mechanisms and role in cardiovascular disease. *Circulation*. 2011;123(19):2145–56.

49. Liu Y, Lu C, Yang Y et al. Influence of histone tails and H4 tail acetylations on nucleosome-nucleosome interactions. *J Mol Biol*. 2011;414(5):749–64.

50. Peng L, Seto E. Deacetylation of nonhistone proteins by HDACs and the implications in cancer. *Handb Exp Pharmacol*. 2011;206:39–56.

51. Werner M, Ruthenburg AJ. The united states of histone ubiquitylation and methylation. *Mol Cell*. 2011;43(1):5–7.

52. Arpanahi A, Brinkworth M, Iles D et al. Endonuclease-sensitive regions of human spermatozoal chromatin are highly enriched in promoter and CTCF binding sequences. *Genome Res*. 2009;19(8):1338–49.

53. Jones EL, Zalensky AO, Zalenskaya IA. Protamine withdrawal from human sperm nuclei following heterologous ICSI into hamster oocytes. *Protein Pept Lett*. 2011;18(8):811–16.

54. Gan Q, Yoshida T, McDonald OG et al. Concise review: epigenetic mechanisms contribute to pluripotency and cell lineage determination of embryonic stem cells. *Stem Cells*. 2007;25(1):2–9.

55. Rangasamy D, Berven L, Ridgway P et al. Pericentric heterochromatin becomes enriched with H2A.Z during early mammalian development. *Embo J*. 2003;22(7):1599–607.

56. Wu SF, Zhang H, Cairns BR. Genes for embryo development are packaged in blocks of multivalent chromatin in zebrafish sperm. *Genome Res*. 2011;21(4):578–89.

57. Carrell DT. Epigenetic marks in zebrafish sperm: insights into chromatin compaction, maintenance of pluripotency, and the role of the paternal genome after fertilization. *Asian J Androl*. 2011;13(4):620–1.

58. Portela A, Esteller M. Epigenetic modifications and human disease. *Nat Biotechnol*. 2010;28(10):1057–68.

59. Ng HH, Bird A. DNA methylation and chromatin modification. *Curr Opin Genet Dev*. 1999;9(2):158–63.

60. Bronner C, Chataigneau T, Schini-Kerth VB et al. The "epigenetic code replication machinery", ECREM: a promising druggable target of the epigenetic cell memory. *Curr Med Chem*. 2007;14(25):2629–41.

61. Deaton AM, Bird A. CPG islands and the regulation of transcription. *Genes Dev*. 2011;25(10):1010–22.

62. Thomson JP, Skene PJ, Selfridge J et al. CpG islands influence chromatin structure via the CpG-binding protein CFP1. *Nature*. 2010 Apr 15;464(7291):1082–6.

63. Illingworth RS, Bird AP. CpG islands – 'a rough guide'. *FEBS Lett*. 2009;583(11):1713–20.

64. Molaro A, Hodges E, Fang F et al. Sperm methylation profiles reveal features of epigenetic inheritance and evolution in primates. *Cell*. 2011;146(6):1029–41.

65. Jenkins TG, Carrell D. Sperm epigenetics before and after fertilization. *Frontiers in Genetics*. (Submitted).

66. Li E. Chromatin modification and epigenetic reprogramming in mammalian development. *Nat Rev Genet*. 2002 Sep;3(9):662–73.

67. Reik W, Dean W, Walter J. Epigenetic reprogramming in mammalian development. *Science*. 2001;293(5532):1089–93.

68. Abdalla H, Hirabayashi M, Hochi S. Demethylation dynamics of the paternal genome in pronuclear-stage bovine zygotes produced by in vitro fertilization and ooplasmic injection of freeze-thawed or freeze-dried spermatozoa. *J Reprod Dev*. 2009;55(4):433–9.

69. Hales BF, Grenier L, Lalancette C et al. Epigenetic programming: from gametes to blastocyst. *Birth Defects Res A Clin Mol Teratol*. 2011;91(8):652–65.

70. Meehan RR. DNA methylation in animal development. *Semin Cell Dev Biol*. 2003;14(1):53–65.

71. Rougier N, Bourc'his D, Gomes DM et al. Chromosome methylation patterns during mammalian

preimplantation development. *Genes Dev.*
1998;**12**(14):2108–13.

72. Mayer W, Niveleau A, Walter J *et al.* Demethylation of
the zygotic paternal genome. *Nature.* 2000 Feb
3;**403**(6769):501–2.

73. Young LE, Beaujean N. DNA methylation in the
preimplantation embryo: the differing stories of the
mouse and sheep. *Anim Reprod Sci.* 2004;**82–83**:61–78.

74. Zaitseva I, Zaitsev S, Alenina N *et al.* Dynamics of
DNA-demethylation in early mouse and rat embryos
developed in vivo and in vitro. *Mol Reprod Dev.*
2007;**74**(10):1255–61.

75. Dean W, Santos F, Stojkovic M *et al.* Conservation of
methylation reprogramming in mammalian
development: aberrant reprogramming in cloned
embryos. *Proc Natl Acad Sci USA.*
2001;**98**(24):13,734–8.

76. Odom LN, Segars J. Imprinting disorders and assisted
reproductive technology. *Curr Opin Endocrinol
Diabetes Obes.* 2010;**17**(6):517–22.

77. Owen CM, Segars JH Jr. Imprinting disorders and
assisted reproductive technology. *Semin Reprod Med.*
2009;**27**(5):417–28.

78. Rajender S, Avery K, Agarwal A. Epigenetics,
spermatogenesis and male infertility. *Mutat Res.*
2011;**727**(3):62–71.

79. Marques CJ, Costa P, Vaz B *et al.* Abnormal
methylation of imprinted genes in human sperm is
associated with oligozoospermia. *Mol Hum Reprod.*
2008;**14**(2):67–74.

80. Kobayashi H, Sato A, Otsu E *et al.* Aberrant DNA
methylation of imprinted loci in sperm from
oligospermic patients. *Hum Mol Genet.*
2007;**16**(21):2542–51.

81. Minor A, Chow V, Ma S. Aberrant DNA methylation
at imprinted genes in testicular sperm retrieved from
men with obstructive azoospermia and undergoing
vasectomy reversal. *Reproduction.*
2011;**141**(6):749–57.

82. Poplinski A, Tuttelmann F, Kanber D *et al.* Idiopathic
male infertility is strongly associated with aberrant
methylation of MEST and IGF2/H19 ICR1. *Int J
Androl.* 2010;**33**(4):642–9.

83. Hammoud SS, Purwar J, Pflueger C *et al.* Alterations in
sperm DNA methylation patterns at imprinted loci in
two classes of infertility. *Fertil Steril.*
2010;**94**(5):1728–33.

84. Nanassy L, Carrell DT. Analysis of the methylation
pattern of six gene promoters in sperm of men with
abnormal protamination. *Asian J Androl.*
2011;**13**(2):342–6.

85. Nanassy L, Carrell DT. Abnormal methylation of the
promoter of CREM is broadly associated with male
factor infertility and poor sperm quality but is
improved in sperm selected by density gradient
centrifugation. *Fertil Steril.* 2011;**95**(7):2310–14.

86. Ashton KI, Punj V, Liu L *et al.* Genome-wide DNA
methylation is altered in some men with abnormal
chromatin packaging or poor IVF embryogenesis. *Fertil
Steril.* 2012;**97**(2):285–92

87. Hammoud SS, Nix DA, Hammoud AO *et al.* Genome-
wide analysis identifies changes in histone retention and
epigenetic modifications at developmental and
imprinted gene loci in the sperm of infertile men. *Hum
Reprod.* 2011;**26**(9):2558–69.

88. Carone BR, Fauquier L, Habib N *et al.* Paternally
induced transgenerational environmental
reprogramming of metabolic gene expression in
mammals. *Cell.* 2010;**143**(7):1084–96.

89. Ng SF, Lin RC, Laybutt DR *et al.* Chronic high-fat diet
in fathers programs beta-cell dysfunction in female rat
offspring. *Nature.* 2010;**467**(7318):963–6.

90. Kaati G, Bygren LO, Pembrey M *et al.*
Transgenerational response to nutrition, early life
circumstances and longevity. *Eur J Hum Genet.*
2007;**15**(7):784–90.

91. Pembrey ME, Bygren LO, Kaati G *et al.* Sex-specific,
male-line transgenerational responses in humans. *Eur J
Hum Genet.* 2006;**14**(2):159–66.

92. Jenkins TG, Aston KI, Carrell D, editors.
Global changes to 5-methylcytosine and 5-
hydroxymethylcytosine levels associated with aging
and oligozoospermia. American Society of Andrology
Annual Meeting; 2012 April 22–24; Tuscon, AZ.

93. Puleo CM, Schmeidler J, Reichenberg A *et al.*
Advancing paternal age and simplex autism. *Autism.*
2012;**16**(4):367–80.

94. Lu Y, Ma H, Sullivan-Halley J *et al.* Parents' ages at birth
and risk of adult-onset hematologic malignancies
among female teachers in California. *Am J Epidemiol.*
2010;**171**(12):1262–9.

95. Yip BH, Pawitan Y, Czene K. Parental age and risk of
childhood cancers: a population-based cohort study
from Sweden. *Int J Epidemiol.* 2006;**35**(6):1495–503.

Imprinted gene anomalies in sperm

Cristina Joana Marques and Mário Sousa

Introduction

Spermatogenesis is the process by which a spermatogonial stem cell gives rise to a spermatozoon [1]. It can be divided into three distinct phases. The first phase involves the proliferation of spermatogonia, maintaining their number by self-renewal but also giving rise to spermatocytes. The second phase involves the primary and secondary spermatocytes, which go through the process of reductional or meiotic divisions leading to the formation of haploid cells, the spermatids. The third phase concerns the spermatids, which go through a complex series of cytological transformations leading to the production of the spermatozoon (Figure 4.1). The entire process, from primary spermatocytes to spermatozoa, takes approximately 64 days in humans [2].

Mitosis

The undifferentiated germ cells, termed spermatogonia, start to divide mitotically at puberty, giving rise to a clone of cells. Additionally to mitosis, some differentiation occurs, giving rise to primary spermatocytes [3]. Two types of spermatogonia have been described in man: type A, divided into dark (stem) and pale (progenitor) varieties, which differ by nucleus chromatin staining, and type B spermatogonia. Type A and B spermatogonia can be distinguished by their morphology although this can be difficult since morphological characters alter through the life cycle of the cells. It is only during their long S phase and in G_2 phase that they acquire their characteristic nuclear morphology [1]. Type A spermatogonia belong to the stem cell pool of spermatogenesis whereas type B represent the onset of germ cell development up to spermatids [4].

Meiosis

Spermatocytes are the cells that undergo meiosis, i.e. the two successive divisions leading to the production of the haploid cells, the spermatids. Interphasic spermatocytes, or preleptotene spermatocytes, give rise to leptotene spermatocytes in which chromatin becomes clearly filamentous [1]. After the leptotene step, primary spermatocytes enter the zygotene step, during which there is pairing of the homologous chromosomes. As the chromosomes shorten and become thicker, the cell enters the pachytene stage. The chromatin stays in this condition for a long period of time, during which the nuclear and cellular volumes progressively increase. In pachytene spermatocytes, homologous chromosomes are paired and exchange DNA segments through a process of homologous recombination (or meiotic crossing-over). This is helped by a number of proteins, which are localized at the sites of recombination along the paired chromosomes, in structures called synaptonemal complexes [5] and is followed by the short diplotene stage, during which the chromosomes partly split. Finally, the nucleus goes through metaphase, anaphase, and telophase of the first maturation division to yield secondary spermatocytes. These cells have a short lifespan, and without duplicating their DNA they enter the second maturation division, resulting in the formation of the haploid spermatids.

Spermiogenesis

The final phase of spermatogenesis is the differentiation of spermatids into spermatozoa. This process involves extensive cell remodeling, including elongation, but no further cell divisions. During spermiogenesis, three processes take place: condensation of the nuclear

Paternal Influences on Human Reproductive Success, ed. Douglas T. Carrell. Published by Cambridge University Press.
© Cambridge University Press 2013.

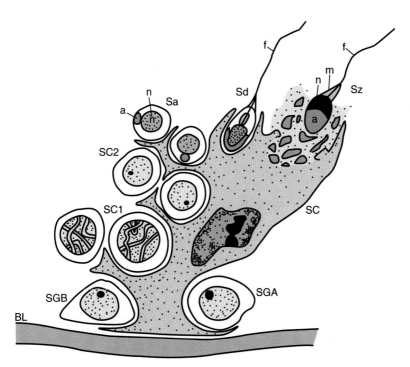

Figure 4.1. Schematic representation of human spermatogenesis in the germinal epithelium. Basal Lamina (BL); Sertoli cell (SC); Spermatogonia A (SGA) and B (SGB); Primary spermatocytes (SC1); Secondary spermatocytes (SC2); Round spermatids (Sa) with round nucleus (n) and acrosomic vesicle (a); Elongated spermatids (Sd) with a flagellum (f); Spermatozoa (Sz) with mitochondria (m) in the midpiece. This figure is presented in color in the color plate section.

chromatin, formation of the enzyme-filled acrosomal vesicle and development of flagellum structures [4]. The head of a sperm consists almost entirely of the nucleus, which contains the DNA bearing the sperm's genetic information. The tip of the nucleus is covered by the acrosomal vesicle, a protein-filled vesicle containing several enzymes that play an important role in the entrance of sperm into the oocyte by digesting the zona pellucida. Most of the tail is a flagellum – a group of contractile microtubules that produce whip-like movements capable of propelling the sperm at a velocity of 1–4 mm/min. The sperm's mitochondria form the midpiece of the sperm and provide the energy for the sperm's movement [3]. The delivery of testicular spermatozoa from the germinal epithelium is called spermiation and is managed by the Sertoli cells.

One important process occurring during spermiogenesis is the compaction of the sperm genome into the sperm head, achieved through the replacement of histones by protamines [6]. During spermatogenesis, there is a replacement of somatic histones by testis-specific variants, followed by the replacement of most histones (85% in human sperm) by transition proteins and then with protamines [7]. Some histone variants were found to be crucial for spermatogenesis to develop normally, mainly phosphorylated H2AX (γH2AX) and

H3.3 which are involved in the mechanism of MSCI (Meiotic Sex Chromosome Inactivation) which occurs to silence transcription in the XY body during the pachytene stage of meiotic prophase [8]. H2AX is an important part of the nucleosome of meiotic cells and it gets phosphorylated in response to double-strand breaks (DSB) in DNA [9]. During spermatogenesis, it accumulates in the sex (XY) body in leptotene/diplotene spermatocytes and allows efficient accumulation of DNA repair proteins [10]. H3.3 incorporation into the XY body promotes extensive chromatin remodeling and is essential for gene silencing on the XY body during the later stages of MSCI and the post-meiotic stages of spermatogenesis [11]. Histone-to-protamine exchange is associated with core histone acetylation, as acetyl groups turn the basic state of histones into a neutral one which, as a consequence, decreases the affinity of histones for DNA and allows protamines to interact with DNA [12]. After meiosis, the beginning of spermiogenesis is characterized by a massive wave of transcriptional activity, which results in the activation of a number of essential post-meiotic genes in early haploid cells [6].

Genomic imprinting

Genomic imprinting is a parental effect mechanism that was first described back in 1984, after experiments of nuclear transplantation in the mouse showing that embryos with two paternal genomes (androgenotes) or two maternal genomes (gynogenotes) were not viable [13, 14]. Moreover, the two conditions seemed to have an opposite phenotype: although gynogenotes gave rise to a relatively normal embryo, albeit small, with severely deficient extraembryonic tissues, androgenotes exhibited embryos very retarded, even though the trophoblast developed relatively well. These results indicated that while the paternal genome was essential for normal development of extraembryonic tissues, the maternal genome might be essential for some stages of embryogenesis [15]. It was thus suggested that specific imprinting of the paternal and maternal genomes occurred during gametogenesis rendering the maternal and paternal contributions not equivalent, so that both a male and female pronucleus is essential in an egg for full-term development.

Imprinted genes show monoallelic expression that is dependent on the parental origin. They usually acquire methylation in one of the germlines, at the differentially methylated regions (DMRs), with the methylated allele being repressed most of the time [16]. Although active genome-wide demethylation occurs in early development, with the paternal pronucleus undergoing a very rapid loss of methylation upon fertilization, this was shown not to affect germline imprints that were previously established [16]. Active DNA demethylation might be achieved by two main candidate pathways: (a) deamination of 5-methylcytosine to thymine by AID and/or APOBEC families of cytidine deaminases, followed by replacement by the mismatch or base excision repair machinery or (b) hydroxylation of the 5-methylcytosine (5mC) into 5-hydroxymethylcytosine (5hmC) by enzymes of the TET family with subsequent enforced passive demethylation due to loss of recognition by DNMT1 or active demethylation by spontaneous or enzymatic removal of the methyl group or by specialized DNA repair proteins recognizing hmC [17].

Establishment of imprinting marks in the male germline

In order to reset imprinting marks in the germline, erasure of previous DNA methylation somatic imprints must occur before the cells undergo gametogenesis. It has been shown in mice that genome-wide erasure of DNA methylation occurs in primordial germ cells (PGCs), between 11.5 and 13.5 dpc (days post-coitum), after the cells migrate into the genital ridge [18, 19]. This erasure was shown to occur in single-copy genes and DMRs of imprinted genes. However, repetitive elements such as intracisternal A particles (IAPs) seemed to be more resistant to this demethylating activity. This process of DNA demethylation in PGCs was shown to be accompanied by an extensive erasure of several histone modifications and exchange of histone variants [20]. Based on their observations, the authors proposed that loss of DNA methylation occurred before histone replacement and that both events were crucial for the acquisition of totipotency in PGCs. A more recent study characterized genome-wide methylation of wild-type and AID-deficient PGCs at embryonic day 13.5 [21]. The authors showed that wild-type PGCs are clearly devoid of methylation, with female PGCs showing methylation levels of 20% while male PGCs had even less methylation, around 10%. For comparison, the authors observed methylation levels in sperm to be around 80–90%. Interestingly, AID-deficient PGCs were up to three times more methylated than wild-type ones, with hypermethylation occurring throughout the genome, with introns, intergenic regions and transposons being relatively more methylated than exons. These results point to an important role for AID in the erasure of methylation in primordial germ cells.

Remethylation of the paternally methylated H19 imprinted gene was shown to start soon after the process of erasure occurs, with mouse 15.5 dpc prospermatogonia already showing a high level of methylation on the paternally inherited alleles [22]. Surprisingly, the maternally inherited alleles start to become remethylated later, at 18.5 dpc and are only completely methylated after completion of meiosis I [23]. These interesting observations show that acquisition of H19 methylation occurs differentially in male germ cell development, which indicates that parental alleles are still distinguishable even when devoid of methylation.

The other two paternally methylated imprinted genes, Gtl2 and Rasgrf1, were shown to become remethylated in mice between embryonic days E12.5 and E17.5 and were already completely methylated in mature sperm [24].

Notably, although methylation levels at CpGs seem to be high in sperm, methylation in a CpG island context is markedly lower [25]. In fact, concerning promoter methylation, sperm were shown to be remarkably similar to embryonic stem (ES) and embryonic germ (EG) cells suggesting that promoters in sperm are already epigenetically reprogrammed and resemble those in pluripotent cell types.

Additionally to DNA methylation marks, histone modifications were also shown to mark imprinted genes in murine spermatogenesis [26]. Specifically, the authors observed that, in stages preceding the global histone-to-protamine exchange (spermatocytes, round and elongating spermatids), H3 lysine 4 methylation and H3 acetylation activating marks are enriched at maternally methylated ICRs (namely *Igf2r* and KvDMR1) but are absent at paternally methylated ICRs. More recently, in an attempt to uncover what signals paternal imprint acquisition in male germ cells, Henckel and collaborators have shown that in PGCs at 13.5 dpc, before acquisition of imprints, H3 lysine-9 and H4 lysine-20 trimethylation are depleted from Imprinting Control Regions (ICRs) in male PGCs, indicating that these modifications do not signal subsequent imprint acquisition [27]. Additionally, H3 lysine-4 trimethylation becomes biallelically enriched at 'maternal' ICRs which are protected against DNA methylation and whose promoters are active in male germ cells. The authors suggest that differential histone modifications linked to transcriptional events may signal the specificity of imprint acquisition in the male germline.

DNA methyltransferases expression

DNA methyltransferases (DNMTs) establish and maintain methylation patterns by adding methyl groups to the carbon 5 position of cytosines located at CpG dinucleotides. Five DNMTs have been described so far – DNMT1, DNMT2, DNMT3A, DNMT3B, and DNMT3L – and characterized in terms of their function [28]: DNMT1 has been shown to act preferentially on hemimethylated DNA and to associate with replication foci during S-phase of mitotic divisions, maintaining methylation during DNA replication preceding cell divisions; on the other hand, DNMT3A and DNMT3B encode essential *de novo* methyltransferases that are responsible for establishing new patterns of DNA methylation. Both DNMT3A and DNMT3L, a co-factor without enzymatic activity but that might be involved in the acquisition of germ cells methylation, have been shown to be essential for normal spermatogenesis to occur [29, 30].

In the male germline, DNMT1 and DNMT3B were shown to be downregulated in gonocytes between 14.5

and 18.5 days of gestation; on the other hand, DNMT3A and DNMT3L are highly expressed in these cells suggesting that they interact to establish *de novo* methylation in prenatal male germ cell development [31]. In adult murine spermatogenesis, these same authors observed that *Dnmt1*, *Dnmt3a*, and *Dnmt3b* transcripts were at their highest level in type A spermatogonia, decreased in type B spermatogonia and preleptotene spermatocytes, increasing again in leptotene/zyotene spermatocytes and in round spermatids [32]. These results suggest that DNA methyltransferases are tightly regulated during spermatogenesis and may contribute differentially to the establishment and maintenance of methylation patterns in male germ cells.

Establishment of imprinting marks in human spermatogenesis

The study of imprinting marks in human spermatogenic cell stages has been described in two reports [33, 34]. The first report, in 2000, analyzed *H19* and *MEST* imprinted genes methylation in individual microdissected cells (from frozen testicular biopsies) at different stages of male germ cell differentiation – fetal spermatogonia, adult spermatogonia, primary spermatocytes, round spermatids, elongated spermatids, and spermatozoa [33]. The authors observed that *H19* and *MEST* were completely unmethylated at fetal spermatogonia, suggesting that the erasure of previous imprints had already taken place, in line with observations in mice where imprints are erased in primordial germ cells. *MEST* genes remained unmethylated in the subsequent stages whereas *H19* started to become remethylated in adult spermatogonia and was completely methylated in primary spermatocytes and subsequent stages up to the spermatozoa stage.

In a more recent report, we have analyzed DNA methylation of *H19* and *MEST* imprinted genes together with DNMTs expression in all stages of human adult spermatogenesis – spermatogonia, primary spermatocytes, secondary spermatocytes, round spermatids and elongated spermatids/spermatozoa [34]. The cells were isolated by micromanipulation from fresh testicular biopsies of three individuals with normal spermatogenesis, undergoing intracytoplasmic sperm injection (ICSI) treatments due to spinal cord injuries. We observed that *H19* was already methylated at the spermatogonial level, with the exception of a few CpGs (maximum three unmethylated CpGs). This high level of methylation was kept in subsequent stages up to the elongated spermatid/spermatozoa stage. Concordantly, *MEST* was found to be unmethylated at all cell stages analyzed with a maximum of 3 CpGs methylated. Regarding DNMTs expression, we observed that maintenance (*DNMT1*) and *de novo* (*DNMT3A and 3B*) methyltransferases were present at all stages of spermatogenesis, with higher mRNA expression at the primary spermatocyte stage and cell-stage specific shuttling between the nucleus and the cytoplasm. Additionally, mRNA levels were increased in ejaculated spermatozoa for all DNMTs, showing distinct localizations – DNMT1 localized in the equatorial region of the sperm head, DNMT3A in the midpiece and DNMT3B in the anterior half of the sperm head. These interesting observations show that DNMTs are present throughout spermatogenesis and particularly at the ejaculated spermatozoa stage, possibly preventing transmission of DNA methylation errors by the male gamete.

Imprinted gene anomalies in human sperm

Abnormal methylation of imprinted genes has been observed in sperm from infertile patients presenting impaired spermatogenesis. A summary of all the studies is described below and depicted in Table 4.1.

Ejaculated sperm

The first imprinting analysis in spermatozoa from men with abnormal sperm count, undergoing ICSI, concluded that there were no methylation defects comparing with normal controls [35]. The authors analyzed methylation at the *SNRPN* imprinted gene, using methylation-specific PCR (M-PCR), and although they had some amplification of maternal specific imprints using an hemi-nested M-PCR, they attributed this fact to possible contamination by diploid cells or incomplete sodium bisulfite treatment.

However, in a subsequent study, our group has shown that *H19* imprinted gene was hypomethylated in sperm from oligozoospermic patients comparing with normal controls [36]. In this study, we used a more sensitive analysis of methylation, by bisulfite genomic sequencing, and analyzed two imprinted genes, one paternally methylated (*H19*) and one unmethylated on the paternal allele (*MEST/PEG1*), on 27 normozoospermic males comparing with 46

moderate oligozoospermic (5–20 million sperm/mL) and 49 severe oligozoospermic (< 5 million sperm/mL) patients. We observed that, although *MEST* gene was correctly unmethylated in all cases, *H19* was hypomethylated in 17% of moderate oligozoospermic and 30% of severe oligozoospermic patients while normozoospermic males presented complete methylation of *H19* on their sperm. Additionally, the CTCF binding site 6 was affected in 11% of the oligozoospermic patients. CTCF is an insulator protein that binds to the unmethylated *H19* DMR in the maternal allele, preventing the *H19/IGF2* common enhancers from activating another imprinted gene, the paternally expressed *IGF2* [37]. The methylation status of the human CTCF binding site 6 was observed to correlate with *IGF2* expression [38]. Following these observations, we hypothesized that sperm from infertile patients could carry an increased risk of transmitting imprinting errors to their offspring.

Indeed, a later study by Kobayashi and collaborators [39], analysing methylation of seven imprinted genes, using a combined bisulfite-PCR restriction analysis and sequencing, in sperm from 97 infertile men, found an abnormal paternal methylation imprint in 14% of the patients and an abnormal maternal imprint in 20% of the patients. Specifically, the imprinted genes that were found to have abnormal methylation were *H19* and *GTL2* (paternally methylated) and *PEG1* (also known as *MEST*), *ZAC* and *SNRPN* (maternally methylated). Additionally, the authors reported that methylation changes were specific to imprinted loci since global DNA methylation, at repetitive DNA elements such as LINE1 and Alu, was normal in these samples.

Another study, using MethyLight and Illumina assays, enabling the analysis of a larger set of sequences, described that methylation levels were generally elevated in DNA from poor-quality sperm, including in maternally imprinted genes *PLAGL1* and *MEST* [40].

We then analyzed methylation of *H19* and *MEST* at the single sperm level, using bisulfite and cloning sequencing [41]. We observed that sperm from patients with less than 10 million sperm per mL carried severe imprinting errors such as *H19* complete unmethylation and *MEST* complete methylation. Although we could observe some methylation changes at a few CpGs in normozoospermic males, both in *H19* and *MEST*, the extent of methylation changes were much more pronounced in sperm from oligozoospermic patients. These methylation changes seemed to be

Table 4.1 Summary of imprinting errors described in sperm from infertile patients.

References	Genes/Regions	Patients	Alterations in DNA methylation
Marques et al., 2004 [36]	H19, MEST	27 NZ 96 OZ	Hypomethylation of H19 (and CTCF-6) in 24% OZ
Kobayashi et al., 2007 [39]	H19, GTL2, PEG1, LIT1, ZAC, PEG3, SNRPN	79 NZ 18 OZ	Hypomethylation in 14% and hypermethylation in 21% patients
Houshdaran et al., 2007 [40]	Repetitive elements, promoter CpG islands, and DMRs of imprinted genes	65[a]	Hypermethylation in nine regions associated with decreased sperm concentration and motility
Marques et al., 2008 [41]	H19, MEST, LINE1	5 NZ 20 OZ	Hypomethylation of H19 (and CTCF-6) and/or hypermethylation of MEST in 47% of patients with sperm count below 10×10^6 Sz/mL
Poplinski et al., 2010 [43]	IGF2/H19 (ICR1), MEST	33 NZ 148 idiopathic infertile	Hypomethylation at ICR1 and hypermethylation of MEST associated with low sperm counts. MEST hypermethylation associated with low sperm motility and abnormal morphology
Marques et al., 2010 [51]	H19, MEST	24 AZ	Hypomethylation of H19 (and CTCF-6) in SAZ and hypermethylation of MEST in OAZ
Boissonnas et al., 2010 [45]	IGF2 (DMR0 and DMR2), H19 (CTCF-3 and CTCF-6), PEG3, LINE1	17 NZ 19 T 22 OAT	Loss of methylation of IGF2-DMR2 and/or CTCF-6 in 58% T patients and loss of methylation of CTCF-6 in 73% of OAT patients
Hammoud et al., 2010 [42]	LIT1, MEST, SNRPN, PLAGL1, PEG3, H19, IGF2	5 fertile 10 OZ 10 APR	Alterations in OZ and APR in all imprinted genes except IGF2
El Hajj et al., 2011 [49]	H19, GTL2, LIT1, MEST, NESPAS, PEG3, ALU, LINE1	35 NZ 106 abnormal	Aberrant methylation of imprints and repetitive elements in association with abnormal semen parameters
Sato et al., 2011 [46]	ZDBF2, H19, GTL2, PEG1, LIT1, ZAC, PEG3, SNRPN	209 NZ 128 OZ	A total of 47 cases showed abnormal methylation at one or more imprinted genes
Minor et al., 2011 [52]	H19, GTL2, MEST	18 AZO 17 VR 9 fertile	Significant decrease in H19 methylation in AZO and VR patients
Aston et al., 2012 [50]	Genome-wide, >27,000 CpGs	15 APR 13 'abnormal embryogenesis' 15 NZ	2 APR and one 'abnormal embryogenesis' patients displayed significantly altered methylation patterns; imprinted regions were more prone to deregulation

NZ, normozoospermia; OZ, oligozoospermia; AZO, azoospermia; SAZ, secretory azoospermia (germinal hypoplasia); OAZ, obstructive azoospermia; T, teratozoospermia; OAT, oligozoospermia and/or asthenozoospermia and/or teratozoospermia; APR, abnormal protamine replacement; VR, vasectomy reversal.
[a]Patients were not classified in terms of spermiogram results.

restricted to the imprinted genes analyzed since we did not observe altered methylation levels at LINE1 retrotransposons, as described before by Kobayashi and collaborators [39]. An important observation was that patients presenting sperm with imprinting errors also had sperm with normal methylation at both imprinted genes, which could justify the low frequency of imprinting errors seen in children born after IVF treatments [42]. Again, we observed unmethylation at the CTCF binding site 6 which could lead to aberrant

IGF2 repression on the paternal allele and be linked to decreased embryo quality and low birth weight, often associated with assisted reproduction technology (ART).

Another study, by Poplinski and colleagues [43], reported that low sperm counts were clearly associated with *IGF2/H19* ICR1 hypomethylation and, even stronger, with *MEST* hypermethylation. Additionally, these authors sequenced the CTCFL gene in 20 men with severe methylation defects but no bona fide mutation was found. CTCFL (also known as BORIS) is present only in the testis and is thought to be involved in the erasure of methylation marks in the male germline [44].

Boissonnas and collaborators [45] analyzed DNA methylation at DMRs of *IGF2* and *H19* imprinted genes, including the sixth CTCF binding site, in human sperm from patients with teratozoospermia (T) and oligoasthenoteratozoospermia (OAT).

In the teratozoospermia group, 11 of 19 patients presented a loss of methylation at variable CpG positions either in the *IGF2* DMR2 or in both the *IGF2* DMR2 and the sixth CTCF binding site of the *H19* DMR. In the OAT group, 16 of 22 patients presented a severe loss of methylation of the sixth CTCF binding site, closely correlated with sperm concentration. The authors concluded that epigenetic perturbations of the sixth CTCF site of the H19 DMR might be a relevant biomarker for quantitative defects of spermatogenesis in humans, consistent with our previous observations [36, 41].

Concerning other causes of male infertility such as abnormal protamine replacement, Hammoud and colleagues [42] studied methylation patterns at seven imprinted loci (*LIT1*, *MEST*, *SNRPN*, *PLAGL1*, *PEG3*, *H19*, and *IGF2*) in patients with abnormal replacement of nuclear proteins by protamine 1 and protamine 2 together with oligozoospermic patients. They observed that at six of the seven imprinted genes analyzed, the overall DNA methylation was significantly altered in both infertile patient populations. The oligozoospermic patients were significantly affected at mesoderm-specific transcript (*MEST*), whereas abnormal protamine patients were affected at KCNQ1, overlapping transcript 1 (*LIT1*), and at small nuclear ribonucleoprotein polypeptide N (*SNRPN*). Therefore, this study also provided evidence that an association between male factor infertility and alterations in sperm DNA methylation at imprinted loci occur.

The study of Sato and colleagues [46] used an automated high-throughput procedure (BPL-bisulfite polymerase chain reaction Luminex), for the detection of alterations in DNA methylation in a total of 337 men, including oligozoospermia and normozoospermia. They observed that a total of 47 cases showed abnormal methylation at one or more imprinted loci, albeit 11 of these had normal sperm counts. The most frequent error in oligozoospermic patients was seen at the *PEG1/MEST* DMR, as described by others [42, 43].

MEST deficiency in mice causes embryonic growth retardation as well as abnormal maternal behavior in females [47]. Therefore, alterations on imprinted genes methylation and expression could be related to the low birth weight in ART children [48].

Another study suggested that hypomethylation at repetitive element ALU is associated with male infertility and/or poor sperm quality, but more importantly also with a poor ART outcome [49].

A more recent study analyzed genome-wide sperm DNA methylation, at more than 27,000 CpGs, in abnormal protamination patients and in patients who have undergone IVF/ICSI resulting in abnormal embryogenesis [50]. Two men with abnormal protamine 1/protamine 2 ratio and one abnormal embryogenesis patient displayed significantly altered methylation patterns across a large number of CpGs, particularly in sites located in imprinted regions. The authors suggest that broad disruption in sperm DNA methylation may be an important signature in some infertile men.

Testicular sperm

To date, only two reports have analyzed methylation of imprinted genes in testicular sperm retrieved from testicular biopsies of azoospermic patients [51, 52]. We analyzed a total of 24 azoospermic patients, five with anejaculation (mainly due to spinal cord injuries), five with secondary obstructive (inflammatory) azoospermia, five with primary obstructive azoospermia (with congenital absence of vas deferens) and nine with secretory azoospermia (due to hypospermatogenesis) [51]. We observed that *H19* methylation, including the sixth CTCF binding site, was significantly reduced in the secretory azoospermia group, in line with previous observations in oligozoospermic patients. Additionally, *MEST* methylation seemed to be more perturbed in the anejaculation and secondary obstructive azoospermia.

A subsequent report isolated testicular sperm from men undergoing vasectomy reversal and from men with azoospermia, both obstructive and non-obstructive. They have shown a decrease in *H19* methylation in patients with azoospermia, albeit this was also observed in the obstructive azoospermic and vasectomy reversal patients [52]. However, the authors did not see any significant changes in *MEST* methylation levels, although some *MEST* clones were completely methylated in two patients, one with vasectomy reversal and the other with azoospermia. The authors suggest that imprinting errors may arise also in response to testicular environment and not only due to spermatogenic failure.

Another study, in spermatogonia and primary spermatocytes isolated from tubules with spermatogenic arrest, claims that there is no evidence for *H19* imprinting errors in these patients; however, the technique the authors used to analyze methylation (SSCA – single strand conformation analysis) only allows the analysis of one CpG in the region, which might account for the lack of evidence for methylation errors [53]. In fact, our unpublished observations show that there are methylation errors at *H19* and *MEST* imprinted genes in primary spermatocytes from patients with impaired spermatogenesis.

Altogether, the studies on ejaculated and testicular sperm from patients with perturbations in spermatogenesis show that abnormal methylation is present at several imprinted genes suggesting that further studies should be undertaken when evaluating sperm quality before using these sperm cells for ART procedures.

Methylenetetrahydrofolate reductase anomalies

Methylenetetrahydrofolate reductase (MTHFR) is one of the main regulatory enzymes involved in folate metabolism, DNA synthesis and remethylation reactions, catalyzing the reduction of 5,10-methylenetetrahydrofolate to 5-methylenetetrahydrofolate, which is the methyl donor for remethylation of homocysteine to methionine. Methionine is in turn converted to S-adenosylmethionine, a methyl donor used in many reactions whereby substrates such as DNA, RNA, hormones and lipids are methylated. In adult male mice, it has been shown that MTHFR levels are highest in the testis suggesting an important role for MTHFR in spermatogenesis. Indeed, *MTHFR* deficiency in mice has been shown to result in abnormal spermatogenesis and infertility [54]. In humans, hypermethylation of the *MTHFR* promoter has been observed in sperm from infertile patients, including oligozoospermic males and in the testis of infertile patients presenting non-obstructive azoospermia [55, 56]. These observations suggest that epigenetic silencing of *MTHFR* could play a role in infertility and may underlie the occurrence of hypomethylation imprinting errors in sperm from infertile patients.

ART consequences of epigenetic defects in the gametes

Imprinting disorders, especially Beckwith–Wiedemann syndrome (BWS) and Angelman syndrome (AS), have been described in a higher frequency in ART children [57]. Importantly, the majority of these children had an imprinting defect as the underlying cause, usually hypomethylation of the maternal allele. This led to the speculation that hormonal ovarian stimulation and/or embryo culture could disrupt the acquisition and maintenance of maternal imprinting marks. Although imprinting errors arising from the paternal allele are less frequent in disease, Silver–Russell syndrome (SRS) has been linked with hypomethylation of *H19* and to be more frequent in ART children [58]. This suggests that the transmission of imprinting errors might be related not only to ART techniques but also to the underlying infertility that could result in the gametes carrying imprinting defects. Indeed, a study analyzing paired samples of ART conceptuses (aborted samples) and parental sperm has shown that abnormal methylation present in the ART sample frequently arose from the parental sperm, especially in the form of abnormal hypomethylation at *H19* and *GTL2* [59]. However, another study analyzing *H19* methylation in day 3 discarded human embryos reported that 19% of the embryos exhibited a hypomethylation pattern that was not observed in the original sperm samples, suggesting that embryo culture could have resulted in the loss of methylation observed [60]. Indeed, a subsequent study has corroborated these findings in developmentally arrested embryos that also showed hypomethylation of *H19* imprinted gene although the matching sperm had normal methylation [61]. Therefore, the authors suggested that the hypomethylation of the paternal allele observed in the embryo could be due to instability of the imprinting mark during the demethylation process that takes place in the early embryo.

Conclusions

Abnormal spermatogenesis leading to oligozoospermia or non-obstructive azoospermia seems to be intrinsically linked to the appearance of methylation errors at imprinted genes in human sperm. The consequences of such errors are still poorly understood but the fact that IVF/ICSI children only rarely exhibit imprinting syndromes related to paternal methylation errors is reassuring. In fact, only

Silver–Russell syndrome (SRS) has been linked to *H19* hypomethylation on the paternal allele and it is still uncertain whether the frequency of this syndrome is increased in ART children. One possible explanation, based on our observations, is that infertile patients that carry imprinting errors in their sperm usually also have normally methylated sperm and these might be more "fit" for fertilizing the oocyte. Another explanation might be that embryos inheriting *H19* hypomethylation from the paternal allele might show developmental delay or arrest since this will result in *IGF2* decreased expression. However, increasing evidence of imprinting errors in sperm from patients with abnormal spermatogenesis is indisputable, recommending that caution should be taken when using these sperm cells in ART procedures, and more research is needed in order to better understand the possible causes and consequences of these epigenetic anomalies.

References

1. Clermont Y. Kinetics of spermatogenesis in mammals: seminiferous epithelium cycle and spermatogonial renewal. *Physiolog Rev.* 1972;**52**(1):198–236.

2. Heller CG, Clermont Y. Spermatogenesis in man: an estimate of its duration. *Science* 1963;**140**:184–6.

3. Vander A, Sherman J, Luciano D. Spermatogenesis. In Kane KT, editor. *Human Physiology: The Mechanisms of Body Function.* New York, NY: WCB/McGraw-Hill; 1998, pp. 635–87.

4. Holstein AF, Schulze W, Davidoff M. Understanding spermatogenesis is a prerequisite for treatment. *Reprod Biol Endocrinol.* 2003;**1**:107.

5. Rousseaux S, Caron C, Govin J *et al.* Establishment of male-specific epigenetic information. *Gene.* 2005;**345**(2):139–53.

6. Sassone-Corsi P. Unique chromatin remodeling and transcriptional regulation in spermatogenesis. *Science* 2002;**296**(5576):2176–8.

7. Kimmins S, Sassone-Corsi P. Chromatin remodelling and epigenetic features of germ cells. *Nature.* 2005;**434**(7033):583–9.

8. Zamudio NM, Chong S, O'Bryan MK. Epigenetic regulation in male germ cells. *Reproduction.* 2008;**136**(2):131–46.

9. Celeste A, Petersen S, Romanienko PJ *et al.* Genomic instability in mice lacking histone H2AX. *Science* 2002;**296**(5569):922–7.

10. Mahadevaiah SK, Turner JM, Baudat F *et al.* Recombinational DNA double-strand breaks in mice precede synapsis. *Nat Genet.* 2001;**27**(3):271–6.

11. van der Heijden GW, Derijck AA, Posfai E *et al.* Chromosome-wide nucleosome replacement and H3.3 incorporation during mammalian meiotic sex chromosome inactivation. *Nat Genet.* 2007;**39**(2):251–8.

12. Biermann K, Steger K. Epigenetics in male germ cells. *J Androl.* 2007;**28**(4):466–80.

13. McGrath J, Solter D. Completion of mouse embryogenesis requires both the maternal and paternal genomes. *Cell.* 1984;**37**(1):179–83.

14. Surani MA, Barton SC, Norris ML. Development of reconstituted mouse eggs suggests imprinting of the genome during gametogenesis. *Nature.* 1984;**308**(5959):548–50.

15. Barton SC, Surani MA, Norris ML. Role of paternal and maternal genomes in mouse development. *Nature.* 1984;**311**(5984):374–6.

16. Reik W, Walter J. Genomic imprinting: parental influence on the genome. *Nat Rev.* 2001;**2**(1):21–32.

17. Branco MR, Ficz G, Reik W. Uncovering the role of 5-hydroxymethylcytosine in the epigenome. *Nat Rev.* 2012;**13**(1):7–13.

18. Hajkova P, Erhardt S, Lane N *et al.* Epigenetic reprogramming in mouse primordial germ cells. *Mechanisms Develop.* 2002;**117**(1–2):15–23.

19. Lee J, Inoue K, Ono R *et al.* Erasing genomic imprinting memory in mouse clone embryos produced from day 11.5 primordial germ cells. *Development* 2002;**129**(8):1807–17.

20. Hajkova P, Ancelin K, Waldmann T *et al.* Chromatin dynamics during epigenetic reprogramming in the mouse germ line. *Nature.* 2008;**452**(7189):877–81.

21. Popp C, Dean W, Feng S *et al.* Genome-wide erasure of DNA methylation in mouse primordial germ cells is affected by AID deficiency. *Nature.* 2010;**463**(7284):1101–5.

22. Davis TL, Yang GJ, McCarrey JR *et al.* The H19 methylation imprint is erased and re-established differentially on the parental alleles during male germ cell development. *Hum Mol Gen.* 2000;**9**(19):2885–94.

23. Davis TL, Trasler JM, Moss SB *et al.* Acquisition of the H19 methylation imprint occurs differentially on the parental alleles during spermatogenesis. *Genomics.* 1999;**58**(1):18–28.

24. Li JY, Lees-Murdock DJ, Xu GL *et al.* Timing of establishment of paternal methylation imprints in the mouse. *Genomics.* 2004;**84**(6):952–60.

25. Smallwood SA, Tomizawa S, Krueger F *et al.* Dynamic CpG island methylation landscape in oocytes and

preimplantation embryos. *Nat Genet.* 2011;**43** (8):811–14.

26. Delaval K, Govin J, Cerqueira F *et al.* Differential histone modifications mark mouse imprinting control regions during spermatogenesis. *EMBO J.* 2007;**26** (3):720–9.

27. Henckel A, Chebli K, Kota SK *et al.* Transcription and histone methylation changes correlate with imprint acquisition in male germ cells. *EMBO J.* 2012;**31** (3):606–15.

28. Bestor TH. The DNA methyltransferases of mammals. *Hum Mol Gen.* 2000;**9**(16):2395–402.

29. Bourc'his D, Bestor TH. Meiotic catastrophe and retrotransposon reactivation in male germ cells lacking DNMT3L. *Nature.* 2004;**431**(7004):96–9.

30. Kaneda M, Okano M, Hata K *et al.* Essential role for *de novo* DNA methyltransferase DNMT3A in paternal and maternal imprinting. *Nature.* 2004;**429**(6994):900–3.

31. La Salle S, Mertineit C, Taketo T *et al.* Windows for sex-specific methylation marked by DNA methyltransferase expression profiles in mouse germ cells. *Dev Biol.* 2004;**268**(2):403–15.

32. La Salle S, Trasler JM. Dynamic expression of DNMT3A and DNMT3B isoforms during male germ cell development in the mouse. *Dev Biol.* 2006;**296** (1):71–82.

33. Kerjean A, Dupont JM, Vasseur C *et al.* Establishment of the paternal methylation imprint of the human H19 and MEST/PEG1 genes during spermatogenesis. *Hum Mol Gen.* 2000;**9**(14):2183–7.

34. Marques CJ, Joao Pinho M, Carvalho F *et al.* DNA methylation imprinting marks and DNA methyltransferase expression in human spermatogenic cell stages. *Epigenetics.* 2011;**6**(11):1354–61.

35. Manning M, Lissens W, Liebaers I *et al.* Imprinting analysis in spermatozoa prepared for intracytoplasmic sperm injection (ICSI). *Int J Androl.* 2001;**24**(2):87–94.

36. Marques CJ, Carvalho F, Sousa M *et al.* Genomic imprinting in disruptive spermatogenesis. *Lancet.* 2004;**363**(9422):1700–2.

37. Bell AC, Felsenfeld G. Methylation of a CTCF-dependent boundary controls imprinted expression of the Igf2 gene. *Nature.* 2000;**405**(6785):482–5.

38. Takai D, Gonzales FA, Tsai YC *et al.* Large scale mapping of methylcytosines in CTCF-binding sites in the human H19 promoter and aberrant hypomethylation in human bladder cancer. *Hum Mol Gen.* 2001;**10**(23):2619–26.

39. Kobayashi H, Sato A, Otsu E *et al.* Aberrant DNA methylation of imprinted loci in sperm from oligospermic patients. *Hum Mol Gen.* 2007;**16** (21):2542–51.

40. Houshdaran S, Cortessis VK, Siegmund K *et al.* Widespread epigenetic abnormalities suggest a broad DNA methylation erasure defect in abnormal human sperm. *PLoS One.* 2007;**2**(12):e1289.

41. Marques CJ, Costa P, Vaz B *et al.* Abnormal methylation of imprinted genes in human sperm is associated with oligozoospermia. *Mol Hum Reprod.* 2008;**14**(2):67–74.

42. Hammoud SS, Purwar J, Pflueger C *et al.* Alterations in sperm DNA methylation patterns at imprinted loci in two classes of infertility. *Fertil Steril.* 2010;**94** (5):1728–33.

43. Poplinski A, Tuttelmann F, Kanber D *et al.* Idiopathic male infertility is strongly associated with aberrant methylation of MEST and IGF2/H19 ICR1. *Int J Androl.* 2010;**33**(4):642–9.

44. Loukinov DI, Pugacheva E, Vatolin S *et al.* Boris, a novel male germ-line-specific protein associated with epigenetic reprogramming events, shares the same 11-zinc-finger domain with CTCF, the insulator protein involved in reading imprinting marks in the soma. *Proc Natl Acad Sci USA.* 2002;**99**(10):6806–11.

45. Boissonnas CC, Abdalaoui HE, Haelewyn V *et al.* Specific epigenetic alterations of IGF2-H19 locus in spermatozoa from infertile men. *Eur J Hum Gen.* 2010;**18**(1):73–80.

46. Sato A, Hiura H, Okae H *et al.* Assessing loss of imprint methylation in sperm from subfertile men using novel methylation polymerase chain reaction luminex analysis. *Fertil Steril.* 2011;**95**(1):129–34, 34 e1–4.

47. Lefebvre L, Viville S, Barton SC *et al.* Abnormal maternal behaviour and growth retardation associated with loss of the imprinted gene mest. *Nat Genet.* 1998;**20**(2):163–9.

48. Schieve LA, Meikle SF, Ferre C *et al.* Low and very low birth weight in infants conceived with use of assisted reproductive technology. *N Engl J Med.* 2002;**346** (10):731–7.

49. El Hajj N, Zechner U, Schneider E *et al.* Methylation status of imprinted genes and repetitive elements in sperm DNA from infertile males. *Sex Dev.* 2011;**5** (2):60–9.

50. Aston KI, Punj V, Liu L *et al.* Genome-wide sperm deoxyribonucleic acid methylation is altered in some men with abnormal chromatin packaging or poor in vitro fertilization embryogenesis. *Fertil Steril.* 2012;**97**(2):285–92.

51. Marques CJ, Francisco T, Sousa S *et al.* Methylation defects of imprinted genes in human testicular spermatozoa. *Fertil Steril.* 2010;**94** (2):585–94.

52. Minor A, Chow V, Ma S. Aberrant DNA methylation at imprinted genes in testicular sperm retrieved from men

with obstructive azoospermia and undergoing vasectomy reversal. *Reproduction*. 2011; **141**(6):749–57.

53. Hartmann S, Bergmann M, Bohle RM *et al.* Genetic imprinting during impaired spermatogenesis. *Mol Hum Reprod*. 2006;**12**(6):407–11.

54. Kelly TL, Neaga OR, Schwahn BC *et al.* Infertility in 5,10-methylenetetrahydrofolate reductase (MTHFR)-deficient male mice is partially alleviated by lifetime dietary betaine supplementation. *Biol Reprod*. 2005;**72**(3):667–77.

55. Khazamipour N, Noruzinia M, Fatehmanesh P *et al.* MTHFR promoter hypermethylation in testicular biopsies of patients with non-obstructive azoospermia: the role of epigenetics in male infertility. *Hum Reprod*. 2009;**24**(9):2361–4.

56. Wu W, Shen O, Qin Y *et al.* Idiopathic male infertility is strongly associated with aberrant promoter methylation of methylenetetrahydrofolate reductase (MTHFR). *PLoS One*. 2010;**5**(11):e13884.

57. Manipalviratn S, DeCherney A, Segars J. Imprinting disorders and assisted reproductive technology. *Fertil Steril*. 2009;**91**(2):305–15.

58. Amor DJ, Halliday J. A review of known imprinting syndromes and their association with assisted reproduction technologies. *Hum Reprod*. 2008;**23**(12):2826–34.

59. Kobayashi H, Hiura H, John RM *et al.* DNA methylation errors at imprinted loci after assisted conception originate in the parental sperm. *Eur J Hum Gen*. 2009;**17**(12):1582–91.

60. Chen SL, Shi XY, Zheng HY *et al.* Aberrant DNA methylation of imprinted H19 gene in human preimplantation embryos. *Fertil Steril*. 2010;**94**(6):2356–8, 8 e1.

61. Ibala-Romdhane S, Al-Khtib M, Khoueiry R *et al.* Analysis of H19 methylation in control and abnormal human embryos, sperm and oocytes. *Eur J Hum Gen*. 2011;**19**(11):1138–43

Has the renewed interest in sperm RNA led to fresh insights? A critical review and hypothesis

David Miller and David Iles

Introduction

The mammalian spermatozoon and those from many other classes is a terminally differentiated cell in which all (except mitochondrial) gene expression has ceased. This change from an active to an inactive nucleus is accompanied by a genome-wide switch in DNA packaging from an exclusively nucleosomal configuration to one comprising a small proportion of 'residual' nucleosomes embedded within a bulk of toroidal, protamine-based chromatin [1–3]. In the human, the ratio of nucleosomal to toroidal chromatin is 1:9 [4, 5], while in mouse, it is far lower at 1:99 [6]. The change from a generalized somatic to a specifically paternal chromatin conformation occurs during spermatid condensation when canonical histones become hyperacetylated on H3 and H4 and gene expression switches to translation of stored mRNAs [7, 8]. Condensation of the spermatid nucleus is highly efficient such that the volume of the spermatozoon nucleus is essentially no greater than the volume of chromatin it contains [9].

The sperm nucleus may be silent, but there is good evidence that it retains a structural integrity resembling an actively expressing cell where individual chromosomes occupy distinct territories within a nuclear lamina that is part of a structural scaffold of protein and RNA [10, 11]. The RNA is of particular interest because over the years, it has courted controversy over its composition and significance since there should be no requirement for it in a silent nucleus [12–16]. Because of the general shutting down of gene expression during spermatogenesis, sperm RNA was thought to be residual and the various reports showing its presence within the nucleus lent weight to the notion that it is a trapped remnant of the post-haploid transcription apparatus that is not removed in the residual

body along with the bulk cytoplasm [17]. However, since the late 1990s and particularly with the advent and development of more sophisticated molecular techniques, it has become increasingly clear that sperm RNA is unlikely to be residual [18]. Perhaps the best indicator for this is its compositional complexity with many hundreds of intact, full-length mRNAs coexisting alongside a mix of partially degraded ribosomal RNAs among many other non-coding RNA types (see below). We are now in a far better position than ever to consider whether sperm RNA has a purpose and if so, what that might be. It is against this backdrop that the most recent reports on sperm RNA composition are considered in this chapter.

Preparation for shutdown

Sperm RNA at least partially originates as a consequence of the switch from a histone-based, nucleosomal to a protamine-based toroidal chromatin configuration [7]. We know that post-meiotic transcription occurs for a large number of genes during this transitional phase and that inter-spermatocyte/ spermatid RNA sharing ensures that all spermatids have equal access to gene products, effectively eliminating the effects of potential allelic imbalances in gene expression on individual cells [19]. Although much of this transcription is directly coupled to translation during this period, a large number of transcripts are also stored for relatively long periods in RNP complexes and are only made available for translation later on in spermiogenesis after the transition has completed [8]. The uncoupling of transcription from translation is necessary to ensure that protein synthesis can continue after transcription has finally ceased. The process of chromatin reconfiguration

Paternal Influences on Human Reproductive Success, ed. Douglas T. Carrell. Published by Cambridge University Press.
© Cambridge University Press 2013.

commences with acetylation of histones H3 and H4, which in normally active cells facilitates the local displacement of nucleosomes favoring the binding of transcription factors; see [20] for recent review. In spermiogenesis, however, hyperacetylation is more of a genome-wide phenomenon that may aid the removal of bulk nucleosomes en masse [21–23]. Under "normal" circumstances, such unmasking could lead to illegitimate transcription of the genome through permissive transcription factor and RNA Pol II binding. Whether this occurs in the spermatid is unknown, although the recently reported presence of a significant cargo of RNAs transcribed from medium reiteration repetitive elements (MER), short (SINE) and long interspersed nucleotide elements (LINE) in human sperm lends credence to this possibility [24].

Given that the late spermatid is transcriptionally inert and relies solely on stored mRNAs to support protein synthesis, it must follow that germ cell proteins required for spermatid condensation and spermiation arise from stored and translated mRNAs. Unlike the cumulus cells of the follicle, there is no evidence that Sertoli cells can contribute large molecules such as mRNAs or proteins to the spermatid (not that the possibility can be excluded altogether). Hence, once spermiation is completed and the sperm are deposited in the epididymis, sperm RNA is unlikely to be functional in the sperm itself. It is for this reason that although widely accepted, the persistence of mRNA in sperm is also generally assumed to be a remnant of the post-haploid support for protein synthesis in the elongating and condensing spermatid. Certainly, its main location embedded within or located peripherally around the nucleus suggests a passive "trapping" of the RNA during condensation rather than an active sequestration [25]. In this respect, it does make energetic sense for the male to "allow" sperm RNA to remain alongside other sperm components for the zygote to dispose of following fertilization. However, as we shall see, evidence is mounting that counters these assumptions.

Characteristics of sperm RNA

Like all scientific endeavors, investigating sperm RNA has depended on the availability of techniques. Its earliest descriptions made use of electron microscopy and simple electrophoresis [26–28]. Hence, bulk RNA was first described in fern, bovine, and human sperm

nuclei using in situ hybridization (ISH) with RNase colloidal gold or on denaturing acrylamide gels. In situ hybridization with ^{35}S-labeled probes has also been used to detect specific transcripts in sperm nuclei and of course, conventional RT-PCR-based strategies have detected many more transcripts in the sperm from various species, including higher plants [29, 30]. The complexity of sperm RNA was focused initially on mRNA and there are now many microarray-based inventories from human, bovine, porcine, and fly sperm but oddly, not from murine sperm (although mRNA has been detected by standard RT-PCR and in situ hybridization) in the public domain [31–36]. The mRNA is frequently full-length although there is also evidence for the persistence of fragmented transcripts [33, 37]. The failure thus far to detect precursor hnRNAs in the sperm nucleus indicates that the genome is indeed transcriptionally silent by the time the mRNA becomes lodged in the nucleus. Visually, following electrophoresis, sperm RNA does not normally show the characteristic 28S and 18S rRNA bands that dominate somatic cell and spermatid RNA preparations [33, 38]. Further evidence that rRNAs are at least partially degraded using standard extraction procedures has been described in reports based on more stringent isolation protocols suggesting that the fragmentation is partially inherent and partially an artifact of the extraction process [39]. Using a commercial chaotropically based dual capture affinity column process that does not rely on DNase 1, Cappallo-Obermann et al. were able to remove residual genomic DNA (eliminating RNA loss by contaminating RNase in so-called RNase free DNase), and allow the visualization of both 18S rRNA and to a lesser extent, 28S rRNA in human sperm RNA ([39] and Figure 5.1). The report also suggested that these dominant rRNAs were not detected in sperm previously either because of inefficient RNA extraction or loss of the residual droplets while processing semen in standard density gradient-based procedures and/or their extraction from the sperm was masked by genomic DNA contaminants. A second report using new generation sequencing (NGS) showed that ribosomal RNA indeed makes up the bulk of human sperm RNA (>75%) but that it is highly fragmented [40]. This report concluded that the fragmentation of rRNA (but not mRNA) is evidence for selective processing of the former (perhaps by protective sequestration into the nucleus) to prevent illegitimate translation of the latter in the zygote. These two reports appear to resolve the conundrum

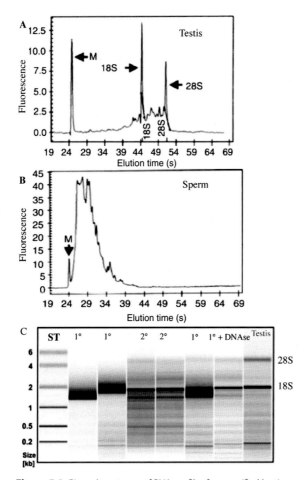

Figure 5.1. Bioanalyser traces of RNA profiles from purified bovine spermatids (A) and spermatozoa (B) and human sperm and testis samples (C). Note the prominent 28S and 18S rRNA peaks in spermatid RNA. These rRNAs are essentially lost when RNA is isolated under identical conditions from bovine (B) and human spermatozoa (not shown). However by carefully processing human sperm samples through RNA spin columns (2° or two rounds of columns) such that the DNA is completely removed, the 18S rRNA is mostly recovered while 28S rRNA is partially recovered. Similar recovery is possible using one round (1°) of columns followed by RNAse-free DNAse treatment. Adapted with permission from Gilbert *et al.* (2007) [33] and Cappallo-Obermann *et al.* (2011) [39].

of the apparent absence of sperm rRNA and suggest that the major 80S subunits, while present, may be unable to support the assembly of functional polysomes [41]. This would almost certainly make translation *de novo* unlikely but it would not prevent potential translation in the zygote where functional ribosomes are abundant.

It is interesting to note, however, a study reporting the existence of an actinomycin D and

cycloheximide-sensitive capacity for protein synthesis in human sperm cells [42]. More recently, two follow-up investigations revisiting the phenomenon have been reported, both of which sought to confirm a chloramphenicol-sensitive translational capacity in human capacitating spermatozoa. The first used BODIPY and ^{35}S-labeled methionine and lysine to visualize translation *de novo* by both autoradiography and microscopy [41]. The second report identified 44 proteins that were diminished in capacitated sperm exposed to chloramphenicol compared with controls, but *de novo* synthesis was not reported [43]. These reports provide evidence for translation of some sperm mRNAs on extra-mitochondrial 55S ribosomes and Gur and Breitbart also presented evidence for these ribosomes in active polysomal fractions. An earlier report of mictochondrial 16S rRNA subunits in sperm nuclei using ISH supports the potential for cytoplasmic mRNAs to utilize 55S mitochondrial ribosomes [44]. Cappallo-Obermann reported the appearance of polysome-like structures in sperm by both electron microscopy and immunomicroscopy using antibodies to ribosomal proteins [39]. This report indicated the presence of a full complement of ribosomal proteins in sperm cells protected from cytoplasmic loss. Interestingly, of all mRNAs in sperm, those encoding ribosomal proteins appear to be among the most abundant species and the most likely to be shared across diverse classes from mammals to flies [18, 45].

Non-coding sperm RNAs

Microarray surveys of human, bovine, porcine, and fly sperm show that they contain cargos of mRNAs that match the compositional complexity of any actively expressing cell type. However, they also contain anti-sense mRNAs and complex loads of sncRNAs representing all known categories including miRNAs, piRNAs and snoRNAs. The most comprehensive survey of these sncRNAs to date has come from deep sequencing studies on human sperm where ~65% appear to be derived from abundant classes of repetitive elements found in the human genome [24] (Figure 5.2). We reported earlier on the presence of LINE1 transcripts in human sperm RNA [17, 46] and concluded that they must be a very abundant contributor to the RNA pool based on the frequency with which we found them in randomly sequenced RT-PCR amplicons. Expression of these repeats is normally highly repressed, but as suggested above,

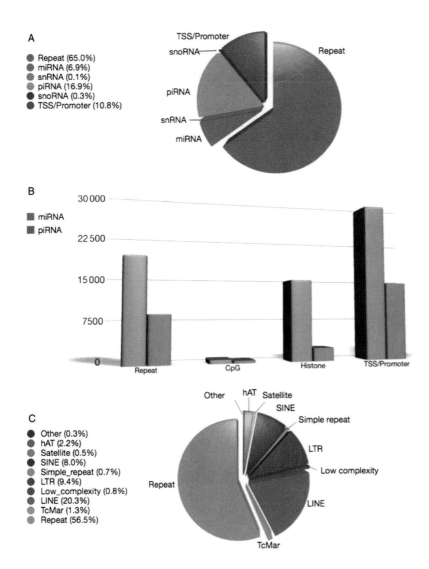

A
● Repeat (65.0%)
● miRNA (6.9%)
● snRNA (0.1%)
● piRNA (16.9%)
● snoRNA (0.3%)
● TSS/Promoter (10.8%)

B
■ miRNA
■ piRNA

C
● Other (0.3%)
● hAT (2.2%)
● Satellite (0.5%)
● SINE (8.0%)
● Simple_repeat (0.7%)
● LTR (9.4%)
● Low_complexity (0.8%)
● LINE (20.3%)
● TcMar (1.3%)
● Repeat (56.5%)

Figure 5.2. Small non-coding (snc) RNAs in human spermatozoa (three donors). (A) Sequences mapping to known genomic elements, Transcription Start Sites (TSS) and promoters. The distribution of sequences mapping to miRNA, piRNA, snoRNA, snRNA, and repeats are shown here. In addition, those sequences that did not map to known genomic elements were analyzed for TSS and promoter association. (B) Sequences mapping to miRNA or piRNA as well as repeats, CpG islands, histones, and TSS or promoters. All sequences associated with miRNA (blue) or piRNA (red) were further analyzed to determine if they also map to repeats, CpG islands, histones, or TSS/promoters. (C) Sequences mapping to known repeat classes. This figure shows the majority of sequences associated with an undefined repeat category. Of the remaining categories, LINE, LTR, and SINE are highly represented. From Krawetz *et al.* (2011) [24] with permission. This figure is presented in color in the color plate section.

the remodeling of the paternal genome may allow permissive windows during which repression is partially lifted. Krawetz *et al.* [24] also reported the presence of miRNAs in human sperm, several of which are linked to the control of fetal development, with four found only in sperm (and zygotes). One of the four, hsa-miR-34c may be required for embryonic genome activation in the mouse (see hypothesis below) and is the first experimental evidence for a sperm-derived RNA that is critical for embryonic development (at least in a naturally reproducing system [47]). Another abundant class of sncRNAs in human sperm are the piRNAs targeting LINE-1 and MER elements among other retrotransposons. Their presence may be

related to the "ping-pong" amplification mechanism of piRNA-PIWI mediated transposon silencing that is active in developing spermatocytes, and their retention in the mature spermatozoon may be related to the maintenance of a repressed state even in the highly compact chromatin of the sperm nucleus [48]. Until recently, piRNAs were assumed to be exclusive to the germline, but a recent report of their expression in the central nervous system of the sea hare indicates that this is not necessarily the case and that they may have other functions beyond transposon surveillance in the germline [49]. The presence of Argonaute proteins (or their mRNAs) has not been confirmed in sperm, but as they are present in oocytes [50], all of the components of an epigenetic mechanism regulating gene expression in the zygote are available. In addition to the human, miRNAs have also been reported in murine and porcine sperm although there are no reports from other mammalian species [35, 51]. A possible explanation for the presence of sncRNAs, including short fragments of repeat element RNAs, is in the maintenance of a repressed state in those sperm chromatin domains that retain an association with nucleosomes rather than protamines. One report demonstrated that the DNA from chromatin released following activation of the endogenous endonuclease activity of murine sperm was dominated by SINE and LINE elements [6]. Perhaps the less compact nucleosomal chromatin of sperm chromatin is "coated" by homologous repetitive RNAs that serve to repress their transcription either in the sperm itself or following fertilization. Moreover, activity of the sperm endonuclease may in part be responsible for the reported fragmentation of ribosomal and other RNAs recovered from sperm preparations [52].

Clinical utility and function of sperm RNA

There are now several reports in the public domain examining the utility of sperm RNA in clinical and veterinary applications and only the more recent findings will be considered here. The original report of mRNA complexity in bovine sperm [53] has been augmented by several more, including the use of subtractive suppression hybridization to uncover over-representation of redundant sperm RNAs (mainly rRNAs) in bulls with very low fertility return rates [31]. Compared with this group, bulls with a high return rate have less "redundant" RNA and greater levels of transcripts with known function. Another report also showed differences in transcript levels between fertile and subfertile animals [53]. The high levels of rRNAs in subfertile bull sperm is worth comparison with the high levels found in human sperm, although there is no suggestion at this stage that higher levels of rRNA in human sperm necessarily correlate with an infertile phenotype. Studies on the human are just beginning to bear fruit in a truly diagnostic setting. For example, Platts *et al.* [54] were able to clearly distinguish between normozoospermic (N = 13) and teratozoospermic (N = 8) samples using cluster and principal component analysis of microarray data. Other reports based on clinical studies have shown clear

differences between the sperm RNA profiles of couples who achieve pregnancies versus those that do not [55, 56]. What is particularly useful about these studies is that they used interventional methods based on standardized treatments that included examining the sperm RNA profiles of partners using intrauterine insemination (IUI) or partners using eggs from the same donor. These studies suggest that the infertile phenotype is associated with more variable transcript profiles than the fertile phenotype, perhaps indicating a generalized deregulation of transcription or transcript retention during spermatogenesis in infertile men. Similar qualitative and quantitative findings have been reported elsewhere for oligozoospermic men [57]. These data may be mechanistically related to alterations in the ratio of PRM1/PRM2 transcripts that have been reported in motile versus immotile sperm [58]. Interestingly, evidence for a potential embryological significance for some sperm mRNAs has arisen from the ontological descriptions of exclusively "expressed" transcripts in fertile samples which are strongly enriched for genes involved in embryological processes [55]. Similar ontological descriptions have been described for DNA sequences associated with modified histones in sperm [5] suggesting a relationship between them. What hampers all of these studies, however, is the absence of scale. For clinical efficacy, one normally expects studies to include hundreds if not thousands of couples. The fact that there are no such studies reported to date is partly for logistical reasons, particularly where donor eggs are concerned, but it also stems from difficulties in deciding precisely what elements of sperm RNA to test for and avoiding the high cost associated with poorly designed studies. The suggestion has been made before that most forms of idiopathic infertility are polygenic in origin and so the sperm RNA profiles of such infertile men may not comprise a definable group with respect to RNA profiling (as indicated above). If this proves to be so, then defining the proven fertile group will be the best way forward for the development of a diagnostic service [32, 37]. Another hurdle to overcome is the misconception of many practitioners who argue that even if we do understand what is wrong in the infertile man, we are powerless to do much about it. We consistently point out to such critics that the more we understand the process, the better equipped we become to develop ameliorative strategies that are in effect, akin to treatment. We know how sensitive spermatogenesis is to the general health and well-being of the individuals concerned; hence it is not beyond the scope of medical practice to suggest simple coping strategies such as changes in occupational circumstances or nutritional standards that could help improve the chances of successful pregnancies in couples seeking help.

Because the sperm delivers its RNA to the egg, it could have roles in the zygote (and beyond). Much has already been written about what these roles may be and the reader is drawn to several recent reviews that consider them in some detail [29, 59]. Suffice to say that evidence has been presented for the translation *de novo* of sperm mRNAs supporting cytoplasmic protein synthesis during capacitation, perhaps to replace essential cellular proteins that are either "consumed" or degraded during this process [41]. Capacitation is a highly dynamic process that involves considerable signaling activity and redistribution of cell components [60, 61]. Turnover of some protein components is therefore likely and replacement could only be accommodated by either mobilization of a precursor protein pool or translational activation of their nascent mRNAs. Considering the importance that such an activity and particularly an intrinsic and unconventional translational capacity would have for furthering our understanding of sperm function, it is frustrating that to date no further progress on the phenomenon has been reported. In particular, the mechanism, if one exists, that permits cytoplasmic mRNAs to be recognized and translated on mitochondrial polysomes requires elucidation. Work by Ward and colleagues and more recently by Yan *et al.* demonstrate the ability of injected mouse sperm nuclei containing intact chromatin to support normal development [62, 63]. Both reports showed that no residual cytoplasmic components are co-injected alongside and so the mRNAs and miRNAs detected in sperm nuclear preparations must be embedded within the chromatin where translation is unlikely to occur. Mohar *et al.* reported a failure of development beyond the one cell zygote if basic proteins were stripped from the nuclei beforehand [64]. Yan *et al.* noted a drop in developmental efficiency in pronase-treated nuclei that they attributed to an enzyme-induced disturbance in sperm DNA binding proteins [62]. While this is certainly possible, the drop in efficiency may also be due to RNase activity found in fresh (unincubated) preparations of pronase [65].

It would be interesting to test the effects of RNase treatment of demembranated nuclei on developmental competence, provided a way could be found for controlling effects of chromatin decondensation that would certainly be required to allow the enzyme access to embedded RNA. Potential roles for sperm RNA carried into the egg by the fertilizing sperm have been demonstrated for coat color and most intriguingly, embryonic genome activation [47, 66]. The former was due to a deregulated c-kit mRNA and the latter to hsa-miR-34c, perhaps operating through similar mechanisms (enhanced rather than repressed expression of the target gene(s)). This latter and at first sight counter-intuitive effect is supported by the likely enhancement of *Sox9* expression in embryos derived from *Prm1* driven *hsa-mir-124* transgenic males [67]. Offspring from such crosses are up to one-third larger than wild types. These miRNA reports are persuasive in that both suggest an epigenetic "enforcement" of phenotype where (for example) one of the most abundant naturally occurring sperm miRNAs, hsa-miR-34c acts perhaps by reinforcement of the paternal germ cell phenotype during spermiogenesis *and* activation of a repressed locus in the zygote leading to ZGA. Moreover, although *Bcl2* was the target zygotic gene of this report and evidence presented for its involvement in the ZGA switch, the involvement of other hsa-miR-34c targets cannot be excluded.

The link between sperm RNA and the developing embryo: a hypothesis

This final section seeks to address the most intriguing and frequently asked question regarding sperm RNA, namely, does it function in the embryo? The question is valid because conventional wisdom suggests that at least within the limits of our current understanding, it should not. For example, a sperm is not required for successful mammalian embryonic development. As elegantly demonstrated by diploid gynogenetic embryos which develop "normally" and at a relatively high efficiency compared with embryos arising from somatic nuclear transfer, altering the imprinting control regions at the H19 and Dlk1 loci of an introduced oocyte nucleus is sufficient to permit full development to term (at least in the mouse, where the paternal centrosome is redundant) [68]. Such constructs partially "mimic" the paternal imprinting status of the zygote but we do not know if the maternal genome is similarly dispensable, as reciprocal experiments have not been reported with diploid androgenotes (probably because of the absence of an X chromosome rather than the presence of two Ys).

One way of reconciling these findings in light of the mounting evidence for transmission of epigenetic information from the sperm is to assume that the information is ornamental rather than essential. In this perspective, sperm RNA could induce both non-heritable and heritable but non-essential trans-generational effects on subsequent progeny. One such heritable effect has already been noted for coat color in the paramutated c-kit phenotype mentioned earlier, which can be replicated by injection of effecter RNAs directly into the oocytes [66]. On the other hand, the report on the transmission of an apparently essential sperm miRNA required to effect embryonic genome activation goes against this perspective but also seems paradoxical in the light of viable gynogenotes. Changing the perspective from "gynocentric" to "androcentric" however, may help reconcile these contradictory findings.

Since the paternal genome is to all intents and purposes dispensable, it is also likely to have evolved strategies aimed at ensuring its survival. Clearly, the development of classic genomic imprinting is one way of achieving this but it need not be the only way. The concept of genome surveillance, conflict and consolidation has recently been applied to sperm–egg interactions, principally in the context of blocking the proliferation of selfish elements that can potentially be introduced to the egg from the sperm [48]. As indicated earlier, control of such elements that include retrotransposons is essential to maintain genomic integrity. Yet we know that these elements have also played an important role in reshaping the genome through both vertical and horizontal routes of transmission [69, 70]. Interestingly, surveys of murine oocytes and cleavage stage embryos show that retrotransposon RNAs make up a high proportion of their transcriptomes and regulatory sequences within their encoding elements can serve as alternative promoters for cellular genes [71, 72]. A limited survey of cDNA libraries generated from cleavage stage embryos revealed many examples of novel transcripts generated from retrotransposon-derived promoters and suggested that many more exist but remain unidentified. These experiments suggest that retrotransposons, (previously regarded as "junk" DNA) may be important in influencing early embryonic development. Perhaps this represents a form of co-opting and adaptation of an undesirable retroviral process into an

essential cellular requirement, similar to that reported for the evolution of the trophoblast-expressed syncytin gene, which was originally derived from the *env* gene of an endogenous retrovirus [73]. A much earlier report on the possible origins of tumor suppressor genes (TSGs) by horizontal and vertical transmission of primitive mating factor genes (MFGs) important in many Protista is another example [74]. This generally overlooked study provided compelling evidence based on sequence comparisons and immunofluorescence studies for an ancient interaction between retro-elements and MFGs leading to the consolidation of the latter in vertebrates as TSGs. This early report predicted much of what is only now being revealed by the resurgence of interest in sperm-mediated trans-generational epigenetic effects. Recent reports (reviewed in [75]) show that genotoxic insult to the germline itself (or even as a bystander effect following exposure of somatic tissues to a potential genotoxin) can be heritably and stably transmitted. These effects have been linked to the ability of an organism to respond to environmental stress far more rapidly than conventional mutational and heritable change can accommodate and provide a connection between the evolution of meiotic recombination (crossing over) and equivalent changes brought about by the mixing and integration of "foreign" DNAs into the genome. The evolutionary connection between MFGs and TSGs provides direct evidence for this phenomenon that is not (to this author's mind) coincidental and essentially predicts the notion of confrontation and consolidation in genomic (and sexual) compatibility that sperm RNAs may play a role in.

From this perspective, sperm RNA can be seen as a vector for rapid and heritable genomic change via an epigenetic pathway. Non-coding sperm RNAs may help to drive this relationship with either heritable changes in the methylation of key zygotic genes or targeted degradation of their mRNAs. It is likely that other paternal and maternal ncRNAs interact to test the "fitness" of the introduced genome prior to syngamy and eventual zygotic genome activation. This can be viewed as a co-opting of the surveillance mechanism that protects the genome from invasion by foreign transposable elements and could help explain the presence of other miRNA and piRNA species in sperm RNA. Corresponding antisense sncRNAs should be found in oocytes and indeed antisense transcripts of many alternatively spliced transcripts driven from alternative retrotransposon-derived promoters

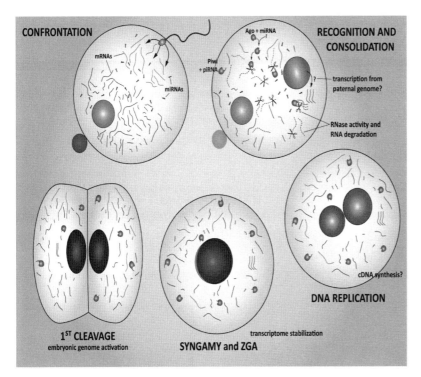

Figure 5.3. Introduction of sperm RNA to the egg leads to possible cytoplasmic confrontation mediated through miRNAs and other RNA types (including piRNAs). This serves mainly as protection against the proliferation of sperm-borne LTR and non-LTR retrotransposons. Assuming that this threat is neutralized, confrontation is defused following compatibility "checking" and the sperm is recognized and consolidated into the early zygote. The compatibility check itself may be driven by oocyte Ago and Piwi proteins using sperm miRNAs as downregulators of key maternal mRNAs. These may be required prior to syngamy and before the first round of DNA replication can commence. DNA replication may offer a window for cDNA synthesis from unknown RNA templates using an endogenous reverse transcriptase present in the ooplasm. The role of RT in the process is implied by the prevention of ZGA in the presence of RT inhibitors. This figure is presented in color in the color plate section.

are present in oocytes, sperm, and cleavage stage embryos [72]. Yet, the viability of gynegenotic mice where no sperm is involved suggests that dependency on sperm RNA is only seen (or required) in a sexually compatible system.

One additional factor where sperm RNA and the concept of conflict and consolidation between gametes may figure is reverse transcriptase. This enzyme has been proposed to play a role in horizontal gene transfer [70] because the transfer mechanism includes an intermediate RNA stage that requires the enzyme for cDNA synthesis and eventual genomic integration. There are three possible sources of RT in eukaryotes, two of which (LINE1 *Orf 2* and the *pol* gene of LTR retrotransposons) are at least occasionally active, even in the testis [76, 77]. Telomerase is not thought to play a role in the transfer mechanism. Several studies over the years have reported RT activity in both oocytes and sperm, and sperm appear to have the ability to absorb RNA containing an intronic sequence and to correctly process the RNA to intronless cDNA [78]. The work by Peaston *et al.* [71] suggests that a similar process may be at work in oocytes. It is possible to hypothesize a mechanism that retains features of this process including an inter-gamete, RNA-based communication signaling

mechanism that checkpoints the mutual compatibility of sperm and egg. If miRNAs and/or reverse transcriptase are involved in this mechanism and are required for ZGA in sexually compatible zygotes, then inhibiting the function of either should inhibit ZGA (Figure 5.3).

In this respect, there are reports on the failure of ZGA in cleavage stage zygotes exposed to inhibitors of reverse transcriptase and of course, to the downregulation of hsa-miR-34c described above [47, 78]. Another report provided evidence of a role for siRNAs in mediating alternative splicing during transcriptional gene silencing [79]. Putting these three elements together in the zygote provides a framework for an epigenetic cross-talk between the gametes that may include the generation of a compatibility "switch" activating ZGA. The switch would be bypassed by gynegenotes or cloned embryos because the (epigenetic) compatibility check that I describe is not encountered. One prediction of this hypothesis is that inter-species hybrids are only possible if their respective gametes can either pass or bypass this compatibility test. It is interesting therefore that in many sterile hybrid marsupials arising from closely related species, there is evidence for a massive expansion of retroelement activity and that this may hold true for eutherian hybrids also [80, 81]. These data suggest that such a check is at best "leaky" but at least ensures that a "minimal" compatibility is achieved before ZGA can go ahead. However the hybrids provide evidence for a connection between the normal repression of retroelement activity in the germline on the one hand and the way that such activity can be usefully directed to both monitor gamete compatibility and promote non-Mendelian changes in genomic structure that may underlie rapid adaptation to environmental changes and perhaps to eventual speciation on the other.

Conclusions

Sperm RNA has had a long and difficult investigational history that is only now beginning to bear fruit with the deployment of more advanced molecular techniques such as high throughput microarraying and new generation sequencing. As a result of these endeavors, we are convinced that the renewed interest in sperm RNA is leading to fresh insights into its function. While roles in the spermatozoon itself are controversial, the RNA is at least fully contained within an intact cell system and is probably a good proxy for the underlying health of the testis. Clinical applications of its examination in an IVF setting are therefore likely to arise as we understand more about the expected RNA profile of a functional sperm and the cost of molecular screening declines. However as the sperm is the only cell that can (legitimately) gain entry to another cell (the oocyte), the function of its RNA in the zygote needs consideration and not without raising its own controversies. Persuasive data are now mounting suggesting that sperm RNA or at least the sncRNA fraction has a function in normal development. This function may be important for triggering embryonic development but only where both parental gametes are involved and where the sperm RNA may serve to "guide" the zygote into accepting the paternal contribution This may be an additional layer of epigenetic information that has arisen through confrontation and consolidation aimed at ensuring the requirement for a paternal genome, while keeping the transmission and proliferation of undesirable transposable elements in check. If this proves indeed to be the case then we can predict that a considerable proportion of failed IVF cycles (particularly ICSI) may be down to dysfunctional sperm RNA. While this may indicate a general dysfunction of the fertilizing sperm, it also suggests a potential salvage pathway for improving ICSI success rates by co-injecting purified miRNA alongside the sperm itself.

References

1. D'Occhio MJ, Hengstberger KJ, Johnston SD. Biology of sperm chromatin structure and relationship to male fertility and embryonic survival. *Animal Reprod Sci.* 2007;**101**(1–2):1–17.

2. Braun RE. Packaging paternal chromosomes with protamine. *Nat Genet.* 2001;**28**(1):10–12.

3. Gu W, Kwon YK, Hecht NB. In postmeiotic male germ cells poly (a) shortening accompanies translation of mRNA encoding gamma enteric actin but not cytoplasmic beta and gamma actin mRNAs. *Mol Reprod Dev.* 1996;**44**(2):141–5.

4. Gardiner-Garden M, Ballesteros M, Gordon M *et al.* Histone- and protamine-DNA association: conservation of different patterns within the beta-globin domain in human sperm. *Mol Cell Biol.* 1998;**18**(6):3350–6.

5. Hammoud SS, Nix DA, Zhang H *et al.* Distinctive chromatin in human sperm packages genes for embryo development. *Nature.* 2009;**460**(7254):473–8.

6. Pittoggi C, Renzi L, Zaccagnini G *et al.* A fraction of mouse sperm chromatin is organized in nucleosomal hypersensitive domains enriched in retroposon DNA. *J Cell Sci.* 1999;**112**(Pt 20):3537–48.

7. Oliva R. Protamines and male infertility. *Hum Reprod Update.* 2006;**12**(4):417–35.

8. Hecht NB. Molecular mechanisms of male germ cell differentiation. *Bioessays.* 1998;**20**(7):555–61.

9. Balhorn R. A model for the structure of chromatin in mammalian sperm. *J Cell Biol.* 1982;**93**(2):298–305.

10. Kramer JA, McCarrey JR, Djakiew D *et al.* Human spermatogenesis as a model to examine gene potentiation. *Mol Reprod Dev.* 2000; **56**(S2):254–8.

11. Johnson GD, Lalancette C, Linnemann AK *et al.* The sperm nucleus: chromatin, RNA, and the nuclear matrix. *Reproduction.* 2011;**141**(1):21–36.

12. Abraham KA, Bhargava PM. Nucleic acid metabolism of mammalian spermatozoa. *Biochem J.* 1963;**86**:298–307.

13. Bhargava PM. Incorporation of radioactive amino-acids in the proteins of bull spermatozoa. *Nature.* 1957;**179**(4570):1120–1.

14. Markewitz M, Graff S, Veenema RJ. Absence of RNA synthesis in shed human spermatozoa. *Nature.* 1967;**214**(86):402–3.

15. MacLaughlin J, Terner C. Ribonucleic acid synthesis by spermatozoa from the rat and hamster. *Biochem J.* 1973;**133**:635–9.

16. Premkumar EB, Bhargava PM. Transcription and translation in bovine spermatozoa. *Nat New Biol*. 1972;**240**:139–43.

17. Miller D, Briggs D, Snowden H *et al*. A complex population of RNAs exists in human ejaculate spermatozoa: implications for understanding molecular aspects of spermiogenesis. *Gene*. 1999;**237**(2):385–92.

18. Fischer BE, Wasbrough E, Meadows LA *et al*. Conserved properties of drosophila and human spermatozoal mRNA repertoires. *Proc Biol Sci*. 2012;**279**(1738):2636–44.

19. Dym M, Fawcett DW. Further observations on the numbers of spermatogonia, spermatocytes, and spermatids connected by intercellular bridges in the mammalian testis. *Biol Reprod*. 1971;**4**(2):195–215.

20. Clayton AL, Hazzalin CA, Mahadevan LC. Enhanced histone acetylation and transcription: a dynamic perspective. *Mol Cell*. 2006;**23**(3):289–96.

21. Oliva R, Bazett-Jones DP, Locklear L *et al*. Histone hyperacetylation can induce unfolding of the nucleosome core particle. *Nucleic Acids Res*. 1990;**18**(9):2739–47.

22. Rousseaux S, Reynoird N, Escoffier E *et al*. Epigenetic reprogramming of the male genome during gametogenesis and in the zygote. *Reprod Biomed Online*. 2008;**16**(4):492–503.

23. Hazzouri M, Pivot-Pajot C, Faure AK *et al*. Regulated hyperacetylation of core histones during mouse spermatogenesis: involvement of histone deacetylases. *Eur J Cell Biol*. 2000;**79**(12):950–60.

24. Krawetz SA, Kruger A, Lalancette C *et al*. A survey of small RNAs in human sperm. *Hum Reprod*. 2011;**26**(12):3401–12.

25. Miller D, Ostermeier GC. Towards a better understanding of RNA carriage by ejaculate spermatozoa. *Hum Reprod Update*. 2006;**12**(6):757–67.

26. Rejon E, Bajon C, Blaize A *et al*. RNA in the nucleus of a motile plant spermatozoid: characterization by enzyme-gold cytochemistry and *in situ* hybridization. *Mol Reprod Devel*. 1988;**1**:49–56.

27. Pessot CA, Brito M, Figueroa J *et al*. Presence of RNA in the sperm nucleus. *Biochem Biophysic Res Comms*. 1989;**158**(1):272–8.

28. Kumar G, Patel D, Naz RK. C-myc messenger-RNA is present in human sperm cells. *Cell Mol Biol Res*. 1993;**39**(2):111–17.

29. Hamatani T. Human spermatozoal RNAs. *Fertil Steril*. 2012;**97**(2):275–81.

30. Miller DJ. Physiology and endocrinology symposium: sperm-oviduct interactions in livestock and poultry. *J Anim Sci*. [*Congresses*]. 2011;**89**(5):1312–14.

31. Lalancette C, Thibault C, Bachand I *et al*. Transcriptome analysis of bull semen with extreme nonreturn rate: use of suppression-subtractive hybridization to identify functional markers for fertility. *Biol Reprod*. 2008;**78**(4):618–35.

32. Lalancette C, Platts AE, Johnson GD *et al*. Identification of human sperm transcripts as candidate markers of male fertility. *J Mol Med*. 2009;**87**(7):735–48.

33. Gilbert I, Bissonnette N, Boissonneault G *et al*. A molecular analysis of the population of mRNA in bovine spermatozoa. *Reproduction*. 2007;**133**(6):1073–86.

34. Feugang JM, Rodriguez-Osorio N, Kaya A *et al*. Transcriptome analysis of bull spermatozoa: implications for male fertility. *Reprod Biomed Online*. 2010;**21**(3):312–24.

35. Curry E, Ellis SE, Pratt SL. Detection of porcine sperm microRNAs using a heterologous microRNA microarray and reverse transcriptase polymerase chain reaction. *Mol Reprod Dev*. 2009;**76**(3):218–19.

36. Yang CC, Lin YS, Hsu CC *et al*. Identification and sequencing of remnant messenger RNAs found in domestic swine (*Sus scrofa*) fresh ejaculated spermatozoa. *Animal Reprod Sci*. 2009;**113**(1–4):143–55.

37. Ostermeier GC, Goodrich RJ, Diamond MP *et al*. Toward using stable spermatozoal RNAs for prognostic assessment of male factor fertility. *Fertil Steril*. 2005;**83**(6):1687–94.

38. Ostermeier GC, Dix DJ, Miller D *et al*. Spermatozoal RNA profiles of normal fertile men. *Lancet*. 2002;**360**:772–7.

39. Cappallo-Obermann H, Schulze W, Jastrow H *et al*. Highly purified spermatozoal RNA obtained by a novel method indicates an unusual 28s/18s rRNA ratio and suggests impaired ribosome assembly. *Mol Hum Reprod*. 2011;**17**(11):669–78.

40. Johnson GD, Sendler E, Lalancette C *et al*. Cleavage of rRNA ensures translational cessation in sperm at fertilization. *Mol Hum Reprod*. 2011;**17**(12):721–6.

41. Gur Y, Breitbart H. Mammalian sperm translate nuclear-encoded proteins by mitochondrial-type ribosomes. *Genes Dev*. 2006;**20**(4):411–16.

42. Naz RK. Effect of actinomycin d and cycloheximide on human sperm function. *Arch Androl*. 1998;**41**(2):135–42.

43. Zhao C, Guo XJ, Shi ZH *et al*. Role of translation by mitochondrial-type ribosomes during sperm capacitation: an analysis based on a proteomic approach. *Proteomics*. 2009;**9**(5):1385–99.

44. Villegas J, Araya P, Bustos-Obregon E *et al*. Localization of the 16s mitochondrial rRNA in the

nucleus of mammalian spermatogenic cells. *Mol Hum Reprod.* 2002;**8**(11):977–83.

45. Zhao Y, Li Q, Yao C *et al.* Characterization and quantification of mRNA transcripts in ejaculated spermatozoa of fertile men by serial analysis of gene expression. *Hum Reprod.* 2006;**21**(6):1583–1590.

46. Miller D. Analysis and significance of messenger RNA in human ejaculated spermatozoa. *Mol Reprod Dev.* 2000;**56**(2 Suppl):259–64.

47. Liu WM, Pang RT, Chiu PC *et al.* Sperm-borne microRNA-34c is required for the first cleavage division in mouse. *Proc Natl Acad Sci USA.* 2012;**109**(2):490–4.

48. Bourc'his D, Voinnet O. A small-RNA perspective on gametogenesis, fertilization, and early zygotic development. *Science.* 2010;**330**(6004):617–22.

49. Rajasethupathy P, Antonov I, Sheridan R *et al.* A role for neuronal piRNAs in the epigenetic control of memory-related synaptic plasticity. *Cell.* 2012;**149**(3):693–707.

50. Lykke-Andersen K, Gilchrist MJ, Grabarek JB *et al.* Maternal argonaute 2 is essential for early mouse development at the maternal-zygotic transition. *Mol Biol Cell.* 2008;**19**(10):4383–92.

51. Amanai M, Brahmajosyula M, Perry AC. A restricted role for sperm-borne microRNAs in mammalian fertilization. *Biol Reprod.* 2006;**75**(6):877–84.

52. Sotolongo B, Huang TT, Isenberger E *et al.* An endogenous nuclease in hamster, mouse, and human spermatozoa cleaves DNA into loop-sized fragments. *J Androl.* 2005;**26**(2):272–80.

53. Bissonnette N, Levesque-Sergerie JP, Thibault C *et al.* Spermatozoal transcriptome profiling for bull sperm motility: a potential tool to evaluate semen quality. *Reproduction.* 2009;**138**(1):65–80.

54. Platts AF, Dix DJ, Chemes HE *et al.* Success and failure in human spermatogenesis as revealed by teratozoospermic RNAs. *Human Mol Genet.* 2007;**16**(7):763–73.

55. Garcia-Herrero S, Garrido N, Martinez-Conejero JA *et al.* Differential transcriptomic profile in spermatozoa achieving pregnancy or not via ICSI. *Reprod Biomed Online.* 2011;**22**(1):25–36.

56. Garcia-Herrero S, Meseguer M, Martinez-Conejero JA *et al.* The transcriptome of spermatozoa used in homologous intrauterine insemination varies considerably between samples that achieve pregnancy and those that do not. *Fertil Steril.* 2010;**94**(4):1360–73.

57. Montjean D, De La Grange P, Gentien D *et al.* Sperm transcriptome profiling in oligozoospermia. *J Assist Reprod Genet.* 2012;**29**(1):3–10.

58. Lambard S, Galeraud-Denis I, Martin G *et al.* Analysis and significance of mRNA in human ejaculated sperm from normozoospermic donors: relationship to sperm motility and capacitation. *Mol Hum Reprod.* 2004;**10**(7):535–41.

59. Boerke A, Dieleman SJ, Gadella BM. A possible role for sperm RNA in early embryo development. *Theriogenology.* 2007;**68**(Suppl. 1):S147–55.

60. Breitbart H. Intracellular calcium regulation in sperm capacitation and acrosomal reaction. *Mol Cell Endocrinol.* 2002;**187**(1–2):139–44.

61. Gadella BM, Tsai PS, Boerke A *et al.* Sperm head membrane reorganisation during capacitation. *Int J Dev Biol.* 2008;**52**(5–6):473–80.

62. Yan W, Morozumi K, Zhang J *et al.* Birth of mice after intracytoplasmic injection of single purified sperm nuclei and detection of messenger RNAs and microRNAs in the sperm nuclei. *Biol Reprod.* 2008;**78**(5):896–902.

63. Ward WS, Kishikawa H, Akutsu H *et al.* Further evidence that sperm nuclear proteins are necessary for embryogenesis. *Zygote.* 2000;**8**(1):51–6.

64. Mohar I, Szczygiel MA, Yanagimachi R *et al.* Sperm nuclear halos can transform into normal chromosomes after injection into oocytes. *Mol Reprod Dev.* 2002;**62**(3):416–20.

65. Tolstoshev P, Wells JR. Nature and origins of chromatin-associated ribonucleic acid of avian reticulocytes. *Biochemistry.* 1974;**13**(1):103–11.

66. Rassoulzadegan M, Grandjean V, Gounon P *et al.* RNA-mediated non-Mendelian inheritance of an epigenetic change in the mouse. *Nature.* 2006;**441**(7092):469–74.

67. Grandjean V, Gounon P, Wagner N *et al.* The mir-124-sox9 paramutation: RNA-mediated epigenetic control of embryonic and adult growth. *Development.* 2009;**136**(21):3647–55.

68. Kawahara M, Wu Q, Takahashi N *et al.* High-frequency generation of viable mice from engineered bi-maternal embryos. *Nat Biotechnol.* 2007;**25**(9):1045–50.

69. Miller D, Brinkworth M, Iles D. The testis as a conduit for genomic plasticity: an advanced interdisciplinary workshop. *Biochem Soc Trans.* 2007;**35**(Pt 3):605–8.

70. Brosius J, Tiedge H. Reverse transcriptase: mediator of genomic plasticity. *Virus Genes.* 1995;**11**(2–3):163–79.

71. Peaston AE, Knowles BB, Hutchison KW. Genome plasticity in the mouse oocyte and early embryo. *Biochem Soc Trans.* 2007;**35**(Pt 3):618–22.

72. Peaston AE, Evsikov AV, Graber JH *et al.* Retrotransposons regulate host genes in mouse oocytes and preimplantation embryos. *Dev Cell.* 2004;**7**(4):597–606.

73. Knerr I, Beinder E, Rascher W. Syncytin, a novel human endogenous retroviral gene in human placenta:

evidence for its dysregulation in preeclampsia and HELLP syndrome. *Am J Obstet Gynecol.* 2002;**186**(2):210–13.

74. Gosden CM, Liloglou T, Nunn J *et al.* The knights of the round table hypothesis of tumour suppressor gene function – noble sacrifice or sexual dalliance: genes, including p53, BRCA1/2 and RB have evolved by horizontal and vertical transmission of mating factor genes and are involved in gametogenesis, implantation, development and tumourigenesis. *Int J Oncol.* 1998;**12**(1):5–35.

75. de Boer P, Ramos L, de Vries M *et al.* Memoirs of an insult: sperm as a possible source of transgenerational epimutations and genetic instability. *Mol Hum Reprod.* 2009;**16**(1):48–56.

76. Branciforte D, Martin SL. Expression of line-1 RNA and protein in mouse testis. *Mol Biol Cell.* 1992;**3**(SS):A101.

77. Kazazian HH Jr., Wong C, Youssoufian H *et al.* Haemophilia A resulting from *de novo* insertion of L1 sequences represents a novel mechanism for mutation in man. *Nature.* 1988;**332**:164–6.

78. Sciamanna I, Vitullo P, Curatolo A *et al.* Retrotransposons, reverse transcriptase and the genesis of new genetic information. *Gene.* 2009;**448**(2):180–6.

79. Allo M, Buggiano V, Fededa JP *et al.* Control of alternative splicing through siRNA-mediated transcriptional gene silencing. *Nat Struct Mol Biol.* 2009;**16**(7):717–24.

80. Metcalfe CJ, Bulazel KV, Ferreri GC *et al.* Genomic instability within centromeres of interspecific marsupial hybrids. *Genetics.* 2007;**177**(4):2507–17.

81. Brown JD, Piccuillo V, O'Neill RJ. Retroelement demethylation associated with abnormal placentation in *Mus musculus* × *Mus caroli* hybrids. *Biol Reprod.* 2012;**86**(3):88.

The role of the sperm centrosome in reproductive fitness

Heide Schatten and Qing-Yuan Sun

Introduction

Male factor infertility accounts for more than 40% of infertility problems experienced by one in eight couples of reproductive age in the Western world [1, 2]. While significant progress has been made in the field of reproduction to identify specific causes for the still high rate of infertility, recent research has focused on understanding infertility problems on cellular and molecular levels.

One of the critically important organelles contributed by sperm in non-rodent mammalian fertilization is the centriole that provides the template for centrioles and their varied functions through all stages of embryo development and in adult somatic cells. It is therefore highly important to understand the centriole and its associated centrosomal material (here referred to as the centriole-centrosome complex), the molecular composition of the centrosomal material and how this complex functions during sperm aster, zygote aster, and mitotic apparatus formation and during symmetric and asymmetric cell divisions that are important for cellular differentiation and for the formation of the primary cilium, a non-motile cilium with chemical and mechanical sensory functions that influences embryo development and plays a critical role in axis determination. Defects and dysfunctions in the centriole-centrosome complex can be causes for male factor infertility and for adulthood diseases such as cancer. New research has begun to identify specific defects of the sperm's centriole-centrosome complex and new therapies are being considered to repair centrosome dysfunctions.

Before getting into a more detailed discussion of the topic it is important to clarify that the mouse is excluded as a suitable model for mammalian fertilization studies, as the centriole-centrosome complex is not contributed by sperm in the mouse system. The mouse is atypical and not suited for mammalian fertilization studies, as it employs completely different fertilization mechanisms and does not even tolerate centrioles in the ooplasm [3, 4]. During the past few years we have written several review papers on centrosome structure and functions [5], oocyte maturation [6], and fertilization [6–9], and some of these papers have highlighted the significant differences between sperm of rodent and non-rodent species which we find important to emphasize because of the enormous functional and structural differences between non-rodent and rodent sperm and the mode of fertilization that are not representative for mammalian fertilization studies. These differences exclude the mouse as a suitable animal model for humans regarding centrosome and cytoskeletal dynamics for at least several cell cycles after fertilization. As pointed out in our previous reviews the porcine and bovine systems are most suitable as models for humans and will be addressed in more detail in this review. The present chapter is structured into three sections to address (1) the centrosome complex and its essential functions during fertilization and its impact on embryo development; (2) nuclear proteins that contribute to centrosome functions and synchronization of centrosome-nuclear cell cycles; and (3) considerations of centrosome dysfunctions for assisted reproductive technology (ART).

The centrosome complex and its essential functions during fertilization and its impact on embryo development

The sperm's centriole-centrosome complex

As shown in Figure 6.1 the centriole-centrosome complex is located within the sperm's connecting piece between the midpiece and the sperm's nucleus.

Paternal Influences on Human Reproductive Success, ed. Douglas T. Carrell. Published by Cambridge University Press.
© Cambridge University Press 2013.

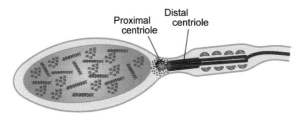

Figure 6.1. Schematic representation of non-rodent sperm showing sperm head with DNA and nuclear matrix proteins and the centriole complex consisting of two centrioles that are in perpendicular orientation to each other. The centriole close to the nucleus (proximal centriole) will become important for microtubule nucleation of sperm aster, zygote aster, and mitotic apparatus in the fertilized oocyte while the centriole associated with the sperm tail (distal centriole) will be destroyed along with the sperm tail after fertilization. This figure is presented in color in the color plate section.

It consists of one proximal centriole surrounded by a small amount of specific centrosomal material, primarily composed of the centrosomal protein γ-tubulin and centriole-associated centrin, and it consists of one tail-associated distal centriole that plays a role in organizing microtubules in the sperm tail. The proximal and distal centrioles are positioned perpendicular to each other. While the distal centriole is thought to degenerate after fertilization along with the sperm tail, the proximal centriole becomes highly functional and accumulates additional centrosomal proteins from the ooplasm during the fertilization process to form the microtubule-based sperm aster and zygote aster that develops into the microtubule-rich mitotic apparatus in preparation for first cell division [8, 10]. Centrins are important for centriole functions and play an essential role in centrosome duplication after fertilization. Other centrosomal proteins are likely to associate with the sperm centriole but detailed studies have not yet been performed to determine the specific centrosome profile before and after fertilization. One other sperm centrosomal protein, speriolin, has been identified in recent studies [11] that may play a role in first division but detailed studies on this and on other specific centrosomal proteins and their functions after fertilization have not yet been pursued.

Because of the importance of the sperm's centriole-centrosome complex for fertilization and embryo development in non-rodent mammalian species the study of this complex is important and recent interest has been focused on its dysfunctions as a contributing factor for male factor infertility (discussed later in this chapter). Its role for the entire program of embryo

development has been emphasized and new studies are emerging in which its functions in establishing asymmetry have been explored [6, 8–10].

Many of the previous studies had been focused on the centriole ultrastructure and produced excellent electron micrographs of human sperm that have been presented in several original papers and review articles [12–23]. These papers describe in detail the clear centriole structure of proximal and distal centrioles and the structural associations between the sperm nucleus and the proximal centriole.

The centrosome complex and centrosome remodeling during the first and subsequent embryonic cell cycles

Fertilization takes place at the MII stage (metaphase of second meiosis) in humans and most mammalian species, which is the stage in which oocytes become arrested after maturation (Figure 6.2A). An early requirement for proximal centriole functions is the disengagement from the sperm tail-connecting piece. Release of the proximal centriole requires proteasome activity [24, 25]. After release of the proximal centriole precise nucleation of microtubules by γ-tubulin and dynamic microtubule growth is important to nucleate precise amounts of microtubules in the rapidly changing sperm aster. For the sperm aster to grow, γ-tubulin needs to be recruited from the oocyte to increase sperm aster size and length that results in the functional zygote aster as an important structure for pronuclear apposition (Figure 6.2B–C). The formation of the sperm aster requires precise regulation, as over-recruitment of γ-tubulin will result in nucleation of too many microtubules while under-recruitment of γ-tubulin will result in reduced aster formation that both will have consequences for developmental potential. We do not yet know the full range of requirements for optimal sperm and zygote aster formation but we do know that the microtubule motor protein dynein is important to carry cargo including additional centrosomal proteins to the centrosome core structure for centrosome enlargement and modification of cell cycle-specific centrosome functions. Detailed analysis of centrosome proteins during this stage of fertilization will be important. Such studies have been generated for somatic cells and similar studies in fertilized eggs may allow determination of individual centrosome profiles to identify specific components that may account for infertility or decrease

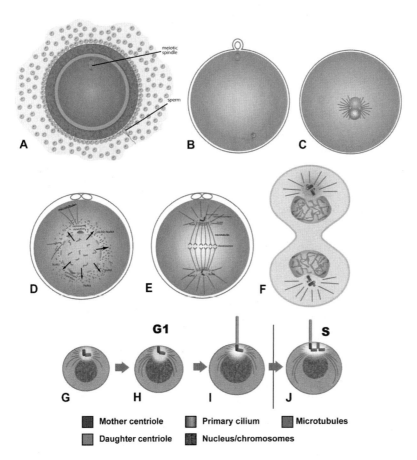

Figure 6.2. Fertilization takes place at the MII stage in most mammalian systems (A); shortly after fertilization a sperm aster becomes nucleated and organized by the sperm's centriole-centrosome complex, indicating successful sperm incorporation and centrosome functions (B). Duplication and subsequent separation of the centriole-centrosome complex occurs at the pronuclear stage (C) followed by nuclear envelope breakdown and dispersion of nuclear proteins including NuMA (D) and maturation of centrosomes into division-competent centrosomes in mitosis (E). The distribution of centrosomal material to the dividing daughter cells may be symmetric or asymmetric (F). During later stages of embryo development there is a close relationship between the older (mother) centriole of the centrosome complex and the formation of the primary cilium (G–J). The assembly of the primary cilium is initiated during G1 (G–H) when the distal end of the mother centriole becomes associated with a membrane vesicle. An axoneme assembles (I) and centrioles duplicate and lengthen during the subsequent S phase (J). Please see text for more detailed description. This figure is presented in color in the color plate section.

- ■ Mother centriole
- ■ Daughter centriole
- ■ Primary cilium
- ▦ Nucleus/chromosomes
- ■ Microtubules

in developmental potential, as will be addressed in more detail later in this chapter.

Specific centrosome proteins that we know to play a critical role in centrosome and sperm functions during fertilization include pericentrin and centrin that have been well explored in somatic cells [5]. We know from studies in somatic cells that pericentrin forms a complex with γ-tubulin and depends on dynein for assembly onto centrosomes [26–28]. Pericentrin gene mutation results in recruitment loss of several other centrosomal proteins. Because of its recruitment of γ-tubulin to the centrosome core structure pericentrin plays a role in the enlargement of the sperm aster during fertilization. It is well known that centrosomal abnormalities play a role in adulthood diseases [29] and pericentrin dysfunctions contribute to loss of centrosome integrity. Centrins are important for centriole functions and are essential for centrosome duplication [30–34]. Our knowledge of other centrosomal proteins and their specific functions during fertilization is still minimal but we know that

duplication of the blended centriole-centrosome complex takes place during the pronuclear stage and during the S phases of subsequent cell divisions which requires regulation by cyclins [35] while cell cycle-specific centrosome remodeling requires protein degradation [36, 37] that is important for centrosome plasticity throughout development [6, 8, 9].

As the centrosome matures from fertilization to mitosis (Figure 6.2B–E) to become a division-competent centrosome the centrosome structure undergoes shape changes that can clearly be detected in sea urchin cells during the first embryonic cell cycle [8]. The centrosomal core material consists of a fibrous scaffolding lattice. This highly dynamic structure composed of centrosome core proteins and cell cycle-specific centrosome-associated proteins is important for the control of cell cycle-specific events. Microtubules are anchored with their minus ends to the centrosome core structure by the γ-tubulin ring complex (γ-TuRC) that is composed of γ-tubulin and several accessory proteins [5]. Microtubule numbers and lengths are regulated and re-organized throughout the cell cycle. Spindle pole centrosomes contain numerous centrosome proteins and centrosome-associated proteins with a special role for the centrosome-associated protein NuMA as will be discussed later in this chapter.

The centriole-centrosome complex as multifunctional organelle, its role in asymmetry and formation of the primary cilium

While we do not yet clearly understand how the proximal centriole duplicates during the first embryonic cell cycle we do know that duplication of the centriole-centrosome complex occurs during the pronuclear stage and during the S phases in subsequent embryonic cell cycles. Centriole and centrosome duplication has been well studied in somatic cells [5] but it is not clear how one proximal centriole can give rise to a centriole pair that is detected at each pole of the bipolar mitotic apparatus. Centriole duplication is semi-conservative referring to a daughter centriole forming perpendicular to the mother centriole. This mechanism of duplication establishes an intrinsic asymmetry and it also establishes an age difference in the centriole pair. The older (mother) centriole contains appendages while the younger (daughter) centriole develops these appendages during the next cell cycle when it becomes a mother centriole [10]. The structural differences also result in functional differences and it has been shown in *Drosophila* male germline stem cells [38, 39] that the mother centriole can nucleate more microtubules than the daughter centriole, thereby establishing a differential system by which transport of cell fate determinants can be established as an important aspect for cell differentiation.

Historically, numerous debates had been centered around the question whether or not the sperm entry site is important for the establishment of asymmetry and it is now clear that this debate can be refocused on the centriole and the centriole's specific structure that introduces asymmetry on cellular and molecular levels [10]. This asymmetry is already established during the pronuclear cycle when the zygote aster forms and centrioles begin to separate and start relocating to the mitotic poles. The morphologically different centrioles in the now duplicated centriole-centrosome complex may accumulate centrosomal components differently

(Figure 6.2F), i.e. a quantitative and qualitative difference in centrosome composition may be established around the mother and daughter centrioles with consequences for microtubule nucleation and subsequent implications for distribution of cellular components and cell fate determinants along microtubules to the centrosome complex which also has implications for signal transduction. The differential accumulation of cellular components is critical for proper development and assures targeted distribution during subsequent cell divisions. It includes cytoplasmic factors such as transcripts of developmental genes which allows different gene activity in different cells; for example, an inheritance of mRNA localized at centrosomes has been described for *Ilyanassa* [40] although studies in mammalian systems await further research. Throughout development the asymmetry in the centriole-centrosome complex allows the mother centriole to assemble centrosomal proteins and microtubule formations different from the daughter centriole which also has consequences for cellular communication throughout cellular differentiation and embryo development. Transport along microtubules to centrosomes is also utilized for protein degradation, as shown for embryonic stem cell divisions; this allows asymmetric inheritance of proteins destined for different degradation in the different dividing daughter cells.

Extensive studies on asymmetric centrosome distribution in non-rodent mammalian embryos have not yet been performed but some data are available for other systems, including early stages of *Drosophila*, *C. elegans*, and the sea urchin system [10]. In recent years, studies of the primary cilium and its role in asymmetry have been pursued when it was recognized that this solitary non-motile single cilium (one per cell) plays important roles in chemical and mechanical sensory functions. While we do not yet exactly know when primary cilia form during mammalian development we do know that they are critically important for adult tissue homeostasis and for the establishment of left-right body asymmetry. In the adult, the primary cilium is found in almost all cells of our body [41]. The primary cilium develops from the mother centriole of the cell's centriole pair and becomes anchored to the cell by the basal body. A close cell cycle-specific relationship exists between primary cilia and the cell's centriole-centrosome complex (Figure 6.2G–J) and plays a role in accurate cell cycle progression. The primary cilium is maintained in the G0 phase of the cell cycle. It is assembled during G1 and becomes disassembled at the entry into mitosis. It reassembles during exit from mitosis with the mother centriole of the cell's centriole-centrosome complex providing the seed material during each cell cycle. The cycle is initiated in G1 when the distal end of the mother centriole becomes associated with a membrane vesicle and the primary cilium's axoneme then assembles directly onto the microtubules of the mother centriole. The axoneme lengthens as the ciliary vesicle enlarges into a sheath and fuses with the plasma membrane to become continuous with the cell surface. Centrioles duplicate and lengthen during the subsequent S phase and mature to full length in late G2/M. Centriole shortening then occurs during G2/M and fully matured centrioles become relocated at the mitotic poles. Several important pathways are coupled through primary cilia-centrosome interactions [10]. These interactions show the power of the centriole-centrosome complex throughout development which can be traced back to the sperm's centriole-centrosome complex.

It is also important to note that the centrosome is a multifunctional organelle and the multifunctional roles of the centrosome have been well studied in somatic cells. This includes a significant role for signal transduction in which the microtubules nucleated by centrosomes serve as railroads to translocate cellular components to the centriole-centrosome complex and modify its configurations for cell cycle-specific requirements. Cellular communication between the centrosome and the cytoplasm is assured by centrosome plasticity and by the absence of a membrane which distinguishes this organelle from most other cellular organelles and allows rapid cell cycle-specific nucleation of microtubules and bidirectional transport along microtubules for centrosome shape changes and for receiving or distributing cellular components to affect cellular metabolism and a diversity of different cell functions.

Centrosome-nuclear interactions to assure cell cycle synchrony

As will be detailed below there is a close association of the centriole-centrosome complex with the nuclear membrane and with nuclear material. As shown in Figure 6.1 the sperm's proximal centriole is closely associated with the sperm nucleus which is important, as nuclear and centrosome functions are tightly synchronized to ensure precise apposition of the two

pronuclei after fertilization and distribution of the genome to the dividing daughter cells. This process is precisely orchestrated involving centrosomes, microtubules, and their attachment to chromosomes. Details of this process will be addressed below. We do not yet know the structural associations of the nuclear membrane and the proximal centriole in sperm before fertilization but data are beginning to emerge on centrosome-nuclear associations and associated functions after fertilization although these studies have not yet been performed in mammalian species. The sperm's nuclear matrix has been investigated more recently [42] and future studies may bring about more information on nuclear proteins that are important for centrosome functions after fertilization. The nuclear mitotic apparatus protein (NuMA) is of specific interest in this context, as it is detected in the decondensing sperm nucleus after fertilization [43] and becomes an essential centrosome-associated protein during mitosis [44]. We do not yet know whether or not NuMA is present in the sperm nucleus before fertilization because studies are more difficult in the extremely compact sperm nucleus and require new methods and new methodological approaches to determine its presence or absence in the sperm nucleus.

Nuclear proteins that contribute to centrosome functions and synchronization of centrosome-nuclear cell cycles

A close structural and functional relationship between nuclear and centrosome proteins is important and becomes particularly apparent after fertilization when centrosome and nuclear maturation takes place and a mitotic apparatus forms prior to cell division. As mentioned earlier, the centriole-centrosome complex is duplicated during the pronuclear phase. In subsequent cell cycles during embryo development synchronized duplication of centrosomes and DNA takes place during the S-phases which ensures synchronized functions during mitosis to separate chromosomes equally to the dividing daughter cells [5, 6, 8, 9].

As mentioned above, a structural connection already exists between the proximal centriole and the nucleus and a structural association persists after fertilization when the proximal centriole remains attached to the male pronucleus to form the sperm aster (Figure 6.2B).

Structural relationships between centrosomes and the nucleus have been described in more detail in different cell systems [45].

Several proteins link nuclear to centrosome functions in which NuMA plays a distinctly important role. NuMA is a 236kDa multifunctional protein that functions as nuclear matrix protein in interphase and as centrosome-associated protein during mitosis [6, 8, 9, 44]. While we do not yet know whether NuMA plays a role in sperm DNA organization and nuclear decompaction in the maturing male pronucleus we know that the nuclear matrix is important for DNA replication in the zygote [42, 46]. Dispersion of NuMA into the cytoplasm after nuclear envelope breakdown (NEBD) (Figure 6.2D) is followed by NuMA association with mitotic centrosomes (Figure 6.2E) which has been shown for somatic cells and for several reproductive cell systems [44, 47, 48]. In sperm, the correlation between nuclear and centrosome proteins has not yet been studied in detail but new data on the nuclear matrix in sperm [42] may indicate that such a relationship between the sperm nucleus and centrosomes may exist. However, we do not yet know whether NuMA plays a role in sperm DNA organization and nuclear decompaction in the zygote embryo but it is clear that the nuclear matrix is important for DNA replication in the zygote [42, 46].

To better understand whether NuMA exists in the sperm nucleus and to analyze possible functions and dysfunctions originating in the sperm nucleus new methods and new methodological approaches are needed to determine whether NuMA is localized in the sperm nucleus. Such studies have not yet been pursued because of the density of the sperm nucleus that presents experimental difficulties. The mature sperm nucleus is distinguished from other nuclei by its extreme chromatin condensation state. The tight compaction is achieved during spermiogenesis when the majority of histones are replaced by protamines [49]. However, new research of the sperm nucleus has revealed more complex contributions by sperm than previously thought which includes epigenetic contributions that influence embryogenesis [50–53]. The existence of the nuclear matrix was controversial when it was first reported but new methods have clearly been able to show its existence and its significant influence on DNA organization and functions. It has clearly been shown that it exists in the sperm nucleus and that it is important from fertilization throughout embryo development [42]. However, the study of sperm components has been difficult because of the special sperm compaction that is not amenable to routine immunofluorescence microscopy or other microscopy methods. Specialized methods are necessary and have been employed for embryonic cells [54].

Nuclear mitotic apparatus protein is an important link in synchronizing nuclear and centrosome maturation events after fertilization. Nuclear mitotic apparatus protein is highly insoluble in the nucleus but during NEBD it becomes hyperphosphorylated which allows its dispersion into the cytoplasm. In somatic cells, NuMA requires precise regulation including regulation by cyclin B to move out of the nucleus into the cytoplasm prior to prophase and to associate with mitotic centrosomes during mitosis [44, 45]. Nuclear-centrosome cell cycle synchronization has been studied in detail for the S phase in somatic cells and critical regulatory processes have been identified including activation of CDK2-cyclin E and other cell cycle-specific proteins [35–37]. Such studies on nuclear-centrosome regulation have not yet been performed in mammalian reproductive systems.

Considerations of centrosome dysfunctions for ART

Worldwide, one in 50 children are born through assisted reproductive technology (ART) [55] and it can be expected that the demand for ART will increase for various reasons, including women who postpone having children until advanced ages in life and are faced with physiological fertility problems. While ART has been enormously helpful to couples experiencing fertility problems the technology still suffers from unexplained failures, some of which may be related to various centrosomal dysfunctions. As outlined above, compromised sperm centrosome functions are associated with decreased fertility and/or male factor infertility. Based on our knowledge of the centriole-centrosome complex as described above, we can now consider several dysfunctions that might contribute to male factor infertility. This knowledge may help to improve the success rate in IVF clinics if centrosome-related dysfunctions are diagnosed as causes for male factor infertility.

It has been known for decades that sperm flagellar abnormalities are associated with motility-related male factor infertility [12, 14–17] and this knowledge led to the highly successful technique of intracytoplasmic sperm injection (ICSI) [56]. Intracytoplasmic sperm injection technology is now being used in up to half of

IVF cycles in many IVF clinics. This technology can further be utilized to determine specific causes for male factor infertility by using heterologous insemination in which human sperm quality is assessed by injecting sperm into either bovine or porcine oocytes to evaluate sperm aster formation and centrosome functions [8]. As mentioned earlier in this chapter the mouse has been excluded from these studies because of the totally different cell and molecular mechanisms used for fertilization [8, 9]. It would potentially be possible to co-inject factors along with ICSI to overcome known defects and dysfunctions associated with infertility which may include intrinsic sperm centrosomal dysfunctions or centrosome regulation dysfunctions within the oocyte.

Several methods are available to determine molecular components that are defective in sperm and it may be possible to repair these defects on molecular levels. For morphological determination electron microscopy and/or immunofluorescence analysis has been used to assess whether sperm tail or centriole dysfunctions are the underlying causes for male factor infertility. Immunoblotting or proteomic determination [7, 57] have been used to determine specific centrosome proteins. Immunoblotting methods have been employed to determine centrosomal dysfunctions in which decreased γ-tubulin and centrin were correlated with lower fertilization success in humans primarily related to oligoasthenozoospermia [58, 59]. These studies showed that the quality but also the quantity of centrosome proteins affected fertilization which confirmed earlier studies using immunofluorescence microscopy in heterologous fertilization experiments in which the size of the sperm aster served as a criterion for centrosome function which also could be correlated to developmental capacity [7, 8, 60, 61].

Although ICSI has been a highly successful technology to overcome male factor infertility in numerous cases it has not yet been possible to overcome cases with severe centriolar defects. However, newer studies in the cat have demonstrated the potential to overcome centrosome defects and offer the possibility that it may become feasible to co-inject centrosomal material to restore complete centrosome function in patients with compromised centrosome functions. These studies in the domestic cat [62, 63] showed short or absent sperm asters after ICSI with testicular spermatozoa while ejaculated spermatozoa produced large sperm asters after ICSI. A decrease in developmental potential was indicated by delays in first cleavage and reduced

development to morulae and blastocyst stages, indicating that the size of the sperm aster may be used to predict developmental competence. These studies further revealed that replacement of the testicular sperm centrosome by a centrosome from an ejaculated spermatozoon resulted in higher rates of embryo development. These data are significant in that it may be possible to restore centrosome functions with donor centrosomes or, to eliminate ethical concerns, to co-inject centrosomal material along with ICSI as therapy for couples in which infertility is a result of centrosome-related sperm dysfunctions. While centrosome maturation during spermatogenesis has not been addressed in this chapter it may be possible to overcome sperm-related centrosome dysfunctions that may be the result of incomplete centrosome maturation during spermatogenesis. For these studies to be applicable to humans more research is necessary to determine the specific centrosome proteins that are involved in sperm aster and zygote aster formation, as our current knowledge is limited to only a few centrosomal proteins as described earlier, primarily related to γ-tubulin and centrin that are both localized to the basal body and can be analyzed by immunofluorescence or immunoblotting in test sperm samples.

As outlined above, except for the centriole-centrosome complex, nuclear factors play critical roles in cell cycle synchronization and in centrosome functions. Of specific interest is NuMA as one of the essential nuclear and centrosome-associated proteins that is important for successful fertilization and all embryonic cell divisions. NuMA dysfunctions can be among the underlying causes for infertility, developmental disorders, or adulthood disease. NuMA abnormalities have been found in human oocytes [25, 43] in which male decondensation was impaired and may have been the result of NuMA defects in the sperm nucleus or misregulation in the fertilized oocyte. Detailed studies on NuMA before and after fertilization will be necessary to determine whether NuMA dysfunctions play a role in male-factor infertility. Such studies fall in a new line of research that proposes a role for nuclear matrix instability in male-factor infertility [42]. Mis-regulation of NuMA can result in abnormal cell divisions with consequences for embryo abnormalities, fetal loss, or diseases including cancer.

It is also worth noting that environmental factors may influence NuMA functions, as extensive modifications have been seen after herpes simplex virus

(HSV) infection which induces solubilization and relocalization of NuMA [64]; it may affect subsequent NuMA dynamics that may play a role in mitotic abnormalities underlying diseases such as cancer.

Research on the sperm's nuclear matrix has become of increasing interest in recent years, and many of the non-genetic male-factor infertility problems may be related to nuclear matrix instability [42] which may include transgenerational non-genetic instability. Environmental influences may include non-genetic factors that affect the nuclear matrix [50]. Detailed studies are available on chronic exposure of sperm to low doses of cyclophosphamide that has been correlated with an altered nuclear matrix protein profile [65, 66] which affects fertilization and may affect nuclear matrix–centrosome interactions.

Conclusions

In recent years, it has clearly been recognized that the centriole-centrosome complex introduced by sperm in non-rodent mammalian species including humans serves critically important functions and provides the template for centrioles and their varied functions through all stages of embryo development and in adult somatic cells. Dysfunctions of this complex have been identified as causes for male-factor infertility and several childhood and adulthood diseases. Centrosome integrity is important for ICSI and new research has identified specific centrosomal proteins that play a role in male-factor infertility, which calls for more research to identify the entire centrosome protein profile in sperm and the developing embryo to determine specific dysfunctions that will be important to allow therapeutic advances.

References

1. Jamsai D, O'Bryan MK. Mouse models in male fertility research. *Asian J Androl.* 2011;**13**(1):139–51.

2. Baker HWG. Clinical management of male infertility. 2008 [accessed June 29, 2012]; available from: http://www.endotext.org/male/male7/maleframe7.htm

3. Schatten H, Schatten G, Mazia D *et al.* Behavior of centrosomes during fertilization and cell division in mouse oocytes and in sea urchin eggs. *Proc Natl Acad Sci USA.* 1986;**83**(1):105–9.

4. Schatten H, Walter M, Mazia D *et al.* Centrosome detection in sea urchin eggs with a monoclonal antibody against drosophila intermediate filament proteins: characterization of stages of the division cycle of centrosomes. *Proc Natl Acad Sci USA.* 1987;**84**(23):8488–92.

5. Schatten H. The mammalian centrosome and its functional significance. *Histochem Cell Biol.* 2008;**129**(6):667–86.

6. Schatten H, Sun QY. Centrosome dynamics during mammalian oocyte maturation with a focus on meiotic spindle formation. *Mol Reprod Dev.* 2011;**78**(10–11):757–68.

7. Schatten H, Sun QY. The role of centrosomes in mammalian fertilization and its significance for ICSI. *Mol Hum Reprod.* 2009;**15**(9):531–8.

8. Schatten H, Sun QY. New insights into the role of centrosomes in mammalian fertilization and implications for art. *Reproduction.* 2011;**142**(6):793–801.

9. Schatten H, Sun QY. The significant role of centrosomes in stem cell division and differentiation. *Microsc Microanal.* 2011;**17**(4):506–12.

10. Schatten H, Sun QY. The role of centrosomes in fertilization, cell division and establishment of asymmetry during embryo development. *Semin Cell Dev Biol.* 2010;**21**(2):174–84.

11. Goto M, O'Brien DA, Eddy EM. Speriolin is a novel human and mouse sperm centrosome protein. *Hum Reprod.* 2010;**25**(8):1884–94.

12. Chemes HE. Phenotypes of sperm pathology: genetic and acquired forms in infertile men. *J Androl.* 2000;**21**(6):799–808.

13. Chemes HE. Sperm centrioles and their dual role in flagellogenesis and cell cycle of the zygote structure, function and pathology. In Schatten H, editor. *The Centrosome.* Totowa, NJ: Humana Press; 2012.

14. Chemes EH, Rawe YV. Sperm pathology: a step beyond descriptive morphology. Origin, characterization and fertility potential of abnormal sperm phenotypes in infertile men. *Hum Reprod Update.* 2003;**9**(5):405–28.

15. Mitchell V, Rives N, Albert M *et al.* Outcome of ICSI with ejaculated spermatozoa in a series of men with distinct ultrastructural flagellar abnormalities. *Hum Reprod.* 2006;**21**(8):2065–74.

16. Rawe VY, Terada Y, Nakamura S *et al.* A pathology of the sperm centriole responsible for defective sperm aster formation, syngamy and cleavage. *Hum Reprod.* 2002;**17**(9):2344–9.

17. Rawe VY, Chemes H. Exploring the cytoskeleton during intracytoplasmic sperm injection in humans. *Methods Mol Biol.* 2009;**518**:189–206.

18. Sathananthan AH. Mitosis in the human embryo: the vital role of the sperm centrosome (centriole). *Histol Histopathol.* 1997;**12**(3):827–56.

19. Sathananthan AH. Human centriole: origin, and how it impacts fertilization, embryogenesis, infertility and cloning. *Indian J Med Res.* 2009;**129**(4):348–50.

20. Sathananthan AH. Human centrosomal dynamics during gametogenesis, fertilization and embryogenesis and its impact on fertility: ultrastructural analysis. In Schatten H, editor. *The Centrosome*. Totowa, NJ: Humana Press; 2012.

21. Sathananthan AH, Kola I, Osborne J *et al.* Centrioles in the beginning of human development. *Proc Natl Acad Sci USA.* 1991;**88**(11):4806–10.

22. Sathananthan AH, Ratnam SS, Ng SC *et al.* The sperm centriole: its inheritance, replication and perpetuation in early human embryos. *Hum Reprod.* 1996;**11**(2):345–56.

23. Sathananthan AH, Ratnasooriya WD, de Silva PK *et al.* Characterization of human gamete centrosomes for assisted reproduction. *Ital J Anat Embryol.* 2001;**106**(2 Suppl. 2):61–73.

24. Rawe VY, Diaz ES, Abdelmassih R *et al.* The role of sperm proteasomes during sperm aster formation and early zygote development: implications for fertilization failure in humans. *Hum Reprod.* 2008;**23**(3):573–80.

25. Schatten H, Rawe VY, Sun Q-Y. Cytoskeletal architecture of human oocytes with focus on centrosomes and their significant role in fertilization. In Agarwal A, Varghese A, Nagy ZP, editors. *Practical Manual of in vitro Fertilization: Advanced Methods and Novel Devices*. Totowa, NJ: Humana Press; 2012.

26. Doxsey SJ, Stein P, Evans L *et al.* Pericentrin, a highly conserved centrosome protein involved in microtubule organization. *Cell.* 1994;**76**(4):639–50.

27. Dictenberg JB, Zimmerman W, Sparks CA *et al.* Pericentrin and gamma-tubulin form a protein complex and are organized into a novel lattice at the centrosome. *J Cell Biol.* 1998;**141**(1):163–74.

28. Young A, Dictenberg JB, Purohit A *et al.* Cytoplasmic dynein-mediated assembly of pericentrin and gamma tubulin onto centrosomes. *Mol Biol Cell.* 2000;**11**(6):2047–56.

29. Badano JL, Teslovich TM, Katsanis N. The centrosome in human genetic disease. *Nat Rev Genet.* 2005;**6**(3):194–205.

30. Salisbury JL. Centrin, centrosomes, and mitotic spindle poles. *Curr Opin Cell Biol.* 1995;**7**(1):39–45.

31. Lutz W, Lingle WL, McCormick D *et al.* Phosphorylation of centrin during the cell cycle and its role in centriole separation preceding centrosome duplication. *J Biol Chem.* 2001;**276**(23):20,774–80.

32. Manandhar G, Schatten H, Sutovsky P. Centrosome reduction during gametogenesis and its significance. *Biol Reprod.* 2005;**72**(1):2–13.

33. Salisbury JL. Thoughts on progress in the centrosome field. In: Schatten H, editor. *The Centrosome*. Totowa, NJ: Humana Press; 2012.

34. Salisbury JL, Suino KM, Busby R *et al.* Centrin-2 is required for centriole duplication in mammalian cells. *Curr Biol.* 2002;**12**(15):1287–92.

35. Boutros R. Regulation of centrosomes by cyclin-dependent kinases. In Schatten H, editor. *The Centrosome*. Totowa, NJ: Humana Press; 2012.

36. Fisk HA. Many pathways to destruction: the centrosome and its control by and role in regulated proteolysis. In Schatten H, editor. *The Centrosome*. Totowa, NJ: Humana Press; 2012.

37. Prosser SL, Fry MA. Regulation of the centrosome cycle by protein degradation. In Schatten H, editor. *The Centrosome*. Totowa, NJ: Humana Press; 2012.

38. Yamashita YM, Mahowald AP, Perlin JR *et al.* Asymmetric inheritance of mother versus daughter centrosome in stem cell division. *Science.* 2007;**315**(5811):518–21.

39. Yamashita YM, Yuan H, Cheng J *et al.* Polarity in stem cell division: asymmetric stem cell division in tissue homeostasis. *Cold Spring Harb Perspect Biol.* 2010;**2**(1):a001313.

40. Lambert JD, Nagy LM. Asymmetric inheritance of centrosomally localized mRNAs during embryonic cleavages. *Nature.* 2002;**420**(6916):682–6.

41. Wheatley DN, Wang AM, Strugnell GE. Expression of primary cilia in mammalian cells. *Cell Biol Int.* 1996;**20**(1):73–81.

42. Johnson GD, Lalancette C, Linnemann AK *et al.* The sperm nucleus: chromatin, RNA, and the nuclear matrix. *Reproduction.* 2011;**141**(1):21–36.

43. Alvarez Sedo C, Schatten H, Combelles CM *et al.* The nuclear mitotic apparatus (NuMA) protein: localization and dynamics in human oocytes, fertilization and early embryos. *Mol Hum Reprod.* 2011;**17**(6):392–8.

44. Sun QY, Schatten H. Role of NuMA in vertebrate cells: review of an intriguing multifunctional protein. *Front Biosci.* 2006;**11**:1137–46.

45. Schatten H, Sun Q-Y. Nuclear-centrosome relationships during fertilization, cell division, embryo development, and in somatic cell nuclear transfer (SCNT) embryos. In Schatten H, editor. *The Centrosome*. Totowa, NJ: Humana Press; 2012.

46. Yamauchi Y, Shaman JA, Ward WS. Non-genetic contributions of the sperm nucleus to embryonic development. *Asian J Androl.* 2011;**13**(1):31–5.

47. Zhong ZS, Zhang G, Meng XQ *et al.* Function of donor cell centrosome in intraspecies and interspecies nuclear transfer embryos. *Exp Cell Res.* 2005;**306**(1):35–46.

48. Liu Z, Schatten H, Hao Y *et al.* The nuclear mitotic apparatus (NuMA) protein is contributed by the donor cell nucleus in cloned porcine embryos. *Front Biosci.* 2006;**11**:1945–57.

49. Delbes G, Hales BF, Robaire B. Toxicants and human sperm chromatin integrity. *Mol Hum Reprod.* 2010;**16** (1):14–22.

50. de Boer P, Ramos L, de Vries M *et al.* Memoirs of an insult: sperm as a possible source of transgenerational epimutations and genetic instability. *Mol Hum Reprod.* 2010;**16**(1):48–56.

51. Jenkins TG, Carrell DT. The paternal epigenome and embryogenesis: poising mechanisms for development. *Asian J Androl.* 2011;**13**(1):76–80.

52. Jenkins TG, Carrell DT. The sperm epigenome and potential implications for the developing embryo. *Reproduction.* 2012;**143**(6):727–34.

53. Chao SB, Guo L, Ou XH *et al.* Heated spermatozoa: effects on embryonic development and epigenetics. *Hum Reprod.* 2012;**27**(4):1016–24.

54. Degrouard J, Hozak P, Heyman Y *et al.* Nucleoskeleton of early bovine embryos and differentiated somatic cells: an ultrastructural and immunocytochemical comparison. *Histochem Cell Biol.* 2004;**121**(6):441–51.

55. Manipalviratn S, DeCherney A, Segars J. Imprinting disorders and assisted reproductive technology. *Fertil Steril.* 2009;**91**(2):305–15.

56. Palermo G, Joris H, Devroey P *et al.* Pregnancies after intracytoplasmic injection of single spermatozoon into an oocyte. *Lancet.* 1992;**340**(8810):17–18.

57. Bohring C, Krause W. Immune infertility: towards a better understanding of sperm (auto)-immunity. The value of proteomic analysis. *Hum Reprod.* 2003;**18** (5):915–24.

58. Hinduja I, Zaveri K, Baliga N. Human sperm centrin levels and outcome of intracytoplasmic sperm injection (ICSI) – a pilot study. *Indian J Med Res.* 2008;**128** (5):606–10.

59. Hinduja I, Baliga NB, Zaveri K. Correlation of human sperm centrosomal proteins with fertility. *J Hum Reprod Sci.* 2010;**3**(2):95–101.

60. Navara CS, First NL, Schatten G. Phenotypic variations among paternal centrosomes expressed within the zygote as disparate microtubule lengths and sperm aster organization: correlations between centrosome activity and developmental success. *Proc Natl Acad Sci USA.* 1996;**93**(11):5384–8.

61. Tachibana M, Terada Y, Ogonuki N *et al.* Functional assessment of centrosomes of spermatozoa and spermatids microinjected into rabbit oocytes. *Mol Reprod Dev.* 2009;**76**(3):270–7.

62. Comizzoli P, Wildt DE. Centrosomal functions and dysfunctions in cat spermatozoa. In Schatten H, editor. *The Centrosome.* Totowa, NJ: Humana Press; 2012.

63. Comizzoli P, Wildt DE, Pukazhenthi BS. Poor centrosomal function of cat testicular spermatozoa impairs embryo development in vitro after intracytoplasmic sperm injection. *Biol Reprod.* 2006;**75** (2):252–60.

64. Yamauchi Y, Kiriyama K, Kimura H *et al.* Herpes simplex virus induces extensive modification and dynamic relocalisation of the nuclear mitotic apparatus (NuMA) protein in interphase cells. *J Cell Sci.* 2008;**121** (Pt 12):2087–96.

65. Codrington AM, Hales BF, Robaire B. Chronic cyclophosphamide exposure alters the profile of rat sperm nuclear matrix proteins. *Biol Reprod.* 2007;**77** (2):303–11.

66. Codrington AM, Hales BF, Robaire B. Exposure of male rats to cyclophosphamide alters the chromatin structure and basic proteome in spermatozoa. *Hum Reprod.* 2007;**22**(5):1431–42.

The male biological clock

Harry Fisch

Introduction

Two cultural and technological trends are driving a rising concern about the impact of age-related changes in paternal reproductive fitness. Couples in many industrialized countries are waiting longer to have children, and advances in reproductive technology are allowing older men and women to consider having children. Both medical professionals and the lay public may not appreciate that men, as well as women, experience a "biological clock" and, hence, they may undervalue the impact that paternal aging can have on fertility and reproductive competency. Age-related changes associated with the male biological clock affect sperm quality, fertility, hormone levels, libido, erectile function, and a host of non-reproductive physiological issues.

This chapter focuses on the potentially adverse effects of the male biological clock on the fertility and health of older men. Advanced paternal age is associated with reduced semen volume, lower percentage of normal sperm, and lower sperm motility. In addition, increased paternal age increases the risk for spontaneous abortion as well as genetic abnormalities in offspring due to DNA damage from abnormal apoptosis and reactive oxygen species. Below-normal testosterone levels may impact reproductive health and are also associated with a range of significant comorbid conditions, which may exact their own toll on health.

In light of the reality of a male biological clock, older men who are considering parenthood should obtain a thorough physical examination focused on their sexual and reproductive capacity. This examination should include disclosure of any sexual dysfunction and the use of medications, drugs, or lifestyle factors that might impair male fertility or sexual response. Older men should also be counseled regarding the effects of paternal age on spermatogenesis and pregnancy.

The reality of the male biological clock

The phrase "biological clock" is commonly understood by physicians and the lay public to refer to the declining fertility, increasing risk for fetal birth defects, and altered hormone levels experienced by women as they age. Abundant scientific evidence, however, suggests that men also experience age-related physiological changes that can accurately be described as a "biological clock" [1, 2]. Men and their physicians must therefore understand the effects of this "clock" on sexual and reproductive health, as well as its potential contributions to significant morbidities such as diabetes, cardiovascular disease, and metabolic syndrome.

The female biological clock is typically obvious and well-defined temporally and biologically, with declining oocyte production in the late 30s to early 40s and cessation of menses in the late 40s and early 50s. Male fertility, in contrast, does not cease abruptly, and, to date, no significant limit to spermatogenesis has been demonstrated. Paternal fertility does change with age, however, and numerous investigators have explored the effect of aging on seminal parameters to determine whether advanced paternal age is associated with diminished semen quality and a higher risk of infertility.

Studies in mice have clearly demonstrated a positive correlation between age, histologic changes in testes, and a decline in semen quality. "Older" mice

Paternal Influences on Human Reproductive Success, ed. Douglas T. Carrell. Published by Cambridge University Press.
© Cambridge University Press 2013.

(age ~18 months) exhibit age-related changes such as an increased number of vacuoles in germ cells and a thinner seminiferous epithelium [3]. By the age of 30 months, extremely thin seminiferous epithelia with very few spermatocytes or spermatids were found. Another study found that total sperm production was significantly reduced in 22- and 30-month-old rats [4]. Other age-related changes found in the murine model include an increased incidence of pre-implantation losses, mutation frequencies, and aneuploidy in the offspring of older male mice [5–7].

Many studies confirm a similar association between aging and compromised male reproductive physiology in humans. For example, a comprehensive review by Kidd *et al.* demonstrated declines in semen volume, sperm concentration, sperm motility, sperm morphology, pregnancy rates, and time to pregnancy/subfecundity in human males [8]. Kidd's meta-analysis of 16 studies of the effect of age on seminal parameters showed that 11 of the 16 reported decreases in semen quality with increasing age. Two of these studies adjusted for the confounder of duration of abstinence and found that a statistically significant correlation still exists between decreasing semen volume and increasing age; they reported decreases of 0.15–0.5% for each increase in year of age [9, 10]. (Out of four studies showing no association between age and semen volume, only one adjusted for duration of abstinence and this study had a maximum patient age of 50 years [11].) Abundant evidence, therefore, links advancing age with reductions in semen volume, and this reduction becomes more significant in men over 50 years of age.

The relationship between increasing age and sperm concentration is less clear. Kidd *et al.* reviewed 21 studies examining the association between age and sperm concentration and found substantial inconsistencies and methodological flaws in many studies [8]. Even the results of the studies adjusting for duration of infertility are conflicting, suggesting no clear association between sperm concentration and increasing paternal age.

A strong association, however, was found between increasing age and declining sperm motility. Thirteen of the 19 studies reviewed by Kidd *et al.* [8] showed this relationship, despite variation in the morphological criteria used to assess sperm abnormalities.

The observed declines in semen volume, sperm motility, and sperm morphology with advancing age may relate to degenerative changes to the prostate, such as a decrease in protein and water content,

which may contribute to the decrease in seminal volume and sperm motility [12]. Additionally, age-related degenerative changes to the germinal epithelium can impact sperm morphology [13].

Kidd *et al.* also examined the impact of advancing male age on pregnancy rate, defined as the percent of male subjects whose partners achieved a pregnancy over a period of time, and subfecundity, defined as the percent of couples remaining infertile at a defined time point. Seven of nine studies reported a correlation between decreasing pregnancy rates and increasing age, and five of them reached statistical significance. However, four of the seven studies did not adjust for female age in the analysis and female age is a well-established independent predictor of achieving pregnancy. Two of the studies that controlled for female partner age found that, after stratifying the study population into men under 30 and men over 50, the pregnancy rate in the cohort of older men was 23–38% lower than the cohort of younger men [14, 15].

Seven of nine studies of the association between male age and subfecundity found a direct correlation between paternal age and time to pregnancy [8]. In these studies, the increased risks of subfecundity with older age groups ranged from 11% to 250%.

The effect of paternal age on the likelihood of delayed conception was also explored by Ford *et al.* in a study of 8515 planned pregnancies [16]. After adjusting for confounding factors such as age of the female partner, body mass index (BMI), smoking, passive smoke exposure, education, duration of cohabitation, duration of oral contraceptive use, and paternal alcohol consumption, increasing paternal age remained highly significantly associated with delayed conception within 6 or 12 months. The study concluded that the probability that a fertile couple will take greater than 12 months to conceive nearly doubles from approximately 8% when a man is less than 25 years old to approximately 15% when he is greater than age 35.

In summary, existing data clearly demonstrate that advanced paternal age is associated with a decline in semen quality and fertility status.

Age-related testosterone decline

The decline in hormone levels experienced by men as they age is not as steep or as sudden as that associated with hormone declines during menopause in women, but the decline itself is real and its effects can be significant. Testosterone levels peak around age 20 [17]. After that, levels begin to decline by about 1% a year [18]. The Massachusetts Male Aging Study (MMAS), a large population-based random-sample cohort, quantified the decreasing testosterone levels as a cross-sectional decline of 0.8%/year of age and a longitudinal decline of 1.6%/year within the 10-year follow-up data. Earlier studies have also reported a longitudinal decline in serum testosterone [19, 20].

Although various levels of testosterone have been suggested over the years as the demarcation between "normal" testosterone and "low" testosterone, a consensus appears now to be forming. The Standards Committee of the International Society for Sexual Medicine and several other professional societies (the International Consultation of Sexual Medicine, International Society of Andrology, International Society for the Study of the Aging Male, European Society of Urology, and the American Society of Andrology) have agreed on the use of two different thresholds of total testosterone for clinical practice: a level of 350 ng/dL, above which symptoms are unlikely and testosterone replacement therapy (TRT) is not usually beneficial nor recommended, and a level of 230 ng/dL, below which symptoms are probable and TRT may be beneficial [21]. Total testosterone (TT) levels between 230 ng/dL and 350 ng/dL are considered borderline, with treatment being guided by clinical experience and the specifics of the individual patient.

In addition to hypogonadism, a variety of terms have been used to describe primarily age-related, below-normal testosterone levels with associated clinical symptoms including "symptomatic androgen deficiency," "andropause," "age-related hypogonadism" and "testosterone deficiency." The term testosterone deficiency (TD) appears to be gaining in popularity as the preferred term to describe age-related testosterone loss. "Hypogonadism," in contrast, is a more general term that refers to any state characterized by reduced testicular function, impaired sperm production, and low testosterone levels.

Available data suggest that the prevalence of biochemical hypogonadism (i.e. low testosterone without considering whether a man is suffering any signs or symptoms) is between 20% and 39% [22, 23]. Biochemical hypogonadism, however, can occur in men who have no signs or symptoms. Clinical hypogonadism is defined as below-normal TT *and* the presence of signs or symptoms related to

hypogonadism. This definition results in much lower prevalence estimates. The MMAS, for example, defined "androgen deficiency" as signs/symptoms in the context of TT levels below 400 ng/dL or free testosterone levels below 8.9 ng/dL [18]. Using this definition in a population-based sample the MMAS found that the prevalence of "androgen deficiency" ranged from 7% in men aged 48–59 to 23% in men aged 70–79 [18]. There appears to be no consistent evidence that the prevalence of hypogonadism differs between racial and ethnic groups [24].

Importantly, the symptoms commonly associated with low testosterone – and thus the diagnosis of TD itself – are highly variable over time in individuals. The MMAS found that 55% of the men who were found to have "androgen deficiency" at baseline were eugonadal when re-tested at a later stage of the study [25]. (Such findings support recommendations for re-testing of borderline testosterone levels and only when the patient is in relatively good health.)

A natural age-related decline in serum testosterone has thus been well established, although there are many other possible causes of below-normal testosterone and there are certainly some younger men who meet the criteria of TD. Varicoceles, for example, can impair sperm production and several studies suggest that they may induce a sub-hypogonadal or hypogonadal state. Animal experiments have demonstrated an association between varicoceles and decreased serum testosterone biosynthesis [19]. Studies in humans suggest a similar association [26, 27]. A study conducted by Shah *et al.* at Columbia University Medical Center retrospectively reviewed testosterone levels of 237 men presenting with male factor infertility and clinical varicoceles between 1994 and 2004 who underwent varicocelectomy [27]. The cohort median age was 36.0 years and the average testosterone level was 389.7 ng/dL; 30.3% (72/237) of patients were found to be hypogonadal (testosterone <300 ng/dL). A similar study by Su *et al.* confirmed this trend and demonstrated that correction of the varicocele can improve testosterone levels for infertile men with varicoceles [28].

In addition to varicocele, many other conditions or insults can cause below-normal testosterone, including congenital anorchidism, cryptorchidism, genetic conditions (i.e. Klinefelter syndrome), pituitary tumors, arious medications (i.e. glucocorticoids and long-acting opioid pain medications), and systemic disease (i.e. liver failure, uremia, sickle-cell disease).

Advanced paternal age and reproductive integrity

As noted earlier, US population studies show that many couples are postponing childbearing until their mid 30s to mid 40s. According to the CDC birth statistics, the average maternal age in 2003 was 25.1 compared with an average maternal age of 21.4 years in 1974. A similar trend is occurring in American men. The birth rate for men 25–44 years has been steadily increasing since the 1970s while the birth rate of men younger than 25 years has been decreasing [29]. These trends are alarming in light of research clearly demonstrating a relationship between increasing paternal age and a host of negative reproductive outcomes. Advanced paternal age, for example, has been linked to increased spontaneous abortions, more autosomal dominant disorders, trisomy 21, and, recently, to an increased risk of schizophrenia.

Of course, it has long been known that women aged 35 years or greater are at higher risk than younger women for adverse reproductive events. And since paternal age often correlates with maternal age, it can be difficult to untangle the independent effects of paternal age. Nonetheless, careful studies have been conducted, starting with research by Yershalmy in 1939 showing a connection between spontaneous abortion and paternal age [30]. This association has been corroborated in more recent studies such as a prospective study of 5,121 American couples that demonstrated a clear link between the risk of spontaneous abortion and advanced paternal age [31]. A prospective analysis of 23,821 women from the Danish National Birth Cohort also demonstrated that pregnancies involving men 50 years or older had almost twice the risk of spontaneous abortion compared with pregnancies involving younger fathers after adjustment for maternal age, reproductive history, and maternal lifestyle during pregnancy [32].

Advanced parental age is also a recognized risk factor for many genetic abnormalities in the developing newborn. This may relate to the previously detailed decreases in semen volume, percent normal sperm, and sperm motility in older men. While these factors adversely affect fertility, they may also degrade the genetic integrity of the sperm. In contrast to oogenesis, spermatozoa are continuously produced and spermatogenic cells undergo lifelong replication and meiosis [33]. This continued replication can introduce spontaneous mutations within the paternal cell line. As men age, the rate of genetic abnormalities that occur during spermatogenesis increases. Investigation of advanced paternal age in the murine model reveals age-dependent effects on the meiotic and premeiotic phase of sperm development. These abnormalities in replication result in both aneuploidy and structural abnormalities in sperm cells [7]. In humans, the frequency of these numerical and structural aberrations in sperm chromosomes increases with increasing paternal age [34]. This age-related increase in sperm cells with damaged DNA results from both increased double-strand DNA breaks and decreased apoptosis during spermatogenesis [35]. (Apoptosis of sperm with damaged DNA is an essential aspect of spermatogenesis that helps raise the percentage of sperm with normal DNA.)

Oxidative stress may also play a role in the observed rise in the frequency of numerical and structural aberrations in sperm chromosomes with increasing paternal age. Spermatozoa have low concentrations of antioxidant scavenging enzymes, which makes them particularly susceptible to DNA damage from reactive oxygen species. A recent study found that seminal reactive oxygen species levels are significantly elevated in men older than 40 years of age [36].

DNA damage in sperm cells is associated with many autosomal dominant disorders such as Apert syndrome, achondroplasia, osteogenesis imperfecta, progeria, Marfan syndrome, Waardenburg syndrome, and thanatophoric dysplasia [37].

In addition to structural errors and resultant autosomal dominant disorders, aneuploidy errors in germ cell lines also occur at higher rates with advanced parental age. Trisomy 21 (Down syndrome) is a common aneuploidy error that affects 1/800 to 1/1000 newborns [38]. Although the association between trisomy 21 and advanced maternal age is well documented, it is only relatively recently that the effects of advanced paternal age on this condition have been elucidated. For example, investigation of the meiotic non-disjunctional error in trisomy 21 reveals the origin of the extra chromosome 21 to be paternal in 5–20% of cases [39].

An evaluation of the Medical Birth Registry of Norway from 1967 to 1978 that included 685,000 total births and 693 cases of Down syndrome revealed an increased risk of Down syndrome with a paternal age of 50 years or greater [40]. An analysis of the

New York State Department of Health congenital malformations registry containing 3,419 trisomy 21 births demonstrated a 111% and 60% increase in the risk of a trisomy 21 birth in women and men over 35 years, respectively [1]. In men and women younger than 35, no effect of parental age was found. A paternal age effect was apparent in association with a maternal age of 35 years or greater and was most pronounced when maternal age was 40 years or greater. The rate of Down syndrome with a combined parental age greater than 40 years was 60/10,000 births, which is a six-fold increase compared with parents less than 35 years. Advanced paternal age in interaction with advanced maternal age significantly increases the risk of trisomy 21 and may possibly explain the exponential increase in trisomy 21 in women older than 35 years.

The genetic changes that occur as part of the male biological clock may also play a role in an observed correlation between paternal age and schizophrenia. Schizophrenia is a complex disease of unclear etiology, however a genetic predisposition does appear to exist [41]. Some early studies suggested an association between advanced paternal age and the development of schizophrenia [42, 43] and more recent studies have confirmed this association [44]. A 12-year evaluation of the Jerusalem birth registry and the Israel psychiatric registry that included 658 individuals with schizophrenia revealed that the risk of schizophrenia increased monotonically with increasing paternal age [45]. This increased risk culminated in a relative risk of 2.96 (95% confidence interval, 1.60–5.47) for offspring of men 50 years or greater. Conversely, maternal age demonstrated no effect on the development of schizophrenia. A Swedish birth registry study revealed that the association between paternal age and schizophrenia was present in families without a previous history of the disorder, but not in those with a family history [46]. Based upon the stronger association between paternal age and schizophrenia in people without a family history the authors suggested that accumulation of *de novo* mutations in paternal sperm contributed to the risk of schizophrenia.

These kinds of deleterious effects associated with advanced paternal age coupled with the trend towards delayed childbirth underscore the importance of appropriate prenatal counseling of older couples about the risks that age may pose to their chances for a successful pregnancy as well as their chances for having a healthy child.

The role of medications and comorbidities

The effects of the male biological clock can be exacerbated by both medications and comorbidities. Pharmacologically mediated fertility declines and/or sexual dysfunction have been demonstrated for antihypertensive drugs, antidepressants, opioid pain medications, and hormonal agents. Seminal emission can be blocked by alpha blocker medications, which are used to treat many symptoms of the lower urinary tract. Gonadotropin-releasing hormone agonists, which are used for prostate cancer treatment, can directly impact sperm production and testosterone levels. High doses of anabolic steroids, sometimes used for athletic performance enhancement, reduce sperm production, sometimes permanently. Erectile dysfunction, ejaculatory disorders, and decreased libido, can be caused by 5-alpha reductase inhibitors.

Sexual function and reproductive function can also substantially decline in males treated for prostate cancer. Treatments such as radiotherapy, surgery, or hormones, alone or in combination may cause impotence, urinary incontinence, reduced libido, or retrograde ejaculation, and the severity of effects increases with age.

Comorbid conditions linked (often bi-causally) to the male biological clock include type II diabetes and metabolic syndrome. Both conditions are strongly associated with below-normal testosterone levels [47]. Grundy found that 40% of men with type II diabetes between the ages of 40 and 49 were hypogonadal – and the rate was nearly 55% among men in their 70s [47]. The low testosterone levels found in males with type II diabetes may be related to the correspondingly high prevalence of erectile dysfunction (ED) among men with diabetes, a rate estimated to range between 35% and 75% [48].

The role of TD in all-cause mortality is unclear. Some epidemiologic studies have found significant associations between lower testosterone levels and higher rates of all-cause mortality in the general population of men [49]. A recent systematic review and meta-analysis of studies exploring the relationship of testosterone and mortality in men, however, found large between-study differences in results and methodological problems that cast doubt on the direction of causality in this association [50]. The study concluded that because concurrent illness is associated with lower testosterone levels, there is a "strong possibility" that previous study results are biased and that low testosterone is simply an epiphenomenon of concurrent or possibly occult illness.

An increasing body of evidence has revealed important associations between ED and three other disease states common among older men: cardiovascular disease (CVD), depression, and benign prostatic hyperplasia (BPH). Assigning causation between hypogonadism and these conditions is not simple, since each disease state can adversely affect the other in reciprocal, complex ways, and the role of declining androgens in ED is similarly complex. Broadly speaking, ED is clearly related to age-related biological changes and, hence, the biological clock is also implicated in these other chronic, frequently progressive, and disruptive conditions.

For example, the prevalence of ED is significantly higher among patients being treated for heart disease and hypertension [51]. Treatments for hypertension may contribute to erectile dysfunction, which may help explain the increased incidence of ED in these patients. But the reverse relationship is also true: ED should be considered a marker for hypertension and other cardiovascular complications [52].

Depression may both contribute to and link erectile dysfunction and cardiovascular disease. Erectile dysfunction is associated with well-established negative psychological effects, primarily depression and anxiety [53]. Several recent studies have described the comorbidity of ED and BPH, which correlate with diminished quality of life [54]. Erectile dysfunction, cardiovascular disease, depression and BPH are all common conditions among older men and since these conditions appear to be strongly correlated, a multidisciplinary approach to future research and clinical practice is warranted.

Testosterone replacement therapy

In recent years several inter-related trends have brought into high relief the relationship of the male biological clock and the use of testosterone replacement therapy (TRT) as a treatment option for the low levels of testosterone that frequently accompany it. New TRT formulations have made treatment more convenient for patients and have generated considerable advertising and promotional efforts on the part of companies marketing these formulations [55]. In addition, men have become more comfortable going

to their physicians for treatment of ED, which can result in discussions of and/or testing for testosterone levels.

Diagnosing TD and treating it effectively, however, can be challenging because testosterone levels are so intimately related to a range of factors such as obesity, lack of exercise, and diabetes, which, themselves, are closely related to lifestyle issues. Behaviors that promote health, such as weight loss with exercise, healthy dietary choices, and avoidance of smoking, may help prevent TD, and they correlate significantly with higher testosterone levels over time in population-based research [56].

Several studies, for example, suggest that testosterone levels rise after weight loss. Niskanen *et al.* found that free testosterone and, to a lesser extent, TT rose significantly during a 9-week rapid weight-loss period in men with abdominal obesity and metabolic syndrome [57]. The increase persisted during a 12-month weight-maintenance period. The proportion of subjects in this study with TD (TT <317 ng/dL) decreased from 48% at baseline to 9% at the end of the weight-loss phase. Such results underscore the importance of addressing health issues to which testosterone levels are related either prior to a trial of testosterone therapy, or concurrent with such therapy.

It is also true, however, that emerging evidence suggests that TRT can have a valuable synergistic effect on therapeutic lifestyle changes. In a study by Heufelder *et al.*, 32 men diagnosed with TD (<345.8 ng/dL) as well as newly diagnosed type II diabetes and metabolic syndrome, were randomly assigned to supervised diet and exercise therapy, either alone or combined with transdermal TRT (gel, 50 mg/day) [58]. No hypoglycemic medications or insulin therapy were used. At the end of the study, mean hemoglobin A_{1C} levels had decreased by $0.5 \pm 0.1\%$ (to $7.1 \pm 0.1\%$) in subjects receiving lifestyle treatment alone and by $1.3 \pm 0.1\%$ (to $6.3 \pm 0.1\%$) in those assigned to lifestyle treatment plus TRT. All patients receiving TRT reached the A_{1C} goal of <7% at 1 year compared with only 30.4% of those receiving lifestyle therapy alone. Nearly two-thirds (62.5%) of patients treated with TRT along with diet and exercise no longer met the criteria for metabolic syndrome at study end. This was true for only 12.5% of those receiving diet and exercise alone. Insulin sensitivity also improved significantly more in the TRT group than in the group receiving diet and exercise alone.

One issue that may have served to inhibit prescriptions of TRT in the past – the fear that TRT might induce prostate cancer – now appears to have been resolved. Early reports of a positive association of testosterone and prostate cancer growth in men with advanced, untreated malignancy were based largely on observations of a very few castrated men [59]. Recent analyses, however, contradict these early, limited reports. For example, pooled data from 18 prospective studies in more than 10,000 men revealed no association between risk of prostate cancer and serum testosterone, calculated free testosterone, or all other sex hormones [60]. Most observational studies have failed to find correlations between circulating testosterone levels and prostate pathology. In fact, case–control studies have found correlations between prostate cancer prevalence and *low* serum testosterone [61].

At the same time, there is unequivocal evidence that testosterone suppression can reduce prostate growth and symptoms in men with locally advanced and metastatic prostate cancer. The explanation for this apparent paradox may be that prostate cancer is very sensitive to changes in serum testosterone when at low concentrations (i.e. near castration levels) but is insensitive at higher concentrations because of saturation of the androgen receptors [24].

There is currently no conclusive evidence that TRT in testosterone-deficient men increases the risk of prostate cancer, and there is no evidence that it will promote sub-clinical cancer to metastatic cancer. There is evidence, however, that testosterone may stimulate the growth of *metastatic* prostatic cancers, which is why TRT is contraindicated in men with existing prostate cancer.

Conclusions

Although it is still not widely known among both physicians and the lay public, men, as well as women, have biological clocks, and the changes induced by these "clocks" significantly affect fertility, reproductive fitness, and a wide range of other physiological conditions. The fact that men and women are waiting longer to have children, and that advances in reproductive technology are allowing older men and women to consider having children, amounts to an unrecognized public health risk in the form of increased infertility and risk for birth defects and other reproductive problems.

This chapter has demonstrated a host of potential reproductive problems among older men, driven by the biological clock. Semen parameters as well as semen genetic integrity decline with age, which lead to an increased risk for spontaneous abortion as well as genetic abnormalities in offspring. The decreasing apoptotic rate and increase in reactive oxygen species among the rapidly replicating spermatogonia are possible mechanisms behind an amplification of errors in germ cell lines of older men. Such errors may account for the observed increases in Down syndrome, schizophrenia, and autosomal dominant disorders in children born to older fathers.

Clinicians who are counseling older men must be fully aware of these dynamics and the potential impact of advanced age on reproductive success. In older men, a complete medical history with attention to medications and prior surgical and medical history is critical. Medications that impair testosterone, ejaculation, or sperm formation may need to be discontinued with approval of their prescribing physician. If the couple is to have IVF, preimplantation genetic screening is more readily available now, especially if there is a concern for a health risk issue in the fetus. If a familial history of genetic defects exists, the couple should consult a genetic counselor about possible risks to the fetus and their decision to pursue a pregnancy.

Future research may elucidate in greater detail the etiology and manifestation of the male biological clock in older men. Novel methods to reverse or slow the clock may be discovered by improved understanding of the cellular and biochemical mechanisms of gonadal aging. This research may diminish potential adverse genetic consequences in offspring and increase the chances that older couples can bear healthy children.

References

1. Fisch H, Hyun G, Golden R *et al.* The influence of paternal age on Down syndrome. *J Urol.* 2003;**169**(6):2275–8.

2. Eskenazi B, Wyrobek AJ, Sloter E *et al.* The association of age and semen quality in healthy men. *Hum Reprod.* 2003;**18**(2):447–54.

3. Tanemura K, Kurohmaru M, Kuramoto K *et al.* Age-related morphological changes in the testis of the BDF1 mouse. *J Vet Med Sci.* 1993;**55**(5):703–10.

4. Wang C, Leung A, Sinha-Hikim AP. Reproductive aging in the male Brown-Norway rat: a model for the human. *Endocrinology.* 1993;**133**(6):2773–81.

5. Serre V, Robaire B. Paternal age affects fertility and progeny outcome in the Brown Norway rat. *Fertil Steril.* 1998;**70**(4):625–31.

6. Walter CA, Intano GW, McCarrey JR *et al.* Mutation frequency declines during spermatogenesis in young mice but increases in old mice. *Proc Natl Acad Sci USA.* 1998;**95**(17):10,015–19.

7. Lowe X, Collins B, Allen J *et al.* Aneuploidies and micronuclei in the germ cells of male mice of advanced age. *Mutat Res.* 1995;**338**(1–6):59–76.

8. Kidd SA, Eskenazi B, Wyrobek AJ. Effects of male age on semen quality and fertility: a review of the literature. *Fertil Steril.* 2001;**75**(2):237–48.

9. Fisch H, Goluboff ET, Olson JH *et al.* Semen analyses in 1,283 men from the United States over a 25-year period: no decline in quality. *Fertil Steril.* 1996;**65**(5):1009–14.

10. Andolz P, Bielsa MA, Vila J. Evolution of semen quality in north-eastern Spain: a study in 22,759 infertile men over a 36 year period. *Hum Reprod.* 1999;**14**(3):731–5.

11. Schwartz D, Mayaux MJ, Spira A *et al.* Semen characteristics as a function of age in 833 fertile men. *Fertil Steril.* 1983;**39**(4):530–5.

12. Schneider E. *The Aging Reproductive System.* New York, NY: Raven Press; 1978.

13. Johnson L. Spermatogenesis and aging in the human. *J Androl.* 1986;**7**(6):331–54.

14. Rolf C, Behre HM, Nieschlag E. Reproductive parameters of older compared to younger men of infertile couples. *Int J Androl.* 1996;**19**(3):135–42.

15. Mathieu C, Ecochard R, Bied V *et al.* Cumulative conception rate following intrauterine artificial insemination with husband's spermatozoa: influence of husband's age. *Hum Reprod.* 1995;**10**(5):1090–7.

16. Ford WC, North K, Taylor H *et al.* Increasing paternal age is associated with delayed conception in a large population of fertile couples: evidence for declining fecundity in older men. The ALSPAC study team (Avon Longitudinal Study of Pregnancy and Childhood). *Hum Reprod.* 2000;**15**(8):1703–8.

17. Bhasin S, Buckwalter JG. Testosterone supplementation in older men: a rational idea whose time has not yet come. *J Androl.* 2001;**22**(5):718–31.

18. Feldman HA, Longcope C, Derby CA *et al.* Age trends in the level of serum testosterone and other hormones in middle-aged men: longitudinal results from the Massachusetts male aging study. *J Clin Endocrinol Metab.* 2002;**87**(2):589–98.

19. Rodriguez-Rigau LJ, Weiss DB, Zukerman Z *et al.* A possible mechanism for the detrimental effect of varicocele on testicular function in man. *Fertil Steril.* 1978;**30**(5):577–85.

20. Morley JE, Kaiser FE, Perry HM, 3rd *et al.* Longitudinal changes in testosterone, luteinizing hormone, and follicle-stimulating hormone in healthy older men. *Metabolism.* 1997;**46**(4):410–13.

21. Buvat J, Maggi M, Guay A *et al.* Standard operating procedures for diagnosing and treating testosterone deficiency in men. *J Sex Med.* Online 12 Sep 2012. DOI: 10.1111/j.1743-6109.2012.02783.x

22. Araujo AB, O'Donnell AB, Brambilla DJ *et al.* Prevalence and incidence of androgen deficiency in middle-aged and older men: estimates from the Massachusetts male aging study. *J Clin Endocrinol Metab.* 2004;**89**(12):5920–6.

23. Mulligan T, Frick MF, Zuraw QC *et al.* Prevalence of hypogonadism in males aged at least 45 years: the HIM study. *Int J Clin Pract.* 2006;**60**(7):762–9.

24. Dandona P, Rosenberg MT. A practical guide to male hypogonadism in the primary care setting. *Int J Clin Pract.* 2010;**64**(6):682–96.

25. Travison TG, Shackelton R, Araujo AB *et al.* The natural history of symptomatic androgen deficiency in men: onset, progression, and spontaneous remission. *J Am Geriatr Soc.* 2008;**56**(5):831–9.

26. Younes AK. Low plasma testosterone in varicocele patients with impotence and male infertility. *Arch Androl.* 2000;**45**(3):187–95.

27. Shah JB, Masson P, Schlegel PN *et al.* Is there an association between varicoceles and hypogonadism in infertile men? *J Urol.* 2005;**449**(S):1656.

28. Su LM, Goldstein M, Schlegel PN. The effect of varicocelectomy on serum testosterone levels in infertile men with varicoceles. *J Urol.* 1995;**154**(5):1752–5.

29. Hamilton BE, Martin JA, Sutton PD. Births: preliminary data for 2002. *Natl Vital Stat Rep.* 2003;**51**(11):1–20.

30. Yershalmy J. Age of father and survival of offspring. *Hum Biol.* 1939;**11**:346–56.

31. Slama R, Bouyer J, Windham G *et al.* Influence of paternal age on the risk of spontaneous abortion. *Am J Epidemiol.* 2005;**161**(9):816–23.

32. Nybo Andersen AM, Hansen KD, Andersen PK *et al.* Advanced paternal age and risk of fetal death: a cohort study. *Am J Epidemiol.* 2004;**160**(12):1214–22.

33. Evans HJ. Mutation and mutagenesis in inherited and acquired human disease. The first Eems Frits Sobels prize lecture, Noordwijkerhout, the Netherlands, June 1995. *Mutat Res.* 1996;**351**(2):89–103.

34. Sartorelli EM, Mazzucatto LF, de Pina-Neto JM. Effect of paternal age on human sperm chromosomes. *Fertil Steril.* 2001;**76**(6):1119–23.

35. Singh NP, Muller CH, Berger RE. Effects of age on DNA double-strand breaks and apoptosis in human sperm. *Fertil Steril.* 2003;**80**(6):1420–30.

36. Cocuzza M, Athayde KS, Agarwal A *et al.* Age-related increase of reactive oxygen species in neat semen in healthy fertile men. *Urology.* 2008;**71**(3):490–4.

37. Lian ZH, Zack MM, Erickson JD. Paternal age and the occurrence of birth defects. *Am J Hum Genet.* 1986;**39**(5):648–60.

38. Cunningham F, Gant N, Leveno K *et al. Williams Obstetrics.* 21st edn. New York, NY: McGraw-Hill; 2001.

39. Jyothy A, Kumar KS, Mallikarjuna GN *et al.* Parental age and the origin of extra chromosome 21 in Down syndrome. *J Hum Genet.* 2001;**46**(6):347–50.

40. Erickson JD, Bjerkedal TO. Down syndrome associated with father's age in Norway. *J Med Genet.* 1981;**18**(1):22–8.

41. Kendler KS, Diehl SR. The genetics of schizophrenia: a current, genetic-epidemiologic perspective. *Schizophr Bull.* 1993;**19**(2):261–85.

42. Hare EH, Moran PA. Raised parental age in psychiatric patients: evidence for the constitutional hypothesis. *Br J Psychiatry.* 1979;**134**:169–77.

43. Gregory I. An analysis of family data on 1000 patients admitted to a Canadian mental hospital. *Acta Genet Stat Med.* 1959;**9**(1):54–96.

44. Zammit S, Allebeck P, Dalman C *et al.* Paternal age and risk for schizophrenia. *Br J Psychiatry.* 2003;**183**:405–8.

45. Malaspina D, Harlap S, Fennig S *et al.* Advancing paternal age and the risk of schizophrenia. *Arch Gen Psychiatry.* 2001;**58**(4):361–7.

46. Sipos A, Rasmussen F, Harrison G *et al.* Paternal age and schizophrenia: a population based cohort study. *Br Med J* 2004;**329**(7474):1070.

47. Grundy SM. Metabolic syndrome: connecting and reconciling cardiovascular and diabetes worlds. *J Am Coll Cardiol.* 2006;**47**(6):1093–100.

48. The Diabetes Control and Complications Trial Research Group. The effect of intensive diabetes therapy on the development and progression of neuropathy. *Ann Intern Med.* 1995;**122**(8):561–8.

49. Traish AM, Miner MM, Morgentaler A *et al.* Testosterone deficiency. *Am J Med.* 2011;**124**(7):578–87.

50. Araujo AB, Dixon JM, Suarez EA *et al.* Clinical review: endogenous testosterone and mortality in men: a systematic review and meta-analysis. *J Clin Endocrinol Metab.* 2011;**96**(10):3007–19.

51. Wei M, Macera CA, Davis DR *et al.* Total cholesterol and high density lipoprotein cholesterol as important predictors of erectile dysfunction. *Am J Epidemiol.* 1994;**140**(10):930–7.

52. Thompson IM, Tangen CM, Goodman PJ *et al.* Erectile dysfunction and subsequent cardiovascular disease. *J Am Med Assoc.* 2005;**294**(23):2996–3002.

53. Araujo AB, Durante R, Feldman HA *et al.* The relationship between depressive symptoms and male erectile dysfunction: cross-sectional results from the Massachusetts male aging study. *Psychosom Med.* 1998;**60**(4):458–65.

54. Calais Da Silva F, Marquis P, Deschaseaux P *et al.* Relative importance of sexuality and quality of life in patients with prostatic symptoms. Results of an international study. *Eur Urol.* 1997;**31**(3):272–80.

55. Eggertson L. Brouhaha erupts over testosterone-testing advertising campaign. *Can Med Assoc J.* 2011;**183**(16): E1161–2.

56. Yeap BB, Almeida OP, Hyde Z *et al.* Healthier lifestyle predicts higher circulating testosterone in older men: the health in men study. *Clin Endocrinol* (Oxf). 2009;**70**(3):455–63.

57. Niskanen L, Laaksonen DE, Punnonen K *et al.* Changes in sex hormone-binding globulin and testosterone during weight loss and weight maintenance in abdominally obese men with the metabolic syndrome. *Diabetes Obes Metab.* 2004;**6**(3):208–15.

58. Heufelder AE, Saad F, Bunck MC *et al.* Fifty-two-week treatment with diet and exercise plus transdermal testosterone reverses the metabolic syndrome and improves glycemic control in men with newly diagnosed type 2 diabetes and subnormal plasma testosterone. *J Androl.* 2009;**30**(6):726–33.

59. Herman LM, Miner MM, Quallich SA. Testosterone deficiency in men: update on treatment strategies. *Pract Clin Exchange.* 2010;**1**(2):1–8.

60. Roddam AW, Allen NE, Appleby P *et al.* Endogenous sex hormones and prostate cancer: a collaborative analysis of 18 prospective studies. *J Natl Cancer Inst.* 2008;**100**(3):170–83.

61. Morgentaler A, Rhoden EL. Prevalence of prostate cancer among hypogonadal men with prostate-specific antigen levels of 4.0 ng/ml or less. *Urology.* 2006;**68**(6):1263–7.

Chapter

8

The role of aging on fecundity in the male

Csilla Krausz and Chiara Chianese

Introduction

In developed countries, delayed parenthood is becoming a widespread phenomenon mainly due to socioeconomic factors. While increased life expectancy would justify the trend of postponing childbearing, from the reproductive standpoint fertility might be affected in a negative manner. It is common knowledge that increased maternal age is the most important risk factor for infertility; in fact, reduced fertility typically occurs in women in the late 30s to early 40s, when there is a progressive impairment of oocyte quality and production. Whether a similar age-dependent effect is also present in the male parent had been relatively scarcely explored. In this chapter, we summarize current data available on male age-related effects on fecundity looking into a number of aspects i.e. natural conception, assisted reproduction technology (ART) outcome, semen quality, chromosomal anomalies, sperm DNA damage, epigenetics, and sperm genome.

Epidemiological aspects of delayed parenthood

Over the last several decades, the mean age of childbearing mothers has had a vertiginous increase that reflects a rising birth rate for women aged 35 and older. Analogously, the paternity rate for 35–49-year-old men has been continuously rising since 1980, in parallel with a decrease of paternity of men aged between 25–29 years old [1]. In fact, the percentage of men fathering children over the age of 35 years old has notably risen from 15% to 25% during the last 40 years. Similarly, the number of men aged between 50–54 desiring to conceive children has remarkably increased [2] and a rise in the number of fathers over age 60 is predicted to happen over the next 10–20 years [3].

Fecundity in the male: epidemiological studies

Unlike women, male reproductive function does not cease abruptly as human spermatogenesis continues well into advanced ages, allowing men to conceive children during senescence; however, some male factors can go through a number of fundamental changes. An effect of paternal age on fecundity of the couple was documented by several studies, the majority of which indicate an association of paternal age with reduced fecundity, especially in couples composed of men older than 35–40 years old and women of at least 35 years old (Table 8.1). The risk of reduced pregnancy onset (failure to conceive within 12 months) was more than doubled in couples with a 35–39-year-old female partner and a ≥ 40-year-old man compared with couples where the male partner was younger [4]. For the same age group, the risk for difficulties in having a baby (infertility and failure in liveborn deliveries) was tripled. Among a total of 10 selected articles focusing on the effect of paternal age on natural conception, seven report a correlation with decreased fecundity evaluated at different end-points. However, it is worth noting that four of these studies might be biased by a number of confounding factors, i.e. the potential overestimation of the paternal age effect because age was evaluated at the time of conception rather than at the beginning of unprotected intercourse [5] and the lack of controlling for maternal age or maternal pathologies associated with infertility [6, 7]. Lastly, the Pregnancy and Lifestyle Study (PALS) [8] was merely based on interviews and considered < 35 years as the reference age class. Two of the three papers that did not report any association are either of low sample size [9] or used an inappropriate

Paternal Influences on Human Reproductive Success, ed. Douglas T. Carrell. Published by Cambridge University Press.
© Cambridge University Press 2013.

Table 8.1 Studies on the effect of paternal age on natural conception.

Reference	Size of study population	Classification by paternal age (y)	Paternal age effect?
Fertility potential			
de La Rochebrochard and Thonneau, 2003 [4]	6,188	< 40 versus ≥ 40	Yes, decline in fertility for men ≥ 40y
Hassan et al., 2003 [59]	2,112	< 25 versus > 45	Yes, decline in fertility for men > 45y, with a five-fold increase in TTP
Dunson et al., 2002 [60]	782	19–26, 27–29, 30–34, 35–39, ≥ 40	Yes, decline in fertility by the late 30s
Ford et al., 2000 [5]	8,515	≤ 24, 25–29, 30–34, 35–39, ≥ 40	Yes, probability of conception within 6 or 12 months decreasing with age. OR (CI) were 0.62 (0.40–0.98), 0.50 (0.31–0.81), 0.51 (0.31–0.86) in men aged 30–34, 35–39 and ≥ 40, respectively
Rolf et al., 1996 [9]	78	> 50, < 30, < 30 selected according to partner's age	No effect neither on pregnancy rate nor on TTP
Joffe and Li, 1994 [10]	2,576	< 30, 30–33, > 30	No significant paternal age effect on TTP when comparing men < 30 y with men > 30y
Ford et al., 1994 [8]	585	< 35 vs ≥ 35	Yes, over 35 y (OR = 2.31; CI = 1.23–3.99)
Olsen, 1990 [11]	10,886	15–19, 20–24, 25–29, 30–34, 35–39, ≥ 40	No effect after adjustment for maternal age
Ducot et al., 1988 [6]	394	≥ 31 versus < 30	Decreased probability of pregnancy for men ≥ 31 y
Stanwell-Smith and Hendry, 1984 [7]	1,025	25–39	Highest pregnancy rate in the age group between 25–29 y
Nieschlag et al., 1982 [61]	43	24–37, 60–88	No
Miscarriage			
de La Rochebrochard and Thonneau, 2002 [12]	3,174 planned pregnancies	20–29, 30–34, 35–39, ≥ 40	Higher risk of miscarriage when the male partner is ≥ 40 y
Wunsch and Gourbin, 2002 [13]	611,000 birth and death certificates	< 35, ≥ 35	Children of older males have significantly higher early neonatal and neonatal mortality rates
al-Ansary and Babay, 1994 [14]	226 miscarriages versus 226 controls	< 30, 30–34, 35–39, 40–49, ≥ 50	Spontaneous miscarriage associated with male age over 50 y
Ford et al.,1994 [8]	484 planned pregnancies	< 35, ≥ 35	Spontaneous miscarriage associated with male age over 35 y
Selvin and Garfinkel, 1976 [15]	1.5 million birth and fetal death certificates	–	Yes, equals maternal age effect
Resseguie, 1976 [17]	Birth and fetal death certificates	–	No

y, years; TTP, Time to pregnancy; OR, odds ratio; CI, 95% confidence interval.

cut-off (< 30 vs > 30 years old) [10]. However, there is also one large study based on 10,886 couples which was unable to demonstrate an independent significant paternal age effect [11]. This contrasting result may derive from the peculiar inclusion criteria (only couples after 36 weeks of pregnancy), which probably resulted in the exclusion or under-representation of couples with reduced fecundity or total sterility.

Concerning the paternal age effect on the miscarriage rate, studies are more convergent. Five of six studies observed a significant increase of miscarriage rate in relationship with male aging in natural conception planning (Table 8.1). Although the categories considered as "advanced age" are markedly heterogeneous, ranging from ≥ 35 to ≥ 50 years old, these studies report a higher risk of miscarriage with increasing fathers' age [8, 12–14]. The fifth study, after controlling for the partner's age [15], obtained an OR of 1.027 for a one-year increase in paternal age, suggesting that the latter has an independent effect on late fetal death. However, the conclusion of this study may be biased by the fact that the effect of age on reproductive failure was assumed to be of a linear nature, whereas it is usually known to follow a J-shaped curve [16]. The only contrasting study focused on the risk of late fetal death (at the 20th week of gestation) [17].

Male aging and ART reproductive outcome

Apart from the reduced fertility potential with respect to natural conception, a number of studies have focused on the paternal age effect in ART [18]. Similarly to natural conception, female age is considered a major proxy for the likelihood of achieving a pregnancy in ART programs. Data are unanimous about the fact that increased maternal age leads to decreased fertility rates and increased miscarriage rates as well as decreased embryo implantation rates [19]. At present, whether paternal age exerts an influence on clinical ART outcomes is still controversial, as reported in Table 8.2. All types of ART procedures have been analyzed in relationship with paternal aging and the results of these studies will be discussed below according to the type of treatment.

Studies related to intrauterine insemination

Mathieu et al. (1995) reported an impressive effect of paternal age on the cumulative pregnancy rate of five cycles (male partner < 30 years old showed 51.7% versus 25% in men over 35) [20]. Similarly, a decline in pregnancy rate was observed in couples with male partner > 40 years old and a female partner > 35 years old [21]. However, the same authors [22] in a subsequent study did not confirm these previous data, observing only a trend of fecundity decline instead of a significant paternal effect. The latest study [23] on this topic was also unable to demonstrate such a negative effect (see discussion of these papers below).

Studies related to intracytoplasmic sperm injection outcomes

One of the first studies had the purpose to investigate any influence of maternal and/or paternal age on gamete characteristics and pregnancy outcomes in intracytoplasmic sperm injection (ICSI) cycles [24]. In all, 821 consecutive ICSI cases were analyzed retrospectively. While a strong negative correlation was found with maternal aging, pregnancy outcomes did not seem to undergo the influence of male age, especially with female partners aged < 35 years. As for embryo quality, the authors noticed an increase in the occurrence of digynous embryos with parental aging.

A more recent study on 454 ICSI cycles observed a significantly lower fertilization rate in men > 50 years old compared with men < 50 years old without a significant difference between the number of high-quality embryos and in pregnancy rates [25].

Another retrospective study focusing on the influence of paternal age on ICSI outcomes in oligozoospermic and normozoospermic patients reached a different conclusion [26]. They found that when sperm concentration was abnormal (i.e. oligozoospermic patients), paternal age had a negative effect on implantation and pregnancy rates, suggesting a 5% decrease of the chance of pregnancy for each additional year of paternal age. On the other hand, in couples where the male partner was normozoospermic, no influence of paternal age was observed. Interestingly, no effect was observed on the high-quality embryo rate between normozoospermic and oligozoospermic subjects.

Studies related to in vitro fertilization

In contrast with ICSI studies, in vitro fertilization (IVF) cycles seem to be more influenced by paternal age. A prospective study including 221 couples undergoing IVF and gamete intrafallopian transfer (GIFT)

Table 8.2 Studies on the effect of paternal age on assisted reproduction technology (ART) outcomes.

Reference	Type of ART	Number of cycles	Paternal age effect?			
			Clinical pregnancy	Miscarriage	Fertilization rate	Embryo development
Intra-uterine insemination (IUI)						
Bellver et al., 2008 [23]	IUI	2,204	No paternal age effect	–	–	–
Brzechffa et al. 1998 [22]	IUI	416	No paternal age effect	–	–	–
Brzechffa and Buyalos, 1997 [21]	IUI	363	Negative effect on pregnancy rates for men ≥ 40 y	–	–	–
Mathieu et al. 1995 [20]	IUI	901	Decreased likelihood of pregnancy for men > 35 y	–	–	–
In vitro fertilization (IVF)						
Bellver et al., 2008 [23]	IVF	1,286	No paternal age effect	No paternal age effect	–	No significant correlations with embryo division and fragmentation after 48 and 72 h
de La Rochebrochard et al., 2006 [28]	IVF	1,938	Decrease	–	–	–
Klonoff-Cohen and Natarajan, 2004 [27]	IVF, GIFT	221	Decrease for each year of paternal age	Not significant	Not significant	–
Intra-Cytoplasmatic Sperm Injection (ICSI)						
Ferreira et al. 2010 [26]	ICSI	1,024	Decrease only in oligozoospermic	NS	–	–
Aboulghar et al, 2007 [25]	ICSI	454	No paternal age effect	–	Higher fertilization rate in men < 50 y	–
Spandorfer et al, 1998 [24]	ICSI	821	Not significant	Not significant	Not significant	Increase in digynous embryos

Table 8.2 (cont.)

Reference	Type of ART	Number of cycles	Paternal age effect?				
			Clinical pregnancy	Miscarriage	Fertilization rate	Embryo development	
Oocyte donation (OD)							
Luna et al., 2009 [31]	IVF, ICSI	672	Not significant	Not significant	Decrease in men > 60 y (IVF)	Decrease at day 3, 5 and 6	
Bellver et al., 2008 [23]	IVF	1,412	No paternal age effect	No paternal age effect	–	Increased embryo fragmentation after 48 and 72 h	
Frattarelli et al., 2008 [19]	IVF, ICSI	1,023	Not significant	Increase	Not significant	Decrease at day 5	
Paulson et al., 2001 [30]	IVF	558	Not significant	–	Not significant	–	
Gallardo et al., 1996 [29]	IVF	345	Not significant	Not significant	Not significant	Not significant	

y, years; GIFT, gamete intrafallopian transfer.

found that pregnancy rates declined as the male aged, and they could estimate that each additional year of paternal age confers a 11% increased risk of not achieving a pregnancy as well as an augmented risk of 12% of not having a successful live birth [27]. When correlating paternal age to the number of attempts, the authors noticed that for subjects undertaking IVF/ GIFT for the first time, each additional year of paternal age was associated with a 5% increased risk of not achieving pregnancy, whereas for men who repeated the ART attempt the risk of negative outcomes was indeed higher (40%).

A rigorous study by de La Rochebrochard et al. [28] analyzed a total of 1,938 IVF cycles and included only men whose female partners were sterile due to bilateral tubal obstruction or absence of both tubes. In this category of couples the risk of clinical pregnancy failure increased considerably with the advancement of paternal age. In detail, they estimated an odds ratio (OR) for paternal age > 40 years old compared with < 30 years of 1.70 (95% confidence interval (CI) 1.14–2.52).

Studies based on IVF/ICSI in the context of oocyte donation

A more appropriate approach to define whether paternal age has an independent effect on IVF is based on the evaluation of IVF/ICSI outcomes with donated oocytes from young women (< 35 years). Although female partner-related biases are excluded by this study design, the male age categories and the semen characteristics of the recruited men largely vary between studies. The first two studies failed to find an effect of paternal age on fecundity parameters [29, 30] whereas in a retrospective cohort analysis of 1,203 men a statistically significant increase of pregnancy loss (decrease in live birth) in men > 50 years old was found [19]. While a decrease in blastocyst formation rate were observed in the same age category, the implantation and pregnancy rates were not influenced by increased paternal age.

Additional information is provided by the retrospective study performed by Luna et al. [31]. The study included 672 oocyte donation (OD) cycles in the frame of IVF and ICSI and were classified as follows: group A, 233 men < 40 years; group B, 323 men 40–49 years; and group C, 116 men > 50 years. While the authors found that laboratory parameters such as fertilization rate and embryo quality were significantly lower for men over 50 years, clinical pregnancy and miscarriage rates were not different in the same age group.

In sharp contrast with the previously discussed data, the largest retrospective study performed on a total of 2,204 intrauterine insemination (IUI) cycles, 1286 IVF cycles and 1412 IVF cycles with donated oocytes did not provide any evidence for a paternal age effect [23]. The mean age of prospective fathers was 34.3 years (ranging between 25–56) for IUI, 34.8 years (ranging between 19–62) for IVF and 41.10 years (ranging between 25–71) for oocyte donation cycles. The comparison of embryo quality, implantation rate, pregnancy, and miscarriage rates between age groups did not reveal any age-related difference in any of the three types of procedures. This strongly contrasting result can be attributed to differences in the study design in respect to previous studies. First of all, this study is based on couples with female partner < 38 years old, only first IVF cycles were considered, and the mean sperm count was largely in the normal range for all types of procedures. Finally, it is also worth noticing that despite the analysis of such a high number of cycles, the proportion of men > 40 years was rather low.

In general, controversies in the literature may well be related to the different age cut-offs used for subgrouping the study populations as well as to the composition of the study populations in terms of: (i) the proportion of male partners > 50 years old with and without > 35 years old female partner; (ii) proportion of oligo/normozoospermic male partners. While the combined maternal–paternal age effect is a rather obvious observation, it is worth paying attention to the proposed concerted action of spermatogenic impairment and increased paternal age. In fact, pregnancy and implantation rates seem to be affected by increased paternal age especially if the men suffer from spermatogenic impairment [26]. Presumably, in the case of men with spermatogenic impairment, the male factor might act as an additional contributor to the negative age-related conditions, thus worsening already compromised sperm-related factors.

In conclusion, although to a much lesser extent than maternal age, it seems that paternal age also exerts a negative effect on fecundity. The biological basis underlying this phenomenon is likely to be multifactorial and may be related to changes in semen quality (sperm number, motility, and morphology) and in genetic/epigenetic features of the aging male gamete. Some of these changes will be discussed in the following paragraphs.

Male aging and semen quality

Although semen quality cannot be considered an absolute marker for a man's fertility potential, it represents an easy-to-evaluate parameter, which therefore has been broadly studied in relation to male aging. Despite efforts, it is still difficult to draw firm conclusions regarding the existence of an eventual age threshold or the type of relationship between age and changes in sperm characteristics, because many of the published large-scale studies are biased by the interference of sometimes underestimated confounding factors (e.g. the duration of abstinence, female age) and selection biases (e.g. subjects should be selected on the basis of their age at the onset of trying for pregnancy and not at conception). Kidd *et al.* [32] provided a thorough review of the literature that collected data from studies published within 1980–1999 focusing on the effects of male age on semen quality and fertility. This paragraph provides a general summary of what is described in the above-mentioned review about the effects of male aging on semen volume, sperm motility, and morphology.

Concerning semen volume, the weight of evidence suggests that there is a decrease in semen volume with increasing age, especially in men > 50 years old. The relative decrease ranges between 3% and 30% for men aged < 30 years old compared with men aged ≥ 50 years old, respectively, and it was estimated to change approximately 20–30%. When it comes to sperm motility the scenario is indeed different; there is strong and consistent evidence of an influence of male aging on this sperm parameter. When comparing men > 50 to those aged 30 or younger, the relative decrease in motility of spermatozoa is estimated to range within 3–37%. As for sperm morphology, good evidence reports a trend toward a decrease in the percent of normally shaped spermatozoa with age, ranging between 4% in men of advanced age (≥ 50 years old) and 22% in those men ≤ 30 years old. As for sperm concentration, the literature is rather controversial about its relationship with paternal age, since most of the studies reach enormously divergent conclusions. Almost 24% of the studies report a decrement of sperm concentration with increased age, whereas another 28% of investigations found very little or even no association between sperm concentration and the man's age. Surprisingly, there are a number of studies reporting that increasing age is associated with an increase in the number of spermatozoa in the ejaculate. Therefore, it still remains extremely difficult not only to determine whether paternal age exerts any effect on sperm concentration but also to define in an absolute manner the nature of such effect (i.e. describing either an inverse or direct relationship).

Conclusively, on the basis of conventional parameters considered for semen quality evaluation, scientific evidence suggests that male aging is associated with a decrease in semen volume, a decrease in sperm motility, and a decrease in the percent of normally shaped spermatozoa, while no firm data from the literature demonstrates that sperm concentration is actually affected by increasing age (for review see [32]). There are several mechanisms that could underlie the age-related effects on semen quality (for review see [33] and references therein). To begin with, a decrease in semen volume might originate from the insufficiency of accessory glands (seminal vesicles and prostate), which are the major contributors to the seminal fluid volume. Since they are androgen-dependent organs, the age-related decrement of testosterone might lead to hypotrophism of the accessory glands and thus reduced seminal fluid. Moreover, in aged males there is a higher probability of chronic prostatitis which is typically associated with reduced semen volume and may also affect sperm motility. In addition, the reduced sperm motility may also be related to alterations at the epididymal level and in this regard an age-dependent reduction of alfa-glucosidase has been reported. However, no data are present about an increased frequency of epididymal infections or inflammations in older men. Age-related degenerative alterations affecting the germinal epithelium might, instead, contribute to alter sperm morphology. Although male aging seems to not affect sperm concentration consistently, cellular or physiological changes depending on age are surely plausible. Sclerosis of the tubular lumen, decreased spermatogenic activity, degeneration of germ cells, and a reduction in the number and function of Leydig cells are some of the age-related histological alterations that might affect sperm concentration. Finally, in older men, the capability to repair both cellular and tissue damage is decreased; therefore, a long-lasting exposure to exogenous environmental agents (including infections, inflammations, toxic substances, etc.) in older subjects is more likely to induce reproductive damage.

Male aging and chromosomal anomalies

In the list of events that may lead to negative reproductive outcomes, alterations of the number and structure of chromosomes in gametes surely occupy a remarkable position. Whether paternal age is associated with an augmented risk of aneuploidy in the offspring is still controversial (for review see [18] and references therein).

Chromosome studies in the male gamete revealed a male age-related increase in XY sperm disomy when 36–60-year-old men were compared with 18–35-year-old men [18]. Moreover, male age seems to be associated with the formation of XX/XY disomy, with a frequency two- to three-fold higher in spermatozoa produced by men > 50 years old. Sperm karyotype analyses based on the hamster-egg penetration method observed that structural chromosomal abnormalities are considerably more frequent compared with aneuploidies [34]. In this regard, it was also demonstrated that the distribution of rearrangements (deletions/duplications) is not linear among all chromosomes, but that larger chromosomes seem to be the most affected [34].

Structural chromosomal anomalies comprise 0.25% of births, 0.4% of stillbirths, and 2% of abortions. In humans, it has been estimated that 80% of structural aberrations detected during embryo development or at birth are of paternal origin (see [34] and references therein). A relationship between men's age and the presence of sperm structural aberrations seems indeed plausible, since a higher frequency of acentric fragments, chromosomal breaks, and rearrangements have been described in the elderly [34–36]. Concerning a structural anomaly of the Y chromosome (AZFa deletion), our laboratory performed an estimate of the meiotic rate of this deletion in sperm-derived DNA of normozoospermic men aged from 20–67 years. All men carried an intact Y chromosome in their genomic DNA whereas the deletion was observed in their spermatozoa with a meiotic rate of the deletion ranging from 0.4 to 4.7 $\times$ 10^{-5}. The highest values were observed in both the younger and older men, indicating the absence of a purely age-related effect on the deletion formation during spermatogenesis (unpublished data).

Paternal age and sperm DNA damage

In spermatozoa, DNA fragmentation, abnormal chromatin packaging, and protamine deficiency are examples of DNA impairment that may lead to spermatogenic arrest, cell death, or mutation. The association between aging and sperm DNA damage has been the object of a number of studies. Higher levels of double-stranded DNA breaks were reported in older men [37] and an inverse relationship has been proposed between DNA fragmentation index and male age [38]. Moreover, paternal age shows a positive correlation with increased DNA damage in sperm donors and in men of infertile couples [35–40].

It is well known that DNA damage negatively affects the reproductive outcome in both natural and ART conception (for review see [41]). Reactive oxygen species (ROS) are considered among the most potent inductors of DNA damage. Since ROS production is likely to increase with age, it is plausible to hypothesize that, in men of advanced age, growing oxidative stress might be responsible for the age-related augment in sperm DNA damage and thus might represent an etiology for ART failures in older men [42]. This phenomenon would become more evident in the case of dysfunctional oocyte repair mechanisms (more frequently found in aged females), which would not fix DNA single-strand breaks after fertilization and could thus lead to poor or even failed blastocyst formation.

Male aging and sperm genome

Paternal aging not only affects the genomic integrity of spermatozoa in terms of DNA fragmentation and numeric and structural chromosomal anomalies, but it has been reported also in relationship with point mutations (for review see [33]). A plausible explanation to such a phenomenon is that spermatozoa undergo many more germline cell divisions compared with oocytes. Furthermore, since sperm production occurs continuously throughout reproductive life, the advancement of paternal age will lead to an increased number of cell divisions and chromosome replications with the consequent acceleration of the mutation rate. By the age of 45 years old, 725 mitotic divisions would have occurred, with the possibility of a DNA copy error at every single replication [43]. This could be due to several mechanisms: first, alterations of age-sensitive processes such as the DNA replication and repair might occur; second, the increased number of cell divisions might represent a compensatory event for cell death at old ages; finally, the accumulation of mutagens from either external or internal sources, which would certainly increase with age, might also contribute. Therefore, paternal aging is considered the major cause of new mutations in human populations leading to the accumulation of mutations that could possibly increase the incidence of recessive genetic disorders in the future [44].

The origin of two diseases, Apert syndrome and achondroplasia, represent the most classic examples of paternally age-driven diseases. Virtually, all mutations in the *FGFR2* gene (causing Apert syndrome) and the *FGFR3* gene (causing achondroplasia, Crouzon and Pfeiffer syndrome) originate in males by *de novo* mutation and are characterized by the strong dependence on paternal age. In both syndromes, an age-dependent increase of the mutation rate in spermatozoa has been observed. However, the magnitude of the age-dependent increase in mutation frequency appears insufficient to explain the incidence of achondroplasia and Apert syndrome in children fathered by older men. In the case of Apert syndrome it has been proposed that *FGFR2* mutations, even though harmful to embryonic development of the affected organism, are paradoxically enhanced because they confer a selective advantage to the male germline in which they arise [45]. In the case of achondroplasia, the positive selection for spermatozoa carrying the mutation may augment their probability of fertilizing the oocyte [46].

Epigenetic aspects of the aging male gamete

Epigenetics encompass a collection of molecular modifications (such as methylation or acetylation) that occur on DNA or histones intimately associated with DNA without causing any alteration of the genomic sequence.

Lately, the scientific interest in the epigenetic mechanisms underlying the paternal influence on offspring development has been importantly increasing. Genome-wide DNA methylation profiling in newborn blood cells showed a general trend towards hypomethylation of CpG islands with advancing parental age, providing evidence of an association of paternal age with congenital differently methylated cytosines [47]. Another interesting finding concerns the paternal general life background where nutritional state, toxicological exposures as well as age seem to influence the offspring, and sometimes the grand-offspring, development [48]. Moreover, it has been amply reported that offspring of older parents are at greater risk of carrying various disorders with possible epigenetic influence, including type I diabetes [47].

An increasing body of evidence shows that specific epigenetic marks in the male gamete are of importance for early embryo development [49]. Consequently, epigenetic modifications may be responsible for impaired embryo development and implantation rate. However, experimental data are still missing about the paternal epigenetic influence on fecundity. It is therefore of major interest to evaluate whether age-related modifications in the sperm epigenome exist and how they could eventually contribute to age-related impaired fecundity.

Telomeres and aging: the bright side of an aged father

Interestingly, in contrast with the general trend that sees paternal aging mainly as an adverse factor to fecundity, fathering at older ages seems also to have a bright side. In fact, emerging data demonstrate that older fathers will transmit to their offspring longer telomeres, a feature which may confer a longer life expectancy to the future generations conceived by aged fathers.

Telomeres consist of a large number of tandem repeats of the (TTAGGG)n tract that caps the ends of all eukaryotic chromosomes. Although the full extent of their function remains still unclear, telomeric involvement in the protection from chromosomal deterioration and maintenance of cellular stability is commonly known [50]. Telomeric repeats are progressively lost in most human cell types that replicate because DNA polymerase is unable to complete the replication of the 3' end of linear DNA at chromosome extremities. As a consequence telomere length (TL) shortens with successive cell divisions and telomeric sequences are then replenished by the activity of telomerase, a reverse transcriptase found in immortal cancer cells, embryonic tissues, lymphocytes, skin and intestinal stem cells, and germ cells [51].

Aging is associated with impaired telomerase activity in somatic cells leading to a progressive shortening of TL. Shorter telomeres in leukocytes are indeed regarded as a biological marker for aging and survival [51, 52]. Based on the above observations, paternal aging has become an object of interest also for studies on TL dynamics and its effects on offspring born from fathers of advanced age. With respect to TL in leukocytes, an advanced age of the father seems to have a positive effect on his offspring [51–53]. In fact, offspring of older fathers display longer leukocytes TL (LTL). This phenomenon might be explained by the fascinating divergent trajectory of TL dynamics in male germ cells, in which TL elongates with age (see [54] and references therein). In addition, a recent study performed on delayed human reproduction found that such an association between paternal age and offspring telomere length (TL) is cumulative across multiple generations, demonstrating that grandchildren of older paternal grandfathers at the birth of their fathers displayed longer telomeres ($P = 0.038$) [55]. The most common explanation for telomere lengthening among offspring of older fathers is the high telomerase activity in the testis [56, 57]. Aston et al. (2012) suggest that sperm TL elongation is dependent on an "over-activation" of telomerase in male germ cells, leading to TL lengthening at every replication cycle (estimated value = 2.48 bp/replication) [54]. However, it remains to be defined why testicular telomerase would lead to the progressive lengthening of sperm telomeres, rather than just maintain a stable length. Kimura et al. proposed that testicular telomerase exerts a preferential effect on long telomeres [56]. This might be dependent on the fact that sperm cells displaying short telomeres undergo a negative selection that with age progressively leads to their disproportional extinction [56].

Conclusions

While the effect of female aging on couple fecundity appears to be a widely confirmed independent negative factor, on the male side, current knowledge does not allow reaching a firm conclusion. The literature is rather controversial and even studies based on oocyte donation programs have reached conflicting results. In a number of ART studies and epidemiological studies, fecundity parameters seem to be affected by advanced paternal age, especially in combination with a > 35-year-old female partner. It has been proposed by de La Rochebrochard et al. [58] that 40 years could be considered as the "amber light" in the reproductive life of a man, however due to the limited number of studies further confirmation is needed. Overall, current data suggest that male aging does not affect couple fecundity as an independent factor but its effect becomes manifest in combination with maternal age or in the presence of altered spermato-genesis. While the paternal age effect on some fecundity parameters such as fertilization rate, embryo quality, and implantation rate is still controversial, there is a rather consistent association between miscarriage and advanced paternal age. This may reflect the higher frequency of numerical and structural chromosomal anomalies, DNA fragmentation, and mutation rate observed in the male gamete of aged men. In fact, it can be hypothesized that

the diffuse negative modifications observed in the sperm genome are probably the most relevant contributors to reduced fecundity.

Given that the trend toward older parenthood is an emerging issue, paternal age effect on fecundity definitely deserves substantial consideration. It is of utmost importance to perform large well-designed studies to assess, in a conclusive manner, the age threshold (if it exists at all) and the entity of the paternal age-related risk for decreased fecundity both in natural and ART conceptions.

References

1. Martin JA, Hamilton BE, Sutton PD et al. Births: final data for 2005. Natl Vital Stat Rep. 2007;**56**(6):1–103.

2. Fisch H. Older men are having children, but the reality of a male biological clock makes this trend worrisome. Geriatrics. 2009;**64**(1):14–17.

3. US Census Bureau; 2005. http://www.census.gov.

4. de La Rochebrochard E, Thonneau P. Paternal age > or = 40 years: an important risk factor for infertility. Am J Obstet Gynecol. 2003;**189**(4):901–5.

5. Ford WC, North K, Taylor H et al. Increasing paternal age is associated with delayed conception in a large population of fertile couples: evidence for declining fecundity in older men. The ALSPAC study team (Avon Longitudinal Study of Pregnancy and Childhood). Hum Reprod. 2000;**15**(8):1703–8.

6. Ducot B, Spira A, Feneux D et al. Male factors and the likelihood of pregnancy in infertile couples. II. Study of clinical characteristics – practical consequences. Int J Androl. 1988;**11**(5):395–404.

7. Stanwell-Smith RE, Hendry WF. The prognosis of male subfertility: a survey of 1025 men referred to a fertility clinic. Br J Urol. 1984;**56**(4):422–8.

8. Ford JH, MacCormac L, Hiller J. PALS (Pregnancy and Lifestyle Study): association between occupational and environmental exposure to chemicals and reproductive outcome. Mutation Res. 1994;**313**(2–3):153–64.

9. Rolf C, Behre HM, Nieschlag E. Reproductive parameters of older compared to younger men of infertile couples. Int J Androl. 1996;**19**(3):135–42.

10. Joffe M, Li Z. Male and female factors in fertility. Am J Epidemiol. 1994;**140**(10):921–9.

11. Olsen J. Subfecundity according to the age of the mother and the father. Danish Med Bull. 1990;**37**(3):281–2.

12. de la Rochebrochard E, Thonneau P. Paternal age and maternal age are risk factors for miscarriage; results of a

multicentre European study. *Hum Reprod.* 2002;**17**(6):1649–56.

13. Wunsch G, Gourbin C. Parents' age at birth of their offspring and child survival. *Social Biol.* 2002;**49**(3–4):174–84.

14. al-Ansary LA, Babay ZA. Risk factors for spontaneous abortion: a preliminary study on Saudi women. *J R Soc Health.* 1994;**114**(4):188–93.

15. Selvin S, Garfinkel J. Paternal age, maternal age and birth order and the risk of a fetal loss. *Hum Biol.* 1976;**48**(1):223–30.

16. Nybo AA, Wohlfahrt J, Christens P *et al.* Is maternal age an independent risk factor for fetal loss? *West J Med.* 2000;**173**(5):331.

17. Resseguie LJ. Paternal age, stillbirths and mutation. *Ann Hum Genet.* 1976;**40**(2):213–19.

18. Wiener-Megnazi Z, Auslender R, Dirnfeld M. Advanced paternal age and reproductive outcome. *Asian J Androl.* 2012;**14**(1):69–76.

19. Frattarelli JL, Miller KA, Miller BT *et al.* Male age negatively impacts embryo development and reproductive outcome in donor oocyte assisted reproductive technology cycles. *Fertil Steril.* 2008;**90**(1):97–103.

20. Mathieu C, Ecochard R, Bied V *et al.* Cumulative conception rate following intrauterine artificial insemination with husband's spermatozoa: influence of husband's age. *Hum Reprod.* 1995;**10**(5):1090–7.

21. Brzechffa PR, Buyalos RP. Female and male partner age and menotrophin requirements influence pregnancy rates with human menopausal gonadotrophin therapy in combination with intrauterine insemination. *Hum Reprod.* 1997;**12**(1):29–33.

22. Brzechffa PR, Daneshmand S, Buyalos RP. Sequential clomiphene citrate and human menopausal gonadotrophin with intrauterine insemination: the effect of patient age on clinical outcome. *Hum Reprod.* 1998;**13**(8):2110–14.

23. Bellver J, Garrido N, Remohi J *et al.* Influence of paternal age on assisted reproduction outcome. *Reprod Biomed Online.* 2008;**17**(5):595–604.

24. Spandorfer SD, Avrech OM, Colombero LT *et al.* Effect of parental age on fertilization and pregnancy characteristics in couples treated by intracytoplasmic sperm injection. *Hum Reprod.* 1998;**13**(2):334–8.

25. Aboulghar M, Mansour R, Al-Inany H *et al.* Paternal age and outcome of intracytoplasmic sperm injection. *Reprod Biomed Online.* 2007;**14**(5):588–92.

26. Ferreira RC, Braga DP, Bonetti TC *et al.* Negative influence of paternal age on clinical intracytoplasmic sperm injection cycle outcomes in oligozoospermic patients. *Fertil Steril.* 2010;**93**(6):1870–4.

27. Klonoff-Cohen HS, Natarajan L. The effect of advancing paternal age on pregnancy and live birth rates in couples undergoing in vitro fertilization or gamete intrafallopian transfer. *Am J Obstet Gynecol.* 2004;**191**(2):507–14.

28. de La Rochebrochard E, de Mouzon J, Thepot F *et al.* Fathers over 40 and increased failure to conceive: the lessons of in vitro fertilization in France. *Fertil Steril.* 2006;**85**(5):1420–4.

29. Gallardo E, Simon C, Levy M *et al.* Effect of age on sperm fertility potential: oocyte donation as a model. *Fertil Steril.* 1996;**66**(2):260–4.

30. Paulson RJ, Milligan RC, Sokol RZ. The lack of influence of age on male fertility. *Am J Obstet Gynecol.* 2001;**184**(5):818–22; discussion 22–4.

31. Luna M, Finkler E, Barritt J *et al.* Paternal age and assisted reproductive technology outcome in ovum recipients. *Fertil Steril.* 2009;**92**(5):1772–5.

32. Kidd SA, Eskenazi B, Wyrobek AJ. Effects of male age on semen quality and fertility: a review of the literature. *Fertil Steril.* 2001;**75**(2):237–48.

33. Sartorius GA, Nieschlag E. Paternal age and reproduction. *Hum Reprod Update.* 2010;**16**(1):65–79.

34. Templado C, Donate A, Giraldo J *et al.* Advanced age increases chromosome structural abnormalities in human spermatozoa. *Eur J Hum Genet.* 2011;**19**(2):145–51.

35. Martin RH, Rademaker AW. The effect of age on the frequency of sperm chromosomal abnormalities in normal men. *Am J Hum Genet.* 1987;**41**(3):484–92.

36. Sartorelli EM, Mazzucatto LF, de Pina-Neto JM. Effect of paternal age on human sperm chromosomes. *Fertil Steril.* 2001;**76**(6):1119–23.

37. Singh NP, Muller CH, Berger RE. Effects of age on DNA double-strand breaks and apoptosis in human sperm. *Fertil Steril.* 2003;**80**(6):1420–30.

38. Wyrobek AJ, Eskenazi B, Young S *et al.* Advancing age has differential effects on DNA damage, chromatin integrity, gene mutations, and aneuploidies in sperm. *Proc Natl Acad Sci USA.* 2006;**103**(25):9601–6.

39. McInnes B, Rademaker A, Martin R. Donor age and the frequency of disomy for chromosomes 1, 13, 21 and structural abnormalities in human spermatozoa using multicolour fluorescence in-situ hybridization. *Hum Reprod.* 1998;**13**(9):2489–94.

40. Vagnini L, Baruffi RL, Mauri AL *et al.* The effects of male age on sperm DNA damage in an infertile population. *Reprod Biomed Online.* 2007;**15**(5):514–19.

41. Zini A, Libman J. Sperm DNA damage: clinical significance in the era of assisted reproduction. *Can Med Assoc J.* 2006;**175**(5):495–500.

42. Shamsi MB, Kumar R, Dada R. Evaluation of nuclear DNA damage in human spermatozoa in men opting for assisted reproduction. *Indian J Med Res*. 2008;**127** (2):115–23.

43. Crow JF. The origins, patterns and implications of human spontaneous mutation. *Nat Rev*. 2000;**1** (1):40–7.

44. Crow JF. Spontaneous mutation in man. *Mutation Res*. 1999;**437**(1):5–9.

45. Goriely A, McVean GA, Rojmyr M *et al*. Evidence for selective advantage of pathogenic FGFR2 mutations in the male germ line. *Science*. 2003;**301**(5633):643–6.

46. Tiemann-Boege I, Navidi W, Grewal R *et al*. The observed human sperm mutation frequency cannot explain the achondroplasia paternal age effect. *Proc Natl Acad Sci USA*. 2002;**99**(23):14,952–7.

47. Adkins RM, Thomas F, Tylavsky FA *et al*. Parental ages and levels of DNA methylation in the newborn are correlated. *BMC Med Genet*. 2011;**12**:47.

48. Curley JP, Mashoodh R, Champagne FA. Epigenetics and the origins of paternal effects. *Hormones Behav*. 2011;**59**(3):306–14.

49. Hammoud SS, Nix DA, Hammoud AO *et al*. Genome-wide analysis identifies changes in histone retention and epigenetic modifications at developmental and imprinted gene loci in the sperm of infertile men. *Hum Reprod*. 2011;**26** (9):2558–69.

50. Chan SR, Blackburn EH. Telomeres and telomerase. *Phil Trans R Soc London*. 2004;**359**(1441):109–21.

51. Unryn BM, Cook LS, Riabowol KT. Paternal age is positively linked to telomere length of children. *Aging Cell*. 2005;**4**(2):97–101.

52. De Meyer T, Rietzschel ER, De Buyzere ML *et al*. Paternal age at birth is an important determinant of offspring telomere length. *Hum Mol Genet*. 2007;**16** (24):3097–102.

53. Arbeev KG, Hunt SC, Kimura M *et al*. Leukocyte telomere length, breast cancer risk in the offspring: the relations with father's age at birth. *Mechan Ageing Develop*. 2011;**132**(4):149–53.

54. Aston KI, Hunt SC, Susser E *et al*. Divergence of sperm and leukocyte age-dependent telomere dynamics: implications for male-driven evolution of telomere length in humans. *Mol Hum Reprod*. 2012; doi: 10.1093/ molehr/gas028.

55. Eisenberg DT, Hayes MG, Kuzawa CW. Delayed paternal age of reproduction in humans is associated with longer telomeres across two generations of descendants. *Proc Natl Acad Sci USA*. 2012;**109** (26):10,251–6.

56. Kimura M, Cherkas LF, Kato BS *et al*. Offspring's leukocyte telomere length, paternal age, and telomere elongation in sperm. *PLoS Genet*. 2008;**4**(2):e37.

57. Baird DM, Britt-Compton B, Rowson J *et al*. Telomere instability in the male germline. *Hum Mol Genet*. 2006;**15**(1):45–51.

58. de La Rochebrochard E, McElreavey K, Thonneau P. Paternal age over 40 years: the "amber light" in the reproductive life of men? *J Androl*. 2003;**24**(4):459–65.

59. Hassan MA, Killick SR. Effect of male age on fertility: evidence for the decline in male fertility with increasing age. *Fertil Steril*. 2003;**79**(Suppl. 3):1520–7.

60. Dunson DB, Colombo B, Baird DD. Changes with age in the level and duration of fertility in the menstrual cycle. *Hum Reprod*. 2002;**17**(5):1399–403.

61. Nieschlag E, Lammers U, Freischem CW *et al*. Reproductive functions in young fathers and grandfathers. *J Clin Endocrinol Metab*. 1982;**55** (4):676–81.

Aging, DNA damage, and reproductive outcome

Aleksander Giwercman and Jens Peter Bonde

Introduction

Due to increasing life expectancy and a number of social factors, at least in the Western world, an increasing proportion of men who are considered to belong to an "older age group" have the wish of becoming fathers. One of the reasons is that many women postpone their first pregnancy, which automatically leads to higher age of the potential fathers. Furthermore, divorce and building new families has become more frequent, which also affects the paternal age.

For those reasons, from a social and a medical point of view, the issue of age-dependent changes in reproductive capacity of the males is receiving increasing attention.

Aging might not only lead to reduced fertility but also to an increase in the occurrence of sperm DNA defects, which potentially might be transmitted to the offspring. Understanding the mechanisms linking paternal age to reproductive outcome is, therefore, crucial not only for understanding this process, but first of all in order to prevent possible negative impact of male aging on fertility and health of the offspring. In this chapter we will focus on the available information regarding age and numerical or structural changes in the DNA. The issue of epigenetic effects will be covered in a separate chapter.

Aging and reproductive outcomes

Age and conventional parameters of semen quality

According to a systematic review more than 20 studies have analyzed age-dependent variation of semen characteristics, but only a few studies include males more than 60 years old (Figure 9.1) [1]. Overall the evidence indicates that semen volume and sperm motility decline gradually with increasing age, even after adjustment for increasing periods of sexual abstinence among elderly men. This is consistent with an earlier histological study of testicular specimens obtained from men suffering a sudden traumatic death which demonstrated a slight decrease in testicular sperm count starting at age above 40 years [2]. Moreover, testis volume – a crude indicator of spermatogenic function – is reduced in men in their 80s and 90s [3] and the proportion of sperm with abnormal morphology seems also to increase slowly and gradually with increasing age. The slow age-dependent decline of testicular function is accompanied by a slight increase in follicle-stimulating hormone (FSH) and a slight decrease in Inhibin B [4].

Age and fecundity

The fecundity of women rapidly declines after 30–35 years of age and reaches a very low level at the age of 45–50 years. Considering this strong age effect on female fecundity and the high age correlation among partners it becomes evident that huge study populations are needed in order to identify effects on fecundity of male aging separately. A large Danish study did indicate that male age above 50 years is associated with a gradual decline of male fecundity taking female age into account, but it is also evident that the effect of female aging is much stronger [5].

The prevalence of erectile dysfunction increases dramatically with age from less than 5% in men less than 25 years of age to more than 35% in men above 74 years of age [6]. This may together with decreasing coital frequency explain some of the reduced fecundity with male aging. An elegant French study that reliably took frequency of sexual intercourse into account indicates that the effect of male aging was limited to

---

Paternal Influences on Human Reproductive Success, ed. Douglas T. Carrell. Published by Cambridge University Press.
© Cambridge University Press 2013.

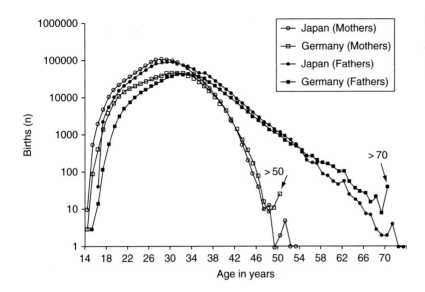

Figure 9.1. Parental age at the time of birth of offspring in Germany (2001) and Japan (2002) (From Kühnert and Nieschlag, 2004 [1] based upon Rolf and Nieschlag, 2000).

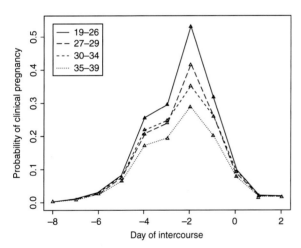

Figure 9.2. Probability of clinical pregnancy following intercourse on a given day relative to ovulation for women of three different age groups (From Dunson *et al.*, 2002 [7].)

partners in which the women were above 35 years of age [7] (Figure 9.2).

Age and embryonal loss and miscarriage

In women the risk of miscarriage increases dramatically with increasing age. In vitro fertilization studies clearly indicate that this is because of reduced ovum quality rather than high age of female reproductive organs [8]. During the past 2 years it has become evident that male age above 40 years is also a risk factor for spontaneous abortion [9]. This is also compatible with findings from an IVF treatment series

indicating a reduced pregnancy rate per embryo transfer in couples with male age over 50 years.

Age and disease in the offspring

It has been known for more than 50 years that certain autosomal dominant diseases, first of all achondroplasia (the most common form of dwarfism) are related to paternal age. Other diseases include syndromes with defects in skull development. Also a few disorders with complex genetic origin such as schizophrenia and Alzheimer's disease have been indicated to occur more frequently with higher paternal age, but data are conflicting. The malignant child disease, retinoblastoma, is in the vast majority of cases of paternal origin and seems to occur more frequently with higher age of the father.

In conclusion, it has become evident during the past decades that male fecundity starts to deteriorate gradually and slowly after 40 years of age, and that reduced fecundity manifests itself as infertility, miscarriage, and increased risk of some congenital information and rare autosomal dominant diseases.

Age and offspring sex ratio

Some studies have indicated a time-related trend in the sex ratio of the offspring with declining proportion of males [10]. The reason for this phenomenon is unknown, but although the data are not unequivocal, the most recent studies indicate that increasing paternal age might play a role. Thus, a synergistic effect of increasing paternal or maternal age causing a decrease in the ratio between male and female offspring has been reported [11]. Other studies demonstrated a more pronounced effect for paternal as compared with maternal age [12].

The data on the associations between paternal age and reproductive outcomes are summarized in Table 9.1.

Aging and sperm genome

The above-mentioned associations between increasing paternal age and the reduced fecundity, higher rate of miscarriages, offspring morbidity and sex ratio might point to effect of male age on the genome of the sperms. Below, we summarize the current knowledge on this issue in relation to different types of genetic outcomes.

Age and sperm DNA integrity

There seems to be quite strong evidence showing an association between male age and the extension of sperm DNA strand breaks. Such an association has

been found using different assays for detection of sperm DNA damage, the sperm chromatin structure assay (SCSA), and Comet [13–15]. Thus, Wyrobek et al. [16] reported an increase in mean DNA fragmentation index (DFI) as measured by SCSA from 13% in the age group 20–29 years to 50% among those 60–80 years old. A DFI above 30% was previously shown to imply a chance of fertility in vivo close to zero, and the percentage of subjects with DFI ≥ 30% was shown to be 10% and 88%, respectively, in the age groups mentioned above.

The mechanisms behind the positive association between age and extension of sperm DNA strand breaks have not been clarified. However, one study has demonstrated age-related decrease in human sperm apoptosis [17] which might lead to decreased removal of spermatozoa with impaired DNA integrity. In *Drosophila*, the relative usage of double-strand break repair mechanisms was shown to change substantially as an organism ages [18], a factor which

Table 9.1 Paternal age and reproductive outcomes.

Reproductive outcome	Association	Comment
Semen quality	↓	Most pronounced effect on seminal volume, motility, and morphology
Fecundity	↓	Weaker effect than seen in women
Embryonal loss/miscarriage	(↑)	
Offspring health	(↓)	Most pronounced in relation to some monogenetic dominant diseases
Offspring sex radio (M:F)	(↓)	May be synergistic to the effect of maternal age

↑, ↓, proven positive/negative association; (↑)/(↓), indication of positive/negative association, conflicting or sparse data.

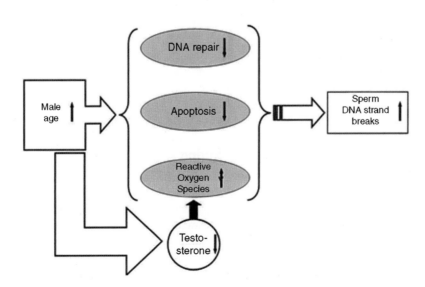

Figure 9.3. Schematic drawing showing possible mechanisms behind DNA-dependent increase in sperm DNA strand breaks.

might also contribute to increased age-related sperm DNA damage. The DNA repair enzyme, topoisomerase II, which is part of the physiological repair of double-strand breaks during spermiogenesis, has been shown to be testosterone dependent [19] and androgen levels decline by age [20]. Finally, even the levels of reactive oxygen species (ROS) were shown to be positively associated with age [21], a factor which may also contribute to the etiology of DNA strand breaks. Interestingly, increased ROS activity in semen was seen to be associated with high body mass index (BMI) [22], which also leads to decrease in testosterone. Therefore, the age-related decline in testosterone might, theoretically, explain at least a part of the increase in sperm DNA strand breaks in older men.

Lifestyle factors may also play a role for explanation of the phenomena mentioned above. Thus, DFI was demonstrated to increase by the length of the abstinence period, which may also be relevant in the context of aging. Consumption of coffee and smoking might also be contributing factors [14, 15].

Age and sperm DNA mutations

Available data indicate that, with increasing age, the frequency of point mutations in the male gamete is much higher than in the female counterpart [23]. This might be a consequence of the fact that the number of cell divisions preceding the production of the mature gamete is much higher in the male. In the female there are 22 cell divisions before meiosis and two during meiosis giving 23 chromosome replications in total, as only one replication occurs during the two meiotic divisions. As the cell divisions are completed before birth, there is no increase with postnatal age. Spermatozoa are produced continuously during life, thus the number of cell divisions and, thereby, chromosome replications increases by age. It has been calculated, that as compared with the female gamete, the number of cell divisions in males is seven times higher at the age of 20 and 25 times higher at the age of 40 [23].

The most extensively studied mutations in sperm are those most frequently occurring, namely single base substitutions in the fibroblast growth factor receptor 3 gene (FGFR3), FGFR2, and the rearranged during transfection (RET) gene leading to syndromes such as achondroplasia, Apert syndrome, multiple endocrine neoplasia 2A and 2B, Crouzon, and Pfeiffer syndrome. Although the evidence of age-dependent increase in the frequency of sperm mutations in sperm is not

completely unequivocal [24], there are strong indications that this, in fact, is true. Wyrobek *et al.* [16] reported a positive association between the age of sperm donor and FGFR3 mutations. The mutation frequency was approximately three times higher in men aged 60 years or more as compared with those in the age span 20–29. When controlling for occupational radiation history it was found that almost 30% of the variance in the frequency of these mutations could be explained by age, there being no "threshold" in this association.

On the other hand no association between age and the occurrence of FGFR2 mutations in the sperm was seen. Such effect of age was, however, seen in other studies [25, 26].

Furthermore, molecular studies in subjects with syndromes caused by mutations in autosomal genes FGFR2, FGFR3, or RET clearly shows that new mutations in the majority, if not all, cases have paternal origin. The predominance of paternal origin has also been seen for X-linked diseases as hemophilia A and B, Lesch–Nyhan disease and ornithine transcarbamylase (OTC) deficiency, for which the male mutation rate is much higher than the female rate. Mutations causing those diseases usually arise in an earlier generation and are transmitted to men through healthy heterozygous mothers [23].

It has been suggested that age dependence in the frequency of single base substitutions is not valid for deletions, which are often large in size. Therefore, small genes such as those mentioned before will become completely deleted, leading to early lethality, and this type of mutation is only seen in larger genes such as those encoding for neurofibromatosis, Duchenne muscular dystrophy, Wilms' tumor or retinoblastoma. Those deletions are often iatrogenic and, therefore, occur by other, non-age-dependent mechanisms. Even those considerations have been supported by clinical molecular data. For Duchenne muscular dystrophy, the vast majority of cases caused by a point mutation were of paternal origin whereas those related to a deletion were derived from the mother. Only a minor proportion of cases of neurofibromatosis, retinoblastoma, and Wilms' tumor is caused by base substitutions and for those diseases only a small effect of paternal age has been seen [23].

Also, for the expansion of the number of units in repeated sequences in a gene, an example being CAG repeat number in the Huntington gene, there seems to be some age dependence, however, the association is more complex than for the single base substitutions [27].

Age and chromosomal aberrations

Using the fluorescence *in situ* hybridization (FISH) technique, it has become possible to screen a large number of sperm for aneuploidy frequency. However, the method is time consuming and most studies are based on relatively small materials, which may be the reason why the results with respect to age dependence are somewhat contradictory.

Griffin *et al.* [28] reported no obvious relationship between increasing age and disomy 18, but the incidence of XY, YY, and XX disomy all were significantly elevated among older men. In the, so far, largest study on age and sperm aneuploidy, including 90 men [16], no association between male age and the aneuploidy or dipoidy frequency in the sperm was seen. Therefore, the issue of male age and the frequency of chromosomal aberrations in the sperm seems still unresolved.

Age-dependent increase in frequency of chromosomal abnormalities in sperm should result in a similar effect of paternal age on aneuploidies in the offspring. However, such effects have not been seen for the autosomal trisomies 13, 18, and 21 nor for Klinefelter syndrome [29]. On the other hand, another study reported both a higher proportion of XY-bearing sperm in older men and higher, in comparison to healthy offspring, mean paternal age for boys diagnosed with Klinefelter syndrome [30].

Age and sex chromosome ratio

In populations where sex-dependent selection of fetuses is not common, the proportion of boys at birth is slightly above 50%. The mechanisms behind this greater proportion of XY subjects and those responsible for possible changes in sex ratio are unknown, but it appears plausible that variation in the proportion of Y- and X-bearing sperm might be involved. However, the available data do not indicate that the proportion of Y-bearing sperm in relation to those carrying a X chromosome changes by age [16, 31] although the studies are few and, mostly, based on relative low numbers of subjects. The data on associations between male age and alterations in sperm genome are summarized in Table 9.2.

DNA damage and reproductive outcome

The impact on reproductive health of some of the numerical or structural changes in sperm DNA, which may be related to male age, seems quite obvious. Mutations and chromosomal aberrations, perhaps with exception of balanced translocation, will often cause distinct syndromes or diseases if transmitted to the offspring. However, in many cases these genetic aberrations may reduce the ability of the couple to conceive or imply an increased risk of abortions. Introduction of preimplantation genetic diagnosis (PGD) may help in increasing chances of fertility and also in selection of embryos not carrying the genetic defect under consideration.

The clinical consequences are less obvious in relation to the impairment of sperm DNA integrity, including DNA strand breaks, which as indicated above was also shown to be strongly age dependent.

Impairment of sperm DNA integrity and fertility

A number of studies have shown an increased proportion of DNA strand breaks in men from infertile couples as compared with those in the general population or proven fertile males [32].

Table 9.2 Male age and alterations in sperm genome.

Outcome	Association	Comments
Sperm DNA integrity	↓	Shown by different methods
Mutations	↑	Shown for single base substitutions but not for deletions. Possibly even for extension of repeat length
Chromosomal aberrations	(↑)	Studies based on few subjects only. Contradictory results
Sperm Y : X chromosome ratio	(↑)	Small studies. So far no evidence

↑, ↓, proven positive/negative association; (↑)/(↓), indication of positive/negative association, conflicting or sparse data.

Two independent, population-based studies have demonstrated that DFI as measured by SCSA is a useful marker in prediction of subfertility in males from non-infertile couples [33, 34]. Both studies have shown that the chance of spontaneous conception starts to decline at DFI levels above 20% and approach zero for DFI above 30–40%. This means that although low DFI (<20%) does not guarantee normal male fertility, high DFI levels are indicative of severely or completely impaired male fertility.

In accordance with the data from non-infertile couples, it was shown that the odds ratio (OR) for infertility is approximately 5 for men having normal standard sperm parameters and DFI levels above 20%. This DFI threshold seems to be even lower (~ 10%) if the sperm concentration is below the level of 20×10^6/mL and/or there is an impairment of sperm motility or morphology (OR for infertility: 16) [35]. The same association was found using an alkaline Comet assay. The OR for infertility was 120 in men having DFI above 25% [36]. A comparison between male infertility patients and donors, using flow cytometric TUNEL assay gave 19% as the cut-off value with no donors and 65% of patients having DNA damage above this level [37]. Thus, in general, for Comet, SCSA, and TUNEL the chance of spontaneous pregnancy seems to be reduced for DFI values exceeding 20%.

For intrauterine insemination (IUI) the results seem to be in agreement with the data on spontaneous pregnancies indicating reduction of chances of pregnancy for SCSA DFI above 20% [38]. For 8-hydroxy-2′-deoxyguanosine (8-OHdG) test the results were similar, with a slightly lower threshold value of 11.5% [39].

Impairment of sperm DNA integrity and in vitro fertilization

The picture seems more blurred concerning the in vitro techniques, in vitro fertilization (IVF) and intracytoplasmic sperm injection (ICSI). It is quite clear that IVF/ICSI can be obtained despite very high DFI levels [38]. A recent meta-analysis by Zini [40] showed a modestly increased pregnancy chance after standard IVF (OR: 1.7) in cases where the proportion of sperm with DNA damage was below a threshold value. Accordingly a Comet-based study showed an OR for clinical pregnancy of 76 for DNA fragmentation below 52% [36]. On the other hand, sperm DNA integrity has, so far, not been found predictive for ICSI pregnancies [38]. One SCSA study [38] for cases with

DFI >30% has shown an OR for clinical pregnancies of 2.0 in favor of ICSI as compared with IVF. However, the couples were not randomized for IVF or ICSI which is why the impact of other factors contributing to the choice of treatment cannot be excluded.

Whether the level of sperm DNA fragmentation has an impact on fertilization rates after IVF and ICSI is still a matter of discussion. Fertilization of oocytes despite DNA damage of sperm was shown in a mouse model [41]. Also human studies have shown that the fertilization rate is independent of the proportion of sperm with damaged DNA as assessed by SCSA [38] or other sperm DNA integrity assays. However, in some other studies, the impairment of sperm DNA integrity was shown to have a significant inverse relationship with fertilization [42]. Thus, the issue of association between sperm DNA damage and fertilization following IVF/ICSI is to be considered as still non-clarified.

It has also been suggested that incomplete or aberrant sperm DNA repair by the oocyte may affect the post-fertilization development of the embryo, and can lead to implantation failure, early miscarriages, or in the worst cases diseases in the offspring [43]. Even here the human data are conflicting. Whilst some authors have reported similar cleavage stage embryo developmental rates between high and low DFI groups as measured by SCSA [44], others have shown that sperm DNA damage is negatively correlated with embryo quality after IVF and ICSI [42]. Two studies have also reported that men with high levels of DNA fragmentation are at increased risk of low blastocyst formation compared with men with a low DFI and consequently, it has been suggested to practice blastocyst culture as a routine in ART [45].

Impairment of sperm DNA integrity and the risk of abortions

Cumulated data indicate that high levels of sperm DNA damage lead to somewhat increased risk of pregnancy loss (OR: 2.5), regardless of the type of in vitro technique applied. Eleven studies have described sperm DNA damage and its association with pregnancy loss after IVF and IVF/ICSI [40]. These pregnancy loss studies are, however, quite heterogeneous in terms of design, inclusion/exclusion criteria, and the sperm DNA damage test employed. These data may provide an additional explanation of cause for pregnancy loss after IVF and IVF/ICSI. It may be speculated that the pregnancy loss (at IVF or

ICSI) is a result of impaired embryo/blastocyst development associated with sperm DNA damage [46].

Impairment of sperm DNA integrity and perinatal characteristics

In vitro fertilization/ICSI is able to overcome the apparent impairment of in vivo fertility caused by sperm DNA damage. Although the risk of transmission of DNA defects and, thereby, the health of the offspring is a potential source of worry, there is a lack of such data. However, a recent study found no impact of high SCSA DFI on gestational length and birth weight of IVF/ICSI-conceived children [47]. So far, there are no follow-up studies of IVF children conceived with sperm from a sample with high load DNA impairment. The data on impairment of sperm DNA integrity and reproductive outcomes are summarized in Table 9.3.

Exposures, sperm DNA damage, and reproductive outcome

It seems quite obvious that increasing male age has a negative impact on reproductive outcome. Although the mechanisms behind this association have not yet been clarified, it is plausible to imagine that some of them might operate through alterations in sperm DNA. The negative effects of environmental, occupational, lifestyle-related and iatrogenic exposures – affecting the genome of the male gamete – may accumulate and act synergistically through the fetal life, infancy, puberty, and adulthood. Below, examples of such exposures, and the available data on their mechanisms of action in relation to the reproductive function, are given.

Iatrogenic exposures

Rodent studies over the past 30 years indicate that male exposure to mutagens, clastogens, and carcinogens before mating can introduce heritable genomic changes that may cause reproductive failures including early and late embryonic loss, structural malformations, heritable disease, and cancer in the offspring. A seminal study in the field demonstrated in 1985 that male rats exposed to the cytostatic drug cyclophosphamide causes post-implantation loss without interfering with fertility [11]. Cytotoxic treatment was shown, temporarily, to increase the proportion of aneuploid sperm [48]. However, aneuploid sperm is not a hereditable risk if aneuploid sperm are disadvantaged at fertilization in comparison with normal sperm. Therefore it is of interest that a study in mice provides strong evidence that such selection at fertilization does not take place [49]. It is not valid to argue that xenobiotics causing aneuploid sperm are of little concern because such sperm have lost the fertilizing capacity. Elevated DFI of sperm was found in men who received radiotherapy for cancer in childhood [50] or young adulthood [51]. Reproductive consequences of high DFI are summarized above.

Environment and occupation

In an early but comprehensive review of birth defects in relation to paternal occupation it was concluded that the risk associated with paternal occupation could not be definitively characterized, but a limited number of published studies suggested associations between various birth defects and occupation as forestry and sawmill workers, auto mechanics, electricians, welders, and building painters [52]. A review addressing miscarriage, stillbirth, low birth weight,

Table 9.3 Impairment of sperm DNA integrity and reproductive outcomes.

Outcome	Association	Comments
Fertility in vivo	↓	Shown in population-based studies and in case–control studies
Fertility in vitro	(↓)	Perhaps an effect in relation to standard IVF but not ICSI
IVF fertilization rate	(↓)	Conflicting results
IVF and embryo quality	(↓)	Conflicting results
IVF and miscarriage	(↑)	Conflicting results but most data indicate such association
Offspring perinatal characteristics	–	Only one study

↑, ↓, proven positive/negative association; (↑)/(↓), indication of positive/negative association, conflicting or sparse data.

and preterm delivery pinpoints some of the most important methodological challenges in this field of reproductive epidemiology [52]. Based upon the extensive body of laboratory research and suggestive epidemiological findings it is concluded that the possible role of paternal influence on fetal development should not be overlooked. Since the early reviews many epidemiological studies have found associations between certain paternal occupational exposures and adverse pregnancy outcomes (for a recent review, see [53]). However, in most cases positive findings obtained in one study have not been corroborated in other studies. It is of interest, however, that a recent meta-analysis based on 14 studies selected by rigorous quality criteria concluded that occupational exposure to organic solvents is associated with an increased risk for neural tube defects, while associations with spontaneous abortion seems less likely [54]. The average relative risk across studies was close to two.

Several studies have investigated the association between paternal occupational exposure and risk of childhood cancer in the offspring, but overall the literature does not provide strong evidence of associations between paternal exposure to hydrocarbons, pesticides, and organic solvents and risk of childhood cancer [55].

Radiation

Ionizing radiation is an environmental and occupational exposure of particular interest, because paternally mediated effects seem highly plausible. It is thus surprising that paternal exposure to ionizing radiation and miscarriage remains virtually unexplored. Only two studies link monitoring data of paternal exposure to ionizing radiation with congenital defects in the offspring and these studies provide no consistent evidence of male-mediated effects [56, 57].

In a UK study of cancer in the offspring of radiation workers, records of more than 34,000 childhood cancer cases were linked with updated dosimetric data among radiation workers. The risk of leukemia and non-Hodgkin lymphoma (but not other childhood cancers) was highly significantly elevated (RR 2.3 (95% CI 1.3–4.2)) if the father had been employed on the date of conception, but not if he had left employment before conception and without any relation to the cumulative preconceptional radiation dose [58]. Since cancer risk was not related to radiation dose the authors suggest that infectious agents in areas with high population mixing might explain the results. However, an effect related to

current exposure during 3–6 months before conception is compatible and partly supported by the findings. Children of fathers exposed in Hiroshima and Nagasaki and after the Chernobyl accident seem not to have increased risk [53].

Smoking

The prevalence of tobacco smoking is still in the range of 10–20% in many populations. The levels of exposure to carcinogens and mutagens are extremely high relative to levels encountered in the workplace or general environment. While the diversity of several hundred constituents makes it difficult to attribute effects to one specific chemical, it does increase the chances that one or more such agents will cause male-mediated developmental toxicity. Moreover, it is a methodological strength that exposure easily and reliably is reported by self-administered questionnaires. Concomitant maternal smoking may be a problem in observational studies that can be addressed by adequate statistical modeling. On this background there are still disappointingly few epidemiological studies linking paternal tobacco smoking with miscarriages, birth defects, childhood cancer, and other end-points.

An early review identified eight studies addressing paternal tobacco use and miscarriages. Only one study reported a moderately increased risk of 1.4 (95% CI 1.2–1.5) [59]. Another study also reported a moderately increased risk, albeit not significantly elevated [60]. In a recent prospective cohort study of more than 525 newly married non-smoking female Chinese textile workers, male smoking before conception was related to an almost doubled risk of early embryonal loss (relative risk 1.8 (95% CI 1.0–3.3)). The risk was not increased in males smoking less than 20 cigarettes a day [61]. It is speculated that paternal smoking might increase the risk of early pregnancy loss by inducing chromosomal damage in sperm or through women's exposure to passive smoke. These results are compatible with findings in another recent study on maternal and paternal tobacco consumption and risk of spontaneous abortion [62].

Few high-quality birth defects research programs have examined paternal tobacco smoking and risk of specific birth defects. Such associations have been reported for ventricular septal defects [63], foot deformities [64], limb reduction defects, and neural tube defects [65]. And a meta-analysis addressing paternal smoking as a risk factor for ano-rectal malformation found an association with this rare congenital anomaly (RR 1.5 (95% CI 1.0–2.3)) [65]. But are these associations causal?

The detoxification capacity of men and women may play a role in the etiology of congenital malformations. Glutathione S-transferase P1 (GSTP1) is part of the superfamily of glutathione S-transferases involved in the detoxification of electrophilic compounds by conjugation. GSTP1 is the only isoform that is expressed in the placenta and in the developing embryo as early as 8 weeks of gestation. Genetic variations in detoxification enzymes may alter their functionality. It has been shown that the glutathione S-transferase theta1 (GSTT1) null genotype is related to a threefold increased risk of orofacial cleft in the offspring among smoking mothers. A comprehensive study did, however, not provide any evidence that paternal smoking at the time of conception is related to increased risk of orofacial cleft – not even in men with the glutathione VAL105 allele. It is known that smokers have higher levels of DNA damage in their sperm [66] and the presence of the GSTP1 enzyme in seminal fluid indicates its role in the protection of sperm against oxidative stress. One reason that paternal smoking was not associated with cleft palate in the offspring may be that DNA damage in the sperm was repaired [67]. Another case referent study addressing congenital heart disease also failed to demonstrate interaction between paternal smoking and glutathione S-transferase polymorphism [68]. In conclusion the evidence regarding paternal smoking and developmental toxicity remains circumstantial.

Conclusions

Thus far, most focus has been given to the association between maternal age and reproductive outcome. However, although not all aspects of the possible link between the age of the father and fertility, risk of miscarriage, perinatal characteristics, and health of the offspring are fully clarified, it seems quite clear that even advanced paternal age has a negative effect on a number of reproductive outcomes. To which degree this is due to accumulation of effects caused by environmental, occupational, and lifestyle-related exposures, and thereby potentially preventable, or the aging per se is the causative factor, is not yet clear. However, the impact of paternal age should be taken into consideration when selecting sperm donors, and also when informing about the possible negative effects of postponing parenthood.

References

1. Kühnert B, Nieschlag E. Reproductive functions of the ageing male. *Hum Reprod Update*. 2004;**10**(4):327–39.

2. Johnson L, Petty CS, Neaves WB. Influence of age on sperm production and testicular weights in men. *J Reprod Fertil*. 1984;**70**:211–18.

3. Handelsman DJ, Staraj S. Testicular size: the effects of aging, malnutrition, and illness. *J Androl*. 1985;**6**:144–51.

4. Mahmoud AM, Goemaere S, El-Garem Y *et al.* Testicular volume in relation to hormonal indices of gonadal function in community-dwelling elderly men. *J Clin Endocrinol Metabol*. 2003;**88**(1):179–84.

5. Olsen J. Subfecundity according to the age of the mother and the father. *Danish Med Bull*. 1990;**37**:281–2.

6. Mirone V, Ricci E, Gentile V *et al.* Determinants of erectile dysfunction risk in a large series of Italian men attending andrology clinics. *Eur Urol*. 2004;**45**(1):87–91.

7. Dunson DB, Colombo B, Baird DD. Changes with age in the level and duration of fertility in the menstrual cycle. *Hum Reprod*. 2002;**17**(5):1399–403.

8. Wilcox A. *Fertility and Pregnancy. An Epidemiologic Perspective*. 1st edn. Oxford: Oxford University Press; 2010.

9. de la Rochebrochard E, Thonneau P. Paternal age and maternal age are risk factors for miscarriage; results of a multicentre European study. *Hum Reprod*. 2002;**17**(6):1649–56.

10. James WH. The human sex ratio. Part 1: A review of the literature. *Hum Biol*. 1987;**59**:721–52.

11. Matsuo K, Ushioda N, Udoff LC. Parental aging synergistically decreases offspring sex ratio. *J Obstet Gynaecol Res*. 2009;**35**(1):164–8.

12. Jacobsen R, Moller H, Mouritsen A. Natural variation in the human sex ratio. *Hum Reprod*. 1999;**14**(12):3120–5.

13. Singh NP, Muller CH, Berger RE. Effects of age on DNA double-strand breaks and apoptosis in human sperm. *Fertil Steril*. 2003;**80**(6):1420–30.

14. Schmid TE, Eskenazi B, Baumgartner A *et al.* The effects of male age on sperm DNA damage in healthy non-smokers. *Hum Reprod*. 2007;**22**(1):180–7.

15. Spano M, Kolstad AH, Larsen SB *et al.* The applicability of the flow cytometric sperm chromatin structure assay as diagnostic and prognostic tool in the human fertility clinic. *Hum Reprod*. 1998;**13**:2495–505.

16. Wyrobek AJ, Eskenazi B, Young S *et al.* Advancing age has differential effects on DNA damage, chromatin

integrity, gene mutations, and aneuploidies in sperm. *Proc Natl Acad Sci USA.* 2006;**103**(25):9601–6.

17. Duty SM, Singh NP, Silva MJ *et al.* The relationship between environmental exposures to phthalates and DNA damage in human sperm using the neutral Comet assay. *Environ Health Perspect.* 2003;**111**(9):1164–9.

18. Preston CR, Flores C, Engels WR. Age-dependent usage of double-strand-break repair pathways. *Curr Biol.* 2006;**16**(20):2009–15.

19. Bakshi RP, Galande S, Bali P *et al.* Developmental and hormonal regulation of type II DNA topoisomerase in rat testis. *J Mol Endocrinol.* 2001;**26**(3):193–206.

20. Wu FC, Tajar A, Pye SR *et al.* Hypothalamic-pituitary-testicular axis disruptions in older men are differentially linked to age and modifiable risk factors: the European Male Aging Study. *J Clin Endocrinol Metab.* 2008;**93**(7):2737–45.

21. Cocuzza M, Athayde KS, Agarwal A *et al.* Age-related increase of reactive oxygen species in neat semen in healthy fertile men. *Urology.* 2008;**71**(3):490–4.

22. Tunc O, Bakos HW, Tremellen K. Impact of body mass index on seminal oxidative stress. *Andrologia.* 2011;**43**(2):121–8.

23. Crow JF. The origins, patterns and implications of human spontaneous mutation. *Nat Rev Genet.* 2000;**1**(1):40–7.

24. Ketterling RP, Vielhaber E, Li X *et al.* Germline origins in the human F9 gene: Frequent G:C→A:T mosaicism and increased mutations with advanced maternal age. *Hum Genet.* 1999;**105**(6):629–40.

25. Glaser RL, Broman KW, Schulman RL *et al.* The paternal-age effect in Apert syndrome is due, in part, to the increased frequency of mutations in sperm. *American J Hum Genet.* 2003;**73**(4):939–47.

26. Yoon SR, Qin J, Glaser RL *et al.* The ups and downs of mutation frequencies during aging can account for the Apert syndrome paternal age effect. *PLoS Genet.* 2009;**5**(7):e1000558.

27. Ellegren H. Microsatellite mutations in the germline: implications for evolutionary inference. *Trends Genet.* 2000;**16**(12):551–8.

28. Griffin DK, Abruzzo MA, Millie EA *et al.* Non-disjunction in human sperm: evidence for an effect of increasing paternal age. *Hum Mol Genet.* 1995;**4**(12):2227–32.

29. Sartorius GA, Nieschlag E. Paternal age and reproduction. *Hum Reprod Update.* 2010;**16**(1):65–79.

30. Lanfranco F, Kamischke A, Zitzmann M *et al.* Klinefelter's syndrome. *Lancet.* 2004;**364**(9430):273–83.

31. Tiido T, Rignell-Hydbom A, Jönsson B *et al.* Exposure to persistent organohalogen pollutants associates with human sperm Y:X chromosome ratio. *Hum Reprod.* 2005;**20**(7):1903–9.

32. Erenpreiss J, Elzanaty S, Giwercman A. Sperm DNA damage in men from infertile couples. *Asian J Androl.* 2008;**10**(5):786–90.

33. Evenson DP, Jost LK, Marshall D *et al.* Utility of the sperm chromatin structure assay as a diagnostic and prognostic tool in the human fertility clinic. *Hum Reprod.* 1999;**14** 1039–49.

34. Spano M, Bonde JP, Hjollund HI *et al.* Sperm chromatin damage impairs human fertility. The Danish first pregnancy planner study team. *Fertil Steril.* 2000;**73**(1):43–50.

35. Giwercman A, Lindstedt L, Larsson M *et al.* Sperm chromatin structure assay as an independent predictor of fertility in vivo: a case-control study. *Int J Androl.* 2010;**33**(1):e221–7.

36. Simon L, Lutton D, McManus J *et al.* Sperm DNA damage measured by the alkaline Comet assay as an independent predictor of male infertility and in vitro fertilization success. *Fertil Steril.* 2011;**95**(2):652–7.

37. Sharma RK, Sabanegh E, Mahfouz R *et al.* Tunel as a test for sperm DNA damage in the evaluation of male infertility. *Urology.* 2010;**76**(6):1380–6.

38. Bungum M, Humaidan P, Axmon A *et al.* Sperm DNA integrity assessment in prediction of assisted reproduction technology outcome. *Hum Reprod.* 2007;**22**(1):174–9.

39. Thomson LK, Zieschang JA, Clark AM. Oxidative deoxyribonucleic acid damage in sperm has a negative impact on clinical pregnancy rate in intrauterine insemination but not intracytoplasmic sperm injection cycles. *Fertil Steril.* 2011;**96**(4):843–7.

40. Zini A. Are sperm chromatin and DNA defects relevant in the clinic? *Systems Biol Reprod Med.* 2011;**57**(1–2):78–85.

41. Ahmadi A, N g SC. Fertilizing capacity of DNA damaged spermatozoa. *J Exp Zool.* 1999;**286**:696–704.

42. Sun JG, Jurisicova A, Casper RF. Detection of deoxyribonucleic acid fragmentation in human sperm: correlation with fertilization in vitro. *Biol Reprod.* 1997;**56**:602–7.

43. Aitken RJ, Baker MA. Oxidative stress and male reproductive biology. *Reprod Fertil Dev.* 2004;**16**(5):581–8.

44. Larson-Cook KL, Brannian JD, Hansen KA *et al.* Relationship between the outcomes of assisted reproductive techniques and sperm DNA fragmentation as measured by the sperm chromatin structure assay. *Fertil Steril.* 2003;**80**(4):895–902.

45. Spano M, Seli E, Bizzaro D *et al.* The significance of sperm nuclear DNA strand breaks on reproductive outcome. *Curr Opin Obstet Gynecol.* 2005;**17**(3):255–60.

46. Seli E, Gardner DK, Schoolcraft WB *et al.* Extent of nuclear DNA damage in ejaculated spermatozoa impacts on blastocyst development after in vitro fertilization. *Fertil Steril.* 2004;**82**(2):378–83.

47. Bungum M, Bungum L, Lynch KF *et al.* Spermatozoa DNA damage measured by sperm chromatin structure assay (SCSA) and birth characteristics in children conceived by IVF and ICSI. *Asian J Androl.* 2011;**13**:68–75.

48. Tempest HG, Ko E, Chan P *et al.* Sperm aneuploidy frequencies analysed before and after chemotherapy in testicular cancer and Hodgkin's lymphoma patients. *Hum Reprod.* 2008;**23**(2):251–8.

49. Marchetti F, Lowe X, Bishop J *et al.* Absence of selection against aneuploid mouse sperm at fertilization. *Biol Reprod.* 1999;**61**(4):948–54.

50. Romerius P, Stahl O, Moell C *et al.* Sperm DNA integrity in men treated for childhood cancer. *Clin Cancer Res.*;**16**(15):3843–50.

51. Stahl O, Eberhard J, Jepson K *et al.* Sperm DNA integrity in testicular cancer patients. *Hum Reprod.* 2006;**21**(12): 3199–3205.

52. Olshan A, Faustman EM. Male-mediated developmental toxicity. *Reprod Toxicol.* 1993;**7**:191–202.

53. Cordier S. Evidence for a role of paternal exposures in developmental toxicity. *Basic Clin Pharmacol Toxicol.* 2008;**102**(2):176–81.

54. Logman JF, de Vries LE, Hemels ME *et al.* Paternal organic solvent exposure and adverse pregnancy outcomes: a meta-analysis. *Am J Industr Med.* 2005;**47**(1):37–44.

55. Colt JS, Blair A. Parental occupational exposures and risk of childhood cancer. *Environ Health Perspect.* 1998;**106**(Suppl. 3):909–25.

56. Green LM, Dodds L, Miller AB *et al.* Risk of congenital anomalies in children of parents occupationally exposed to low level ionising radiation. *Occup Environ Med.* 1997;**54**(9):629–35.

57. Doyle P, Maconochie N, Roman E *et al.* Fetal death and congenital malformation in babies born to nuclear industry employees: report from the nuclear industry family study. *Lancet.* 2000;**356**(9238):1293–9.

58. Sorahan T, McKinney PA, Mann JR *et al.* Childhood cancer and parental use of tobacco: findings from the inter-regional epidemiological study of childhood cancer (IRESCC). *Br J Cancer.* 2001;**84**(1):141–6.

59. Rupa DS, Reddy PP, Reddi OS. Reproductive performance in population exposed to pesticides in cotton fields in India. *Environ Res.* 1991;**55**(2):123–8.

60. Lindbohm ML, Hemminki K, Bonhomme MG *et al.* Effects of paternal occupational exposure on spontaneous abortions. *Am J Public Health.* 1991;**81**(8):1029–33.

61. Venners SA, Wang X, Chen C *et al.* Paternal smoking and pregnancy loss: a prospective study using a biomarker of pregnancy. *Am J Epidemiol.* 2004;**159**(10):993–1001.

62. Blanco-Munoz J, Torres-Sanchez L, Lopez-Carrillo L. Exposure to maternal and paternal tobacco consumption and risk of spontaneous abortion. *Public Health Rep.* 2009;**124**(2):317–22.

63. Savitz DA, Schwingl PJ, Keels MA. Influence of paternal age, smoking, and alcohol consumption on congenital anomalies. *Teratology.* 1991;**44**(4):429–40.

64. Zhang J, Savitz DA, Schwingl PJ *et al.* A case-control study of paternal smoking and birth defects. *Int J Epidemiol.* 1992;**21**(2):273–8.

65. Zwink N, Jenetzky E, Brenner H. Parental risk factors and anorectal malformations: systematic review and meta-analysis. *Orphanet J Rare Dis.* 2011;**6**:25.

66. DeMarini DM. Genotoxicity of tobacco smoke and tobacco smoke condensate: a review. *Mutation Res.* 2004;**567**(2–3):447–74.

67. Krapels IP, Raijmakers-Eichhorn J, Peters WH *et al.* The I,105V polymorphism in glutathione S-transferase P1, parental smoking and the risk for nonsyndromic cleft lip with or without cleft palate. *Eur J Hum Gen.* 2008;**16**(3):358–66.

68. Cresci M, Foffa I, Ait-Ali L *et al.* Maternal and paternal environmental risk factors, metabolizing GSTM1 and GSTT1 polymorphisms, and congenital heart disease. *Am J Cardiol.* 2011;**108**(11):1625–31.

Paternal aging and increased risk of congenital disease, psychiatric disorders, and cancer

Simon L. Conti and Michael L. Eisenberg

Introduction

As couples are increasingly delaying parenthood, the effect of the aging man and woman on reproductive outcomes has been an area of increased interest. Advanced paternal age has been shown to independently affect the entire spectrum of male fertility as assessed by reductions in sperm quality and fertilization (both assisted and unassisted) [1]. Moreover, epidemiological data suggest that paternal age can lead to higher rates of adverse birth outcomes and congenital anomalies. Mounting evidence also suggests increased risk of specific pediatric and adult disease states ranging from cancer to behavioral traits. While disease states associated with advancing paternal age have been well described, consensus recommendations for neonatal screening have not been as widely implemented as have been with advanced maternal age. The clinical significance of this topic is made relevant by a population analysis that found a relative risk of 2.35 (95% confidence interval (CI) 1.42–3.88) for childhood mortality from a congenital anomaly when paternal age is greater than 45 when compared with paternal age 25–29 [2].

A genetic basis for the paternal age effect

The first description linking advanced paternal age and genetic disease was in the setting of achondroplasia. A common cause of dwarfism, achondroplasia is commonly caused by a sporadic mutation in the fibroblast growth factor receptor 3 (FGFR3) gene that leads to abnormal cartilage formation. In 1912, Wilhem Weinberg published his observations on the inheritance of sporadic achondroplasia, noting it had an increased incidence amongst last-born children of a siblingship. It was not until 1955 when Penrose refined this

observation to show that paternal age was the main variable influencing Weinberg's observation [3, 4]. Since that time the epidemiologic, molecular, and epigenetic basis for the paternal age effect have been studied at length and both strong and weak associations with paternal age have been made in a wide range of disease states (Table 10.1).

After recognizing a paternal bias in the origin of autosomal dominant disease, as well as the association with advanced paternal age, Penrose's "copy error" hypothesis was developed.

Single base pair substitutions occurring more frequently in the paternal germline are responsible for sporadic cases of several diseases such as achondroplasia and Apert syndrome. To explain the greater importance of paternal age compared with maternal age on sporadic autosomal dominant congenital diseases, investigators have pointed to differences in gametogenesis between the sexes. Each oocyte produced by a female, regardless of her age, has undergone 22 germ-cell divisions and two meiotic divisions for a total of 23 chromosome replications (the final meiotic division does not require DNA replication). As a female grows older, her oocytes do not undergo any further DNA replication events. In the male, spermatogenesis is continuous so that aging increases the number of chromosome replication events, which depends on the number of cell divisions. This leads to spermatic chromosomes that have undergone an estimated 35 replications by age 15, 150 by age 20, 380 by age 30, 610 by age 40 and 840 by age 50 [5]. Through more cycles of DNA replication come more copy error mutations, and in the setting of impaired DNA replication and DNA repair mechanisms, this may explain the higher rate of causative paternal mutations in congenital disease states.

Paternal Influences on Human Reproductive Success, ed. Douglas T. Carrell. Published by Cambridge University Press.
© Cambridge University Press 2013.

Table 10.1 Congenital, neurocognitive, and psychiatric disease associated with advanced paternal age.

Disease state	Reference
Congenital disease	
Achondroplasia	Weinberg, 1912 [3]
Apert syndrome	Tolarova *et al.*, 1997 [54]
Basal cell nevus syndrome	Jones *et al.*, 1975 [55]
Cardiac defects	Olshan *et al.*, 1994 [56]
Cleft lip or palate	Harville *et al.*, 2007 [57]
Cri-du-chat syndrome	Overhauser *et al.*, 1990 [58]
Crouzon syndrome	Glaser *et al.*, 2000 [21]
Down syndrome	Zhu *et al.*, 2005 [11]
Duchenne muscular dystrophy	Bucher *et al.*, 1980 [59]
Fibrodysplasia ossificans progressiva	Risch *et al.*, 1987 [17]
Huntington's disease	Goldberg *et al.*, 1993 [26]
Klinefelter's syndrome	Lowe *et al.*, 2001 [25]
Marfan's syndrome	Murdoch *et al.*, 1972 [60]
Multiple endocrine neoplasia 2A and 2B	Mulligan *et al.*, 1994 [61], Carlson *et al.*, 1994 [62]
Neurofibromatosis Type 1	Risch *et al.*, 1987 [17]
Neurofibromatosis Type 2	Kluwe *et al.*, 2000 [63]
Osteogenesis imperfecta	Young *et al.*, 1987 [64]
Progeria	Eriksson *et al.*, 2003 [65]
Pfeiffer syndrome	Glaser *et al.*, 2000 [21]
Retinitis pigmentosa	Kaplan *et al.*, 1990 [66]
Retinoblastoma (bilateral)	Mills *et al.*, 2012 [38]
Spinal muscular atrophy	Wirth *et al.*, 1997 [67]
Situs inversus	Lian *et al.*, 1986 [68]
Thanatophoric dysplasia	Martinez-Frias *et al.*, 1988 [69]
Treacher Collins	Splendore *et al.*, 2003 [70]
Tetralogy of Fallot	Lu *et al.*, 1999 [71]
Wilms' tumor	Olson *et al.*, 1993 [72]
Neuropsychiatric disorders	
Alzheimer's disease	Bertram *et al.*, 1998 [73]
Autism	Reichenberg *et al.*, 2006 [42]
Bipolar	Frans *et al.*, 2008 [49]
Dyslexia	Jayasekara and Street, 1978 [74]
Lower intelligence	Saha *et al.*, 2009 [50]
Rett syndrome	Amir and Zoghbi 2000 [75]
Schizophrenia	Brown *et al.*, 2002 [46]

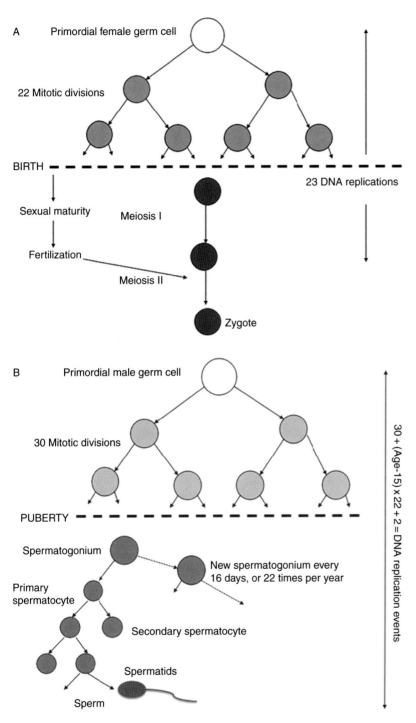

Figure 10.1. Female (A) and male (B) meiosis and DNA replication cycles.

In contrast to germline point mutations, aneuploidy is predominantly maternal in origin [6]. Aneuploidy is defined as an abnormal number of chromosomes and may occur as a result of a mitotic or meiotic error. Indeed, as women age aberrant meiosis leads to higher rates of oocyte aneuploidy [7]. The mechanism of aneuploidy is likely multifactorial, and often debated, but is generally attributed to the mis-segregation of sister chromatids in meiosis I of the oocyte [6]. Some suggest that environmental insults and hormonal changes that occur with maternal aging could affect the fidelity of mechanisms that prevent mis-segregation, such as the spindle accessory checkpoint [8, 9]. Trisomy 21 has been attributed to maternal gamete aneuploidy in 93% of cases [10]. Other trisomies have been shown to have similar rates of maternal origin. The significant role that maternal aging plays in this process has been well described with the incidence of trisomy 21 rising from 1/1250 in a 20-year-old female to 1/100 in a 40-year-old female. Determining the effect of advanced paternal age on aneuploidy has proven more difficult. Nevertheless, there does appear to be an association. In a study by Zhu et al. on a Danish population, investigators found that men who were over 45 had a 4.50- (1.00–20.30) fold higher risk of siring a child with Down syndrome compared with men younger than 30 [11].

Because of the relatively low rates of trisomy, and the confounding effect of maternal age some have turned to sperm DNA content directly to assess the effects of paternal aging. Indeed, Wyrobek et al. describe an increase in sperm chromatin defects and DNA damage in aging men postulating this as an explanation for impaired fertility in older men [12]. Moreover, the same group noted higher rates of mutations in the FGFR3 gene in older men suggesting a 3% increase in the frequency of the mutation with each additional year of age. In contrast, other measures of DNA quality, such as high DNA instability and sperm aneuploidy or diploidy did not appear to vary based on age. However, other studies do show an increased incidence of sperm aneuploidy in men aged over 59 when compared with men under 40 [13]. The mechanisms underlying these observations are not perfectly understood, but as described above, it is likely a product of mis-segregation, most commonly described during meiosis I.

Tarin et al. explore the various mechanisms in effect when comparing advanced maternal age with advanced paternal age. They propose that maternal age-associated trisomy may be multifactorial, but oocytes of middle-aged women suffer more oxidative stress as their mitochondria produce high amounts of reactive oxygen species. The increased oxidative stress may in turn affect the formation of the meiotic spindle leading to mis-segregation and thus aneuploidy. They also note that DNA repair genes monitoring for errors in DNA replication are not affected by maternal age and continue to be functional for the life of the oocyte. On the other hand, elongated spermatids, immature

and mature spermatozoa do not have a DNA repair system leading to the persistence of DNA point mutations in the germline [14].

Autosomal dominant

As previously mentioned, the most completely understood paternal age effect can be seen in the setting of sporadic autosomal dominant diseases. Perhaps the best example of this is the family of autosomal dominant disease affecting the fibroblast growth factor receptor 2 (FGFR2) and FGFR3 which include Apert syndrome and achondroplasia, respectively. Apert syndrome is characterized by acrocephalosyndactyly, or malformations of the skull, face, hands, and feet. In a study by Wilkin et al. it was noted that all 40 patients (100%) affected with achondroplasia had mutations in these receptor genes that were of paternal origin [15]. Interestingly these mutations are single base pair substitutions and nearly all analyzed cases are due to a glycine to arginine substitution at codon 1138. This leads to an alteration in the transmembrane domain of FGFR3 and the achondroplasia phenotype.

Tiemann-Boege et al. provide significant insight to the FGFR3 mutation and the effect of advanced paternal age. They analyzed both birth rates of achondroplasia and rates of the Gly1138Arg mutation in the sperm of older men. While men who are aged 50–54 have a 12-fold increased chance of having a child with achondroplasia, the relative risk of having sperm that carry the mutation is only two-fold [16]. This discrepancy is troubling for the hypothesis that the prevalence of autosomal dominant disease in the setting of APA is solely due to the increasing number of DNA replication cycles (Penrose's copy error hypothesis) in older males and suggests there is more to understand about this observation. It is possible that sperm with this mutation may provide a selective advantage for affected sperm, but a mechanism for this is not known.

A similar discrepancy is found in studies of Apert syndrome, in that the incidence of the phenotype increases exponentially with age starting at age 37 [17, 18]. However the incidence of the mutation in sperm only rises to approximately a 2.5-fold increase in incidence among men older than 65 years old compared with men younger than 30 [18]. As with achondroplasia, over 60% of the cases are due to a single mutation leading to a Ser252Trp mutation, which affects the ligand binding to the receptor [19]. Interestingly, this appears to be a male-specific mutation with one series showing that the culprit mutation in 57 cases was consistently paternally derived [20]. Other diseases with phenotypes that have some similarities to Apert, such as Crouzon and Pfeiffer syndromes, are also associated with increased paternal age, craniosynostoses, and a mutation on the FGFR2 gene. Analyses of the genetic causes of Crouzon and Pfeiffer syndromes show the mutations to be of paternal origin with the average age of men siring affected offspring almost 5 years older than the controls [21].

Multiple endocrine neoplasia type 2A and 2B are generally considered an inherited disease, but sporadic cases have been identified. Many sporadic cases have been attributed to paternal inheritance of mutations in the RET proto-oncogene, with higher risk seen in older fathers, suggesting germline mutation is responsible [22, 23].

While the effect of paternal age on mutation rate has been described as exponential in achondroplasia, Apert syndrome, and MEN2, another autosomal dominant condition, Neurofibromatosis Type 1 (NF1) or Von Recklinghausen disease, exhibits a linear relationship between paternal age and risk. The less dramatic increase with aging is likely due to equal contributions of maternal and paternal mutations to the disease phenotype. Rather than base pair substitutions causing NF1, the disease is attributed to intragenic deletions, which are not thought to arise from repeated DNA replications [23]. In a recent cross-sectional study of a large cohort of patients with NF1 in the Czech republic, it was noted that the average age of fathers of children with the sporadic variant of NF1 was 32.0 in their cohort, whereas the average age of paternity in the general population was 28.8, suggesting a relationship between paternal age and disease susceptibility [24].

Aneuploidy

Advanced paternal age has also been noted to affect aneuploidy in autosomes and sex chromosomes. The autosomal trisomies are difficult to study with respect to paternal age because of the strong influence of maternal age, especially given the fact that partner ages are often similar. Men older than 49 years old have been shown to have a hazard ratio of 4.5 (CI 1–20.3) for having a child with Down syndrome compared with fathers aged 20–29, when adjusted for maternal age [11].

As described above, maternal origin of the aneuploidy is the predominant pattern in most trisomy, with the exception of sex chromosome aneuploidy, where the origin is of equal maternal and paternal

frequency. In fact, there is a 160% increased incidence of having XY-bearing sperm in 50-year-old fathers compared with fathers younger than 30 [25].

Expansion of trinucleotide repeats

Trinucleotide repeat expansions alter normal gene function by leading to abnormal translation or function of protein transcripts. Three disease states that result from expanding trinucleotide repeats are Huntington, myotonic dystrophy (Steinert) and Fragile X syndrome (Martin-Bell syndrome). Huntington's disease is a neurodegenerative disease caused by a CAG expansion within the Huntingtin gene which leads to a mutant form of the protein causing progressive decline in cognition and coordination. Steinert disease (or Type 1 myotonic dystrophy – DM1) is a progressive multisystemic disease causing muscle wasting, cardiac conduction abnormalities, endocrinopathies, and cataracts. Within the responsible gene (DMPK – myotonic dystrophy protein kinase), there is a CTG repeat. Abnormal lengths of the repeat lead to the neuromuscular phenotype. Fragile X syndrome leads to intellectual impairment through expansion of a CGG repeat in the FMR1 (Fragile X mental retardation 1) gene. Rare sporadic cases of these diseases have been shown to be the result of intermediate alleles that undergo expansion in aging males who do not express the phenotype. Indeed, a study of sporadic cases of Huntington's determined all intermediate alleles responsible for the affected child were paternal with expansion of such alleles during gametogenesis associated with advancing age [26].

In addition, genomic imprinting and epigenetic changes in the aging male are also likely to have a role in the transmission and propagation of this class of inherited disease. It is known that there is an inverse relationship between paternal age and onset of Huntington's disease. Importantly, this observation held true even in cases where the Huntington's allele was not of paternal origin, implicating the paternal epigenetic factors [27].

Cancer

There is growing evidence that suggests the lifetime risk of various cancers is associated with both advanced paternal age and advanced maternal age. Not only is the overall incidence of cancer higher, but the onset of malignancies is earlier. Potential causes include increased damage to paternal DNA from prolonged environmental exposures, *de novo* germline mutations, and aberrant epigenetic regulation that activate oncogenes or inactivate tumor suppressor genes [28–30]. For instance, DNA methylation has been shown to be increased in newborns with advanced parental age suggesting that epigenetic mechanisms are corrupted by somatic aging [31]. To date, some data support a small but significantly increased rate of cancer among offspring conceived by older fathers, however, the data is conflicting.

Investigators from Sweden have taken advantage of large birth and cancer registries to demonstrate a 25% increased risk of brain tumors in children born to fathers over 30 compared with those younger than 25 [32]. Importantly, many other solid and hematologic malignancies were also explored in this same study with no consistent relationship.

Childhood leukemia has a risk of 1 in 25,000 in the general population. Epidemiologic studies have shown that when paternal age is greater than 35 this rate increases to 1 in 17,000. The same study calculates the relative risk of developing a childhood leukemia of 1.5 for children of men aged 35 or older [33]. Adult-onset hematologic malignancies such as such as non-Hodgkin's lymphoma also have an association with advanced paternal age. One study of a California database reported a 50% increased risk for paternal age greater than 40 compared with paternal age of 25 [34]. Similar observations have been made in the setting of central nervous system tumors of childhood. A prevalence of 1 in 36,000 exists for this disease state, which increases to 1 in 27,000 with a paternal age of 30–34, 1 in 25,000 with a paternal age of 35–39, and 1 in 21,000 with a paternal age greater than 40 [35].

Breast and prostate cancer have been shown to have similar epidemiologic trends. Using data from the Framingham study, Zhang *et al.* noted that the incidence rate of prostate cancer increased from 1.70 per 1,000 person-years among sons in the lowest quartile of paternal age (paternal age < 27) to 2.00 (27 ≤ paternal age < 32), 2.32 (32 ≤ paternal age < 38), and 2.74 (paternal age ≥ 38) among those of each increased paternal age category, respectively. Overall, the risk of prostate cancer in offspring increased 70% for sons sired by fathers 38 or over compared with those whose fathers were < 27 at birth. Importantly, no relationship existed for maternal age [36]. A Korean case–control study found that paternal age > 40 increases a daughter's lifetime incidence of breast cancer from 1 in 5.3 compared with 1 in 8.5 if the father's age was < 30. In addition to an increase in overall breast cancer incidence, investigators noted a 90% increased odds of earlier onset breast cancer for daughters of older fathers [37].

To date, most of the data examining the relationship between paternal age and malignancies are somewhat conflicting, without consistency between populations. The proposed hypotheses suggest that increased germline mutations (again secondary to the copy-error hypothesis) and epigenetic dysregulation lead to higher cancer incidences. However, given the heterogeneity of the current literature, it is likely that the etiology is multifactorial and heavily influenced by external factors (i.e. environmental). One cancer that does have a sporadic, paternally inherited version is bilateral retinoblastoma. Given the aforementioned notion that most germline mutations are paternally inherited, one study of retinoblastoma survivors found that an offspring's risk of having a sporadic form of retinoblastoma compared with possessing the inherited-familial form increased with paternal age [38].

Neuropsychiatric conditions

Perhaps the largest body of recent literature on advanced paternal age exists on its effect on behavioral and psychiatric conditions. While the evidence linking advanced paternal age and neuropsychiatric diseases is strong, especially in the realm of autism, it is not clear which is cause and which is effect. Does a germline mutation cause autism or are men that have children at an advanced age more likely to carry phenotypes on the autistic spectrum? Some have suggested that traits that lead to siring children at an advanced age, such as aloofness, shyness, and trouble communicating with women may be in part responsible for the association of autism with advanced paternal age [39]. Here we will discuss the evidence for the paternal age effect on neuropsychiatric conditions including autism spectrum disorders, behavioral disorders, cognitive decline, bipolar disorder, and schizophrenia.

Autism

Autism spectrum disorders include a broad range of entities including Asperger syndrome, Rett syndrome, overreactive disorder, childhood disintegrative disorder, and atypical autism that usually affect children by age 3. The three prominent characteristics of autism spectrum disorders (ASDs) are impairments in social interaction, communication and restricted, repetitive, and stereotyped patterns of behavior, interests, and activities. An increase in incidence of autism in the

USA has been noted over the past several decades from 5 per 10,000 in the 1980s to 50 per 10,000 as of 2003 [40]. Diagnostic substitution or overdiagnosis bias is a proposed etiology in the increased incidence, but increasing parental age may also be playing a role [40, 41].

One of the original studies exploring the increased risk of autism in advanced paternal age examined a cohort of nearly 400,000 men and women born in Israel in the 1980s. When analyzing paternal age as a categorical variable they found that paternal age above 40 increased the odds of having a child diagnosed with autism (odds ratio (OR): 5.75, CI 2.65–12.46). Similar findings resulted from examining age as a continuous variable so that for each 10-year increase in age the odds of siring an autistic child more than doubled after adjusting for sociodemographic and maternal factors (OR: 2.14, CI 1.44–3.16). Importantly, the same data were used in a model for advancing maternal age, which showed no significant effect [42].

Another study compared autism to the previously noted sporadic congenital autosomal dominant disorders. Investigators stratified 677 patients with autism from 340 distinct families into either multiplex (having a family history of autism) or simplex (being the only known affected individual in a family). They then found that after controlling for sex, birth order, and family size, there was a linear association with advancing paternal age and probability of being a simplex family. This suggests an interesting correlation with the autosomal dominant diseases that show associations with paternal age in their sporadic forms because of the increased rates of germline mutations [43]. The understanding that germline mutations can affect the autistic phenotype was championed by Sebat and colleagues, who described a stronger than expected association of *de novo* copy number variations (CNVs) with autism in cases of sporadic autism [44]. CNVs are alterations in the number of specific regions of DNA so that cells may contain deletions or duplications of given regions. The authors demonstrated that *de novo* mutations resulting in both gain and loss of DNA region copy number might explain some portion of ASD.

Certainly, the etiology of autism is more complicated than a base pair substitution in a single gene. The genetics of autism spectrum disorders are likely quite complex involving genetic, epigenetic, and environmental factors. Nevertheless, its heritability is established as siblings of autistic children have a 25-fold increased risk of being diagnosed with ASD compared with the general population [44]. Further evidence of the importance of genetics on ASD is revealed by examining the concordance rates of autism in monozygotic (60–90%) and dizygotic (0–10%) twins [45].

Schizophrenia

Schizophrenia and the spectrum of schizophrenia disorders (i.e. schizoaffective personality disorder, schizotypal personality disorder, delusional disorders, or other psychoses) are also associated with older paternal age. In 2002, using over 12,000 participants from the Child Health and Development Study Cohort in the USA, investigators sought to determine the effect of paternal age on the diagnosis of a schizophrenia spectrum disorder. In an analysis of paternal age as a continuous variable in schizophrenia spectrum disorders, each 10-year increase in paternal age had an adjusted rate ratio of 1.86 (CI 1.20–2.87) [46]. The results of this study were similar to an earlier study of Israeli subjects [47]. Investigators examined over 750,000 Swedes, and found that for each 10-year increase in paternal age, the risk of schizophrenia in the offspring increased by nearly 50% (hazard ratio: 1.47, CI 1.23–1.76). Interestingly, the association only existed in those with no family history of schizophrenia suggesting that the accumulation of *de novo* mutations in the sperm contributes to the risk of schizophrenia [48].

Bipolar disorder

Bipolar disorder, a common severe mood disorder, is associated with significant comorbidities including suicidality and substance abuse. In a nested-case control study from Sweden, that controlled for confounders such as maternal age, 13,000 patients with bipolar disorder were identified and matched with five healthy control subjects by sex and year of birth. This study found that the offspring of men 55 years or older were 1.37 (CI 1.02–1.84) times more likely to be diagnosed with bipolar disorder than if the age of the father was less than 25. Moreover, earlier age of disease onset was also associated with advanced paternal age. Interestingly, when analyzed in a similar fashion, maternal age had no significant effect [49].

Behavior and cognitive ability

In their analyses of a cohort from the US Collaborative Perinatal Project, Saha and colleagues have published two studies that elucidate the effect of advanced paternal age on neurocognitive and behavioral outcomes. One examined advanced paternal age and its effect on neurocognitive measures during childhood, while the other showed that advanced paternal age was associated with more "externalizing" adverse behaviors (e.g. aggression, vandalism, disruptive behavior). These researchers found that using five neurocognitive measures (Bayley scales, Stanford Binet Intelligence Scale, Graham–Ernhart Block Sort Test, Wechsler Intelligence Scale for Children, Wide Range Achievement Test) at various developmental ages revealed that children of men with advancing paternal age scored worse. This trend followed a linear pattern when children were grouped into paternal age groups in 5-year intervals. Interestingly maternal age had the opposite effect [50]. In their study of behavioral effects, it was found that for every 5-year increase in paternal age, the odds of higher 'externalizing' behaviors was increased by 12% (OR = 1.12; CI = 1.03, 1.21, $P < 0.0001$) [51]. The notion that cognitive decline exists in the setting of older fathers is not novel, as an animal study of rats from 1983 showed that rats with older fathers exhibited impaired learning and conditioning [52].

Conclusions

Careful examination of the association between paternal age and diseases in the offspring reveals a variety of mechanisms which lead to phenotypic pathology from syndromes caused by single base pair substitutions, genomic imprinting and increasing numbers of trinucleotide repeats, to complex and poorly understood transmission of neuropsychiatric conditions. A recurring theme as one examines the spectrum of disorders that have been linked to advanced paternal age is that heritable germline mutations seem to increase with a father's age. The implications for a society with aging fathers could be quite significant. As many of these diseases do not manifest until after reproductive age, genomic and epigenetic mutations will be passed on to future generations. As might be expected, the associations seem to hold through multiple generations. Indeed, even advanced grandpaternal age has been shown to be associated with increased risk of schizophrenia [53]. As specific genetic targets are identified, it is conceivable that some risks could be mitigated through preimplantation genetic diagnosis. However, while the relative risks of several of these disorders do increase with advanced paternal age, the absolute risk remains low and may render such strategies cost prohibitive.

Currently, no specific treatment can be offered to older patients interested in reproduction, other than sperm cryopreservation and education regarding the potential risks of delayed reproduction.

References

1. Kidd SA, Eskenazi B, Wyrobek AJ. Effects of male age on semen quality and fertility: a review of the literature. *Fertil Steril.* 2001;**75**(2):237–48.

2. Zhu JL, Vestergaard M, Madsen KM *et al.* Paternal age and mortality in children. *Eur J Epidemiol.* 2008;**23**(7):443–7.

3. Weinberg W. Zur vererbung des zwergwuches. *Arch Rassen-u, Gesel Biology.* 1912;**9**:710–18.

4. Penrose LS. Parental age and mutation. *Lancet.* 1955;**269**(6885):312–13.

5. Vogel F, Motulsky AG. *Human Genetics.* Berlin: Springer; 1977.

6. Yoon PW, Freeman SB, Sherman SL *et al.* Advanced maternal age and the risk of Down syndrome characterized by the meiotic stage of chromosomal error: a population-based study. *Am J Hum Genet.* 1996;**58**(3):628–33.

7. Kurahashi H, Tsutsumi M, Nishiyama S *et al.* Molecular basis of maternal age-related increase in oocyte aneuploidy. *Congenit Anom (Kyoto).* 2012;**52**(1):8–15.

8. Jones KT, Lane SI. Chromosomal, metabolic, environmental, and hormonal origins of aneuploidy in mammalian oocytes. *Exp Cell Res.* 2012;**318**(12):1394–9.

9. Khodjakov A, Pines J. Centromere tension: a divisive issue. *Nat Cell Biol.* 2010;**12**(10):919–23.

10. Sartorelli EM, Mazzucatto LF, de Pina-Neto JM. Effect of paternal age on human sperm chromosomes. *Fertil Steril.* 2001;**76**(6):1119–23.

11. Zhu JL, Madsen KM, Vestergaard M *et al.* Paternal age and congenital malformations. *Hum Reprod.* 2005;**20**(11):3173–7.

12. Wyrobek AJ, Eskenazi B, Young S *et al.* Advancing age has differential effects on DNA damage, chromatin integrity, gene mutations, and aneuploidies in sperm. *Proc Natl Acad Sci USA.* 2006;**103**(25):9601–6.

13. Hassold T, Abruzzo M, Adkins K *et al.* Human aneuploidy: incidence, origin, and etiology. *Environ Mol Mutagen.* 1996;**28**(3):167–75.

14. Tarin JJ, Brines J, Cano A. Long-term effects of delayed parenthood. *Hum Reprod.* 1998;**13**(9):2371–6.

15. Wilkin DJ, Szabo JK, Cameron R *et al.* Mutations in fibroblast growth-factor receptor 3 in sporadic cases of

achondroplasia occur exclusively on the paternally derived chromosome. *Am J Hum Genet.* 1998;**63**(3):711–16.

16. Tiemann-Boege I, Navidi W, Grewal R *et al.* The observed human sperm mutation frequency cannot explain the achondroplasia paternal age effect. *Proc Natl Acad Sci USA.* 2002;**99**(23):14,952–7.

17. Risch N, Reich EW, Wishnick MM *et al.* Spontaneous mutation and parental age in humans. *Am J Hum Genet.* 1987;**41**(2):218–48.

18. Glaser RL, Broman KW, Schulman RL *et al.* The paternal-age effect in Apert syndrome is due, in part, to the increased frequency of mutations in sperm. *Am J Hum Genet.* 2003;**73**(4):939–47.

19. Goriely A, McVean GA, Rojmyr M *et al.* Evidence for selective advantage of pathogenic FGFR2 mutations in the male germ line. *Science.* 2003;**301**(5633):643–6.

20. Moloney DM, Slaney SF, Oldridge M *et al.* Exclusive paternal origin of new mutations in Apert syndrome. *Nat Genet.* 1996;**13**(1):48–53.

21. Glaser RL, Jiang W, Boyadjiev SA *et al.* Paternal origin of FGFR2 mutations in sporadic cases of Crouzon syndrome and Pfeiffer syndrome. *Am J Hum Genet.* 2000;**66**(3):768–77.

22. Schuffenecker I, Ginet N, Goldgar D *et al.* Prevalence and parental origin of de novo RET mutations in multiple endocrine neoplasia type 2a and familial medullary thyroid carcinoma. Le groupe d'etude des tumeurs a calcitonine. *Am J Hum Genet.* 1997;**60**(1):233–7.

23. Crow JF. The origins, patterns and implications of human spontaneous mutation. *Nat Rev Genet.* 2000;**1**(1):40–7.

24. Snajderova M, Riccardi VM, Petrak B *et al.* The importance of advanced parental age in the origin of neurofibromatosis type 1. *Am J Med Genet A.* 2012;**158A**(3):519–23.

25. Lowe X, Eskenazi B, Nelson DO *et al.* Frequency of XY sperm increases with age in fathers of boys with Klinefelter syndrome. *Am J Hum Genet.* 2001;**69**(5):1046–54.

26. Goldberg YP, Kremer B, Andrew SE *et al.* Molecular analysis of new mutations for Huntington's disease: intermediate alleles and sex of origin effects. *Nat Genet.* 1993;**5**(2):174–9.

27. Farrer LA, Cupples LA, Kiely DK *et al.* Inverse relationship between age at onset of Huntington disease and paternal age suggests involvement of genetic imprinting. *Am J Hum Genet.* 1992;**50**(3):528–35.

28. Singh NP, Muller CH, Berger RE. Effects of age on DNA double-strand breaks and apoptosis in human sperm. *Fertil Steril.* 2003;**80**(6):1420–30.

29. Crow JF. Development. There's something curious about paternal-age effects. *Science.* 2003;**301**(5633):606–7.

30. Bennett-Baker PE, Wilkowski J, Burke DT. Age-associated activation of epigenetically repressed genes in the mouse. *Genetics.* 2003;**165**(4):2055–62.

31. Adkins RM, Thomas F, Tylavsky FA *et al.* Parental ages and levels of DNA methylation in the newborn are correlated. *BMC Med Genet.* 2011;**12**:47.

32. Hemminki K, Kyyronen P, Vaittinen P. Parental age as a risk factor of childhood leukemia and brain cancer in offspring. *Epidemiology.* 1999;**10**(3):271–5.

33. Murray L, McCarron P, Bailie K *et al.* Association of early life factors and acute lymphoblastic leukaemia in childhood: historical cohort study. *Br J Cancer.* 2002;**86**(3):356–61.

34. Lu Y, Ma H, Sullivan-Halley J *et al.* Parents' ages at birth and risk of adult-onset hematologic malignancies among female teachers in California. *Am J Epidemiol.* 2010;**171**(12):1262–9.

35. Yip BH, Pawitan Y, Czene K. Parental age and risk of childhood cancers: a population-based cohort study from Sweden. *Int J Epidemiol.* 2006;**35**(6):1495–503.

36. Zhang Y, Kreger BE, Dorgan JF *et al.* Parental age at child's birth and son's risk of prostate cancer. The Framingham study. *Am J Epidemiol.* 1999;**150**(11):1208–12.

37. Choi JY, Lee KM, Park SK *et al.* Association of paternal age at birth and the risk of breast cancer in offspring: a case control study. *BMC Cancer.* 2005;**5**:143.

38. Mills MB, Hudgins L, Balise RR *et al.* Mutation risk associated with paternal and maternal age in a cohort of retinoblastoma survivors. *Hum Genet.* 2012;**131**(7):1115–22.

39. Puleo CM, Reichenberg A, Smith CJ *et al.* Do autism-related personality traits explain higher paternal age in autism? *Mol Psychiatry.* 2008;**13**(3):243–4.

40. Fombonne E. The prevalence of autism. *J Am Med Assoc* 2003;**289**(1):87–9.

41. Fombonne E. The epidemiology of autism: a review. *Psychol Med.* 1999;**29**(4):769–86.

42. Reichenberg A, Gross R, Weiser M *et al.* Advancing paternal age and autism. *Arch Gen Psychiatry.* 2006;**63**(9):1026–32.

43. Puleo CM, Schmeidler J, Reichenberg A *et al.* Advancing paternal age and simplex autism. *Autism.* 2012;**16**(4):367–80.

44. Sebat J, Lakshmi B, Malhotra D *et al.* Strong association of *de novo* copy number mutations with autism. *Science.* 2007;**316**(5823):445–9.

45. Geschwind DH. Advances in autism. *Annu Rev Med.* 2009;**60**:367–80.

46. Brown AS, Schaefer CA, Wyatt RJ *et al.* Paternal age and risk of schizophrenia in adult offspring. *Am J Psychiatry.* 2002;**159**(9):1528–33.

47. Malaspina D, Harlap S, Fennig S *et al.* Advancing paternal age and the risk of schizophrenia. *Arch Gen Psychiatry.* 2001;**58**(4):361–7.

48. Sipos A, Rasmussen F, Harrison G *et al.* Paternal age and schizophrenia: a population based cohort study. *Br Med J.* 2004;**329**(7474):1070.

49. Frans EM, Sandin S, Reichenberg A *et al.* Advancing paternal age and bipolar disorder. *Arch Gen Psychiatry.* 2008;**65**(9):1034–40.

50. Saha S, Barnett AG, Foldi C *et al.* Advanced paternal age is associated with impaired neurocognitive outcomes during infancy and childhood. *PLoS Med.* 2009;**6**(3):e40.

51. Saha S, Barnett AG, Buka SL *et al.* Maternal age and paternal age are associated with distinct childhood behavioural outcomes in a general population birth cohort. *Schizophr Res.* 2009;**115**(2–3):130–5.

52. Auroux M. Decrease of learning capacity in offspring with increasing paternal age in the rat. *Teratology.* 1983;**27**(2):141–8.

53. Frans EM, McGrath JJ, Sandin S *et al.* Advanced paternal and grandpaternal age and schizophrenia: a three-generation perspective. *Schizophr Res.* 2011;**133** (1–3):120–4.

54. Tolarova MM, Harris JA, Ordway DE *et al.* Birth prevalence, mutation rate, sex ratio, parents' age, and ethnicity in Apert syndrome. *Am J Med Genet.* 1997;**72** (4):394–8.

55. Jones KL, Smith DW, Harvey MA *et al.* Older paternal age and fresh gene mutation: data on additional disorders. *J Pediatr.* 1975;**86**(1):84–8.

56. Olshan AF, Schnitzer PG, Baird PA. Paternal age and the risk of congenital heart defects. *Teratology.* 1994;**50** (1):80–4.

57. Harville EW, Wilcox AJ, Lie RT *et al.* Epidemiology of cleft palate alone and cleft palate with accompanying defects. *Eur J Epidemiol.* 2007;**22**(6):389–95.

58. Overhauser J, McMahon J, Oberlender S *et al.* Parental origin of chromosome 5 deletions in the Cri-du-chat syndrome. *Am J Med Genet.* 1990;**37**(1):83–6.

59. Bucher K, Ionasescu V, Hanson J. Frequency of new mutants among boys with Duchenne muscular dystrophy. *Am J Med Genet.* 1980;**7**(1):27–34.

60. Murdoch JL, Walker BA, McKusick VA. Parental age effects on the occurrence of new mutations for the Marfan syndrome. *Ann Hum Genet.* 1972;**35**(3):331–6.

61. Mulligan LM, Eng C, Healey CS *et al.* A de novo mutation of the RET proto-oncogene in a patient with men 2a. *Hum Mol Genet.* 1994;**3**(6):1007–8.

62. Carlson KM, Bracamontes J, Jackson CE *et al.* Parent-of-origin effects in multiple endocrine neoplasia type 2b. *Am J Hum Genet.* 1994;**55**(6):1076–82.

63. Kluwe L, Mautner V, Parry DM *et al.* The parental origin of new mutations in neurofibromatosis 2. *Neurogenetics.* 2000;**3**(1):17–24.

64. Young ID, Thompson EM, Hall CM *et al.* Osteogenesis imperfecta type IIA: evidence for dominant inheritance. *J Med Genet.* 1987;**24**(7):386–9.

65. Eriksson M, Brown WT, Gordon LB *et al.* Recurrent de novo point mutations in lamin A cause Hutchinson-Gilford progeria syndrome. *Nature.* 2003;**423**(6937):293–8.

66. Kaplan J, Bonneau D, Frezal J *et al.* Clinical and genetic heterogeneity in retinitis pigmentosa. *Hum Genet.* 1990;**85**(6):635–42.

67. Wirth B, Schmidt T, Hahnen E *et al.* De novo rearrangements found in 2% of index patients with spinal muscular atrophy: mutational mechanisms, parental origin, mutation rate, and implications for genetic counseling. *Am J Hum Genet.* 1997;**61** (5):1102–11.

68. Lian ZH, Zack MM, Erickson JD. Paternal age and the occurrence of birth defects. *Am J Hum Genet.* 1986;**39** (5):648–60.

69. Martinez-Frias ML, Ramos-Arroyo MA, Salvador J. Thanatophoric dysplasia: an autosomal dominant condition? *Am J Med Genet.* 1988;**31**(4):815–20.

70. Splendore A, Jabs EW, Felix TM *et al.* Parental origin of mutations in sporadic cases of Treacher Collins syndrome. *Eur J Hum Genet.* 2003;**11**(9):718–22.

71. Lu JH, Chung MY, Hwang B *et al.* Prevalence and parental origin in tetralogy of Fallot associated with chromosome 22q11 microdeletion. *Pediatrics.* 1999;**104** (1 Pt 1):87–90.

72. Olson JM, Breslow NE, Beckwith JB. Wilms' tumour and parental age: a report from the National Wilms' Tumour Study. *Br J Cancer.* 1993;**67**(4):813–18.

73. Bertram L, Busch R, Spiegl M *et al.* Paternal age is a risk factor for Alzheimer disease in the absence of a major gene. *Neurogenetics.* 1998;**1**(4):277–80.

74. Jayasekara R, Street J. Parental age and parity in dyslexic boys. *J Biosoc Sci.* 1978;**10**(3):255–61.

75. Amir RE, Zoghbi HY. Rett syndrome: methyl-CpG-binding protein 2 mutations and phenotype-genotype correlations. *Am J Med Genet.* 2000;**97**(2):147–52.

Sexual function in the aging male

John R. Gannon, Jeremy B. Myers, and William O. Brant

Introduction

As the population of the world and the western hemisphere ages, naturally the male population ages and therefore the number of men with sexual dysfunction continues to rise. According to the World Health Organization (WHO), as of 2000, the number of people worldwide older than 60 years of age was 700 million. This number is projected to rise to 2 billion people by 2050. Since many of the risk factors for sexual dysfunction are age-related processes, the growing aging population will lead to yet higher numbers of patients with sexual dysfunction. This increasing incidence, along with both the introduction of effective treatments for sexual dysfunction and the more open dialogue engendered between patients and their healthcare providers, has made the subject of sexual dysfunction – once relatively taboo – very commonplace. A simple example of this is the ubiquity of advertisement campaigns for the oral phosphodiesterase inhibitors (PDE-5) as well as for untested and unproven "male supplements" promising a litany of benefits.

Currently 50% of men older than 50 in the US population have underlying sexual dysfunction, based upon the Massachusetts Male Aging Study [1]. This study demonstrated a linear increase in erectile dysfunction, with approximately a 10% increase in prevalence with each increase in decade of life [2]. A similar study from Western Australia [3] found greater than 49% of men had sexual dysfunction after the age of 40. How best to address it as healthcare providers and partners will be an increasingly common question. To appropriately address and treat underlying sexual dysfunction, a multifaceted approach will become the norm. Social circumstances and medical comorbidities will continue to be factors that cannot simply be addressed haphazardly.

Sexual function is often a reflection and barometer of overall health. It combines elements of cardiovascular, neurologic, psychological, and endocrine health. Entering into this mix are libido, social factors, a willing partner, and the physical ability to be sexually active. Sexuality and sexual activity are not limited solely to a sexual act, and it is unfair to define the sexual function of patients based on this limited scope. However, the act and ability to be sexually active plays a central role in sexual health and function in an aging male population.

It also is important that we do not underestimate the importance of erectile and sexual function to a patient's quality of life. The treatments for common medical conditions in the aging male such as hypertension, depression, benign prostatic hyperplasia, and prostate cancer have all been linked to causes of sexual dysfunction. The causes of sexual dysfunction are varied and range from cancer, disability, hypertension to vascular disease. The cause of dysfunction also includes the treatment for other conditions, which are also rising in prevalence as the population ages. The side effects of surgery or medications play a potentially unfortunate but necessary role in an aging population.

Cardiovascular health has been an important factor and a driving force behind many health-related campaigns in the last few decades. Hypertension, diabetes, and end-organ effects of atherosclerosis are significant factors relating to male sexual health. The impacts of these diseases are not the only thing we should all consider in approaching the treatment of male sexual dysfunction. Common therapies such as PDE-5 or vasoactive injection therapy may not be healthy or safe in patients with severe cardiovascular compromise. Prior to treatment of sexual health we need to consider the safety of treating the patient. The

Paternal Influences on Human Reproductive Success, ed. Douglas T. Carrell. Published by Cambridge University Press.
© Cambridge University Press 2013.

consequence of each of these diseases may also lead to severe disability following a heart attack or stroke, having an obvious impact on sexual health and abilities. The incidence of each of these diseases has continued to rise in western populations.

Causes of sexual dysfunction

Cardiovascular health

Approximately 28% of patients greater than 40 years of age in the USA have been diagnosed with hypertension [4]. Hypertension is a vascular disease which causes end-organ effects. It increases the rate of ischemic cardiac disease and renal failure. The root causes of hypertension vary from genetic predisposition, obesity, and other health-related illnesses. Obesity, elevated body mass index, poor diet, and lack of exercise may all contribute to the onset of hypertension as well as concomitant erectile dysfunction.

The treatment of hypertension may cause or contribute to sexual dysfunction. Treatment of hypertension may worsen sexual dysfunction, through direct side effects of the drug interaction. Common first-line medications for hypertension such as non-specific beta-blockers and thiazide diuretics have been especially linked with erectile and sexual dysfunction in several well-controlled studies [5, 6]. In animal studies, propranolol was shown to have peripheral effects increasing the latency for ejaculation, latency to initiate erections, and a reduced number of erectile reflexes [6]. More recent contemporary beta-blocker generations have been shown to be more cardioselective with lower rates of erectile dysfunction. Other commonly utilized antihypertensive agents like angiotension receptor blockers and calcium channel blockers may have less deleterious effects on erections (however, the latter has occasionally been linked to elevated prolactin levels) [5].

In contrast to this early data, a recent study in the cardiology literature has questioned the direct link of antihypertensive therapy and erectile dysfunction that has long been held. In an Italian study in 2003, it was shown that side effects, including erectile dysfunction, in patients on beta-blocker therapy were caused by anxiety, which was felt to be the larger cause of erectile dysfunction than the direct side effects of the medications [7].

In addition to hypertension and its treatment other important factors influencing erectile and sexual function are hyperlipidemia and atherosclerosis. Both these factors have been linked to increasing mortality and morbidity in the aging population. Arterial and venous dysfunction associated with these illnesses stem primarily from plaque formation. Men with cardiovascular disease have been found to have increased rates and earlier incidence of erectile dysfunction. In fact, some view erectile dysfunction as an early harbinger of cardiovascular disease and atherosclerosis [8]. Vascular endothelial health is related to serum nitric oxide (NO) levels. A decrease in NO levels has been associated with coronary artery disease, atherosclerosis, and other vascular diseases [8]. Early work and elucidation of the findings related to NO led to a Nobel prize in 1998 and ultimately the development of PDE-5 inhibitors, the action of which are discussed below.

Nitric oxide supports vascular health by inhibiting platelet aggregation. It additionally prevents adhesion of platelets and inflammatory cells to vascular endothelial lining, helping to prevent or slow atherosclerotic plaque. It lowers vascular muscle tone, allowing vasodilation and works to scavenge free radicals [9]. Not surprisingly, obesity, lack of physical activity, and smoking have each been linked to a decrease in NO levels and increase in vascular disease [8].

Social factors

Smoking and alcohol use each have been studied regarding their effects upon sexual function, and have been linked to erectile dysfunction [10]. Heavy smoking has been linked with vasoconstriction and cardiovascular disease. Alcohol interestingly, but perhaps not surprisingly, has been linked to improved erectile function and libido at low concentrations; however at higher concentrations and with prolonged use this beneficial effect diminishes [11]. In Shakespeare's Macbeth act 2, scene 3, the Porter states to Macduff, "What . . . does drink especially provoke . . . lechery, sir, it provokes, and unprovokes; it provokes the desire, but it takes away the performance."

This observation has been borne out clinically, with smaller amounts of alcohol causing vasodilation and loss of inhibition, whereas larger amounts cause central nervous system depression. Heavy alcohol use and abuse has been linked to erectile dysfunction and delayed ejaculation [11]. A study in 2010 showed decreased penile arterial peak systolic velocity, measured on duplex ultrasound in subjects with moderate to severe alcohol consumption [12]. Additionally, heavy or prolonged alcohol use can cause liver dysfunction and result in elevation of estrogens and decreasing testosterone levels, further compounding erectile and sexual dysfunction [11]. Somewhat contradictory, moderate alcohol consumption has been shown to be cardio-protective [13]. Alcohol may well decrease anxiety and even in moderate amounts decrease the risk of cardiovascular disease, however despite provoking desire it is clearly linked to loss of cardiovascular and erectile health [12, 13].

Diabetes

Diabetes is a rising pandemic. Both type I and type II diabetes have been linked to sexual dysfunction. The rate of type II diabetes is rising in dramatic fashion worldwide. The impact on healthcare and the treatment of this disease will play an important role in the treatment of the aging male and sexual dysfunction. Its effects on end organs such as the retina, the kidney, and peripheral nervous system are well documented. Erectile dysfunction is a very common side effect of diabetes, and approximately 10% of men who present with erectile dysfunction are found to have previously undiagnosed diabetes [14]. The prevalence of diabetes reported in 2010 was 10.9 million, or nearly 27% of US residents greater than 65 years. The rate of erectile dysfunction is more than double in diabetic men; and worsens with aging. Some studies have cited greater than 90% of erectile dysfunction in diabetic men over 65 years of age [15]. Diabetic males have higher rates of peripheral vascular disease and coronary artery disease, which are each risk factors independent of diabetes for sexual and erectile dysfunction [7, 16].

Diabetes likely causes sexual dysfunction through varied pathophysiologies. Diabetes can cause peripheral nerve injury which may lead to decreasing sensation associated with sexual stimuli and activity, as well as worsened orgasmic function and sensation. Additionally, endothelial dysfunction and atherosclerotic lesions are noted in both larger vessels such as the pudendal artery and smaller peripheral vessels. Penile arterial insufficiency was documented in diabetic men on duplex ultrasound with reduction in arterial waveflow and volume [17].

On the biochemical level, there is reduced activity of NO, and reduced smooth muscle relaxation. Structurally, increased collagen deposition in cavernosal

tissues is seen as part of the long-term changes associated with diabetes [18, 19]. Increased collagen content leads to fibrotic changes and decreasing erectile health, leading to long-term erectile dysfunction that is particularly difficult to treat [19].

Diabetes has also been linked to hypogonadism. Hypogonadism in diabetic men may be caused by the presence of peripheral aromatase action associated with obesity, which is highly prevalent in type II diabetics. Aromatase acts to enzymatically convert testosterone to estrogen, which is a strong feedback inhibitor of the hypothalamic-pituitary axis. Although the link between hypogonadism and erectile dysfunction is complex (see below), a eugonadal state is certainly helpful for successful treatment of sexual dysfunction and erectile dysfunction. Hypogonadism is associated with diminution of sexual desire, compounding sexual dysfunction in the setting of erectile dysfunction [20].

Prostate cancer

The incidence of prostate cancer is well documented to rise with age. In 2008 prostate cancer was diagnosed in nearly 900,000 men worldwide, with an estimated 258,000 prostate cancer-related deaths. While the rate of prostate cancer mortality is declining, recently 22.8 per 100,000 in 2008 according to the surveillance epidemiology and end results, SEER database, the number of men seeking treatment of prostate cancer is stable or rising. Sexual function and the side effects of treatment of this disease are at the heart of a current and heated debate regarding prostate cancer. Although the actual rate of erectile dysfunction after surgical treatment of prostate cancer is controversial and depends upon surgeon or patient definitions of sexual dysfunction the improvements in our understanding of pelvic anatomy, surgical techniques, and technological advances have decreased surgical ED from rates of nearly 100% to nearly 30% [21]. Nearly all modern treatments for prostate cancer, regardless of their approach and despite their success at cancer control, cause a decline of sexual function. This decline may be a result of direct damage to the cavernous neurovascular bundle, even in "nerve-sparing" approaches in surgical or radiation therapy. Other causes may include arterial injury or structural changes leading to "venous leak" during erection.

Surgical and radiation therapies may also cause difficulties with urinary control, postoperative pain, or decreasing desire on the part of the male. Many current studies seek to show our improved outcomes from surgery using expanded prostate cancer index composite scores with minimal decline in the postoperative period when compared with the patient's preoperative course [21]. Despite our aggressive efforts to minimize sexual impact, patients are not reporting an increase in their sexual function following modern interventions. Additionally, patients may receive misleading information and expect to have improved outcomes compared with older treatments for prostate cancer with techniques such as robotically assisted prostatectomies, despite a lack of evidence to support this view [22].

Sexual dysfunction in patients treated for prostate cancer is not limited to erectile dysfunction from nerve injury. Other causes of sexual dysfunction include loss of urine with climax (climaturia), decreased libido, decreased penile length, and dyspareunia.

Surgical reconstruction of the bladder neck during radical prostatectomy, via either an open or laparoscopic approach, is associated with urinary incontinence in the postoperative period. The methods used to measure post-prostatectomy continence and urinary function varied markedly in the past, and more recent efforts have been made to uniformly report this data. While the rate of postoperative incontinence has generally declined, from up to 80% to somewhere roughly between 10% and 40%, the number of patients with lower urinary tract symptoms is still significant [23]. The rate of urinary incontinence associated with orgasm is approximately 20% regardless of surgical approach. Climaturia has led to a lower rate of sexual satisfaction post-prostatectomy [23]. In addition to climaturia, prostatectomy has been found to lead to decreased penile length. In one study, up to 71% of patients after prostatectomy had a decrease in penile length. Of these patients 48% had a decrease up to or greater than 1 cm in both stretched and flaccid penile length [24]. This may contribute to patient anxiety, declining libido and sexual dissatisfaction. This combination of structural changes, possible neurovascular bundle injuries, as well as changing patient expectations have profound long-term effects regarding sexual function in the aging male who has been treated for prostate cancer.

Prostate cancer alone is not the sole cancer diagnosis or the sole source of cancer treatment which may cause erectile and/or sexual dysfunction. Surgical resection of colorectal cancers, systemic chemotherapy and other cancer-related treatments have all been linked to declining sexual function from direct causes and damage to erectile mechanisms. Indirect causes such as anxiety and depression associated with cancer diagnosis have a dramatic health and psychosocial impact. The components of anxiety and depression associated with the diagnosis of cancer additionally cause erectile dysfunction. Other procedures with high rates of erectile dysfunction include abdominal-perineal resection for colorectal cancer, retroperitoneal lymph node dissection, pelvic mass resection, as well as surgery for aortic aneurysm and other surgeries that may disturb the delicate neural pathways required for sexual function.

Benign prostate disease

The prostate's relation to sexual and erectile dysfunction is not limited to the treatment of prostate cancer. Medications for the treatment of benign prostatic hyperplasia, as well as the underlying disease process may have a role in a decline in sexual function. The frequency of transurethral resections of the prostate (TURPs) for an enlarged prostate has declined in recent years. The decline of TURPs is due to other common treatments that have become increasingly frequent such as alpha-blocker therapy with terazosin or tamsulosin, or 5 alpha reductase (5AR) treatment with finasteride or dutasteride.

There is an increasing awareness of common pathophysiology in lower urinary tract symptoms (LUTS) and ED [25]. In a recent large study of men undergoing prostate cancer screening there was a correlation between ED and LUTS attributable to benign prostatic hyperplasia [26]. This relationship is reflected in the recent FDA approval of tadalafil, a PDE-5 inhibitor commonly used in ED, as a first-line treatment for LUTS [27]. There are some other factors that are important to consider in relation to the medical treatment of benign prostatic hyperplasia and sexual function. Alpha-blockers improve urinary flow by causing relaxation of the prostatic urethra's muscle layer; they also cause relaxation of the bladder neck. As a result of this, one of the most common side effects of these medications is retrograde ejaculation, which can cause a variable degree of bother with sexual function in men. In addition, 5AR medications decrease the conversion of testosterone to dihydrotestosterone and have been linked with sexual dysfunction and decreased libido, although the mechanism for this decrease remains unclear [28].

Other benign disorders of the prostate that can lead to sexual dysfunction can include chronic pelvic or perineal pain related to prostatitis, orchalgia, and interstitial cystitis. All these problems may cause pain, resulting in erectile or ejaculatory dysfunction. These conditions are commonly linked to chronic inflammation, which may worsen with sexual activity. Additionally they may result in depression and loss of interest in sexual activity, further compounding sexual dysfunction in the aging male [29].

Low testosterone

Hypogonadism is a common ailment in the aging male. Based upon the Massachusetts Male Aging Study, the prevalence in 2004 of hypogonadism was approximately 12.3 per 1000 person years [30]. Another study examining men presenting to their primary care physician's office estimated that the rate of hypogonadism (testosterone levels <300 ng/dL) identified the prevalence at 38.7% [20]. Decline in testosterone production is likely a result of both central and peripheral effects. The exact mechanism of this decline is not completely understood, however it seems to have both a primary (testicular) and central (hypothalamic-pituitary) cause. The number of Leydig cells within the testis decreases in older men. The remaining cells secrete less testosterone during gonadotropin and luteinizing hormone stimulation, resulting in lower serum testosterone. Central production and stimulation occurs within the pituitary. In animal studies, aging males have shown a decrease in the release of gonadotropins, causing secondary decline in testosterone levels [30]. Therefore both peripheral and central factors play a role in the decline of testosterone production.

Testosterone has a multitude of roles in the aging male. Hypogonadism is associated with hyperglycemia, high triglycerides, obesity, and elevated BMI. It has been shown that appropriate treatment with testosterone may improve these conditions [20, 31]. Each of these conditions may be linked to sexual and erectile dysfunction from medical comorbidities independent of testosterone alone.

Men with low testosterone levels frequently experience decreased libido, or hypoactive sexual desire. Low testosterone has been additionally linked to erectile

dysfunction not caused only by a hypoactive desire but rather a failure of the NO mechanism associated with vasodilation and tumescence. Testosterone may be used with supplemental medication such as PDE 5 inhibitors, intercavernosal injection therapy, or urethral suppositories. The success rates of each of these modalities improve in a eugonadal state [31, 32]. Treatment with testosterone, when appropriate, will decrease the rates of metabolic syndrome, cardiovascular incidents, and diabetes. All of these will improve overall health and subsequently sexual health [31].

Fortunately the treatment of the hypogonadal male has become increasingly common. Low testosterone may be treated with a variety of formulations including oral, transdermal patches, topical gels, and intramuscular injections or depots. Other testosterone supplementations include dihydrotestosterone and DHEA, although literature supporting the use of these latter supplements is lacking. Testosterone treatment may boost energy levels and libido and has been shown to decrease osteoporosis rates and increase muscle mass, all positive effects in an aging male population [20]. These positives unfortunately come with numerous possible side effects which must be monitored for and may dissuade a physician from choosing this treatment, such as potential for worsened cardiovascular indices like lipids, fluid retention, polycythemia, and obstructive sleep apnea [33].

In younger males a primary concern is that use of exogenous testosterone suppresses luteinizing and follicle-stimulating hormones leading to decreased spermatogenesis and infertility. Understanding this relationship is very important in treating men seeking fertility with associated sexual or erectile problems, since testosterone therapy will result in a decline in fertility. For patients who are still seeking fertility, there are alternative agents which should be used, such as clomiphene citrate which stimulates a rise in endogenous testosterone production and does not interfere with spermatogenesis.

In older patients testosterone supplementation may cause gynecomastia, erythrocytosis, sleep apnea, and cardiovascular events [32]. These side effects should be considered in each individual patient, and serial examination and laboratory tests can help to prevent and identify some of these issues early on. Testosterone treatment will continue to grow by both subspecialist and primary care providers. As a result of continued use of this medication we must work to use this medication in an effective and safe manner to treat hypogonadism and possibly gain secondary benefits for our patients.

Associated conditions

Medical conditions such as liver or renal failure, thyroid and other endocrine abnormalities each play a role in erectile dysfunction. Elderly men in renal failure have elevated erectile dysfunction rates. Chronic disease, elevation of prolactin levels, systemic uremia, and decreased testosterone levels are all associated with chronic renal disease and hemodialysis [16, 18, 19].

Suppression of the hypothalamic-pituitary axis responsible for the release of luteinizing hormone and follicle-stimulating hormone by GnRH have dramatic impacts on sexual function through decreasing testosterone levels. Central endocrine dysfunction from tumor, pituitary failure, or other reasons may have dramatic secondary impacts on a patient's global health as well as sexual function.

Hyperprolactinemia can be caused by tumor or pharmaceutical treatments. Hyperprolactinemia inhibits the release of GnRH from the pituitary, which results in a decline in central stimulation and peripheral testosterone production. In addition to decreased testosterone, hyperprolactinemia has been linked to gynecomastia, infertility, and erectile dysfunction. Hyperthyroidism has been linked to decreasing libido in older men. Hypothyroidism causes an increased prolactin level. Each of these chronic and systemic diseases is linked to erectile dysfunction beyond their pathologic mechanisms. Each has additionally been linked to anxiety, depression and their respective impacts on sexual function [16, 19].

Disability and psychological aspects

Sexual function is a physical activity. Some underlying disorders with an increased prevalence in the aging population such as cerebral vascular accidents, multiple sclerosis, or other neuropathies may decrease a patient's ability to be sexually active. Sexual dysfunction may result from decreased tactile sensation and stimulation leading to erectile dysfunction, as mentioned earlier with diabetes [19]. Sexual dysfunction may additionally arise from the patient's deteriorated physical state and inability to be mobile enough to be sexually active. Parkinson's disease, stroke, or other neurologic conditions all have increasing incidence with increasing age and related sexual dysfunction secondary to physical disability.

There are many psychological aspects associated with sexual function. Included among these are depression, psychogenic erectile dysfunction, and loss of libido [34]. These are complicated and can be difficult for clinicians to diagnose and treat. They are part of a complex interplay of health and social factors and are at the very heart of sexual function and well-being.

Depression is a common problem in the aging population. The disease and its treatments each may cause erectile and other sexual dysfunction. The Massachusetts Male Aging Study found that the probability of erectile dysfunction in subjects with the most severe depression was approximately 90%, with rates declining in less depressed groups [34]. According to a US Surgeon General Report in 1997 anywhere between 10–30% of the elderly population may suffer from major or minor depressive disorders.

The treatment of depression is ironically linked to erectile dysfunction as well, creating a difficult balancing act with the treatment of the disease and minimizing side effects. Tricyclic antidepressants, one of the most common mainstays for treatment over the past century, have peripheral anticholinergic and beta-adrenergic effects which have been linked to ejaculatory disorders and declining erectile function [35]. Selective serotonin reuptake inhibitors (SSRIs) have been linked with dramatic changes in sexual function including inhibitory effects on erectile reflexes in the peripheral nervous system. In addition, a very common side effect of SSRIs is their known link to anorgasmia [35].

The rates of sexual dysfunction vary depending on the type of medication being used. Atypical agents such as bupropion have been found to have the lowest rates of sexual dysfunction at therapeutic dosing. Approximately 22% of patients had significant sexual dysfunction on bupropion. More typical and older-generation agents such as many SSRIs were linked to sexual dysfunction in 36–43% of patients [35]. The newer generations of antidepressants with mixed receptor blockades have been linked to lower rates of sexual dysfunction and, while the studies are limited, they may in fact be linked to improvement of sexual function in some patients with the overall benefit of declining depression outweighing the side effects of the medication upon sexual function.

While the role of sexual medicine specialists is unlikely to include the initial treatment and evaluation of a patient diagnosed with depression, it is important to be aware of the effects of treatment and the common side effects of these medications. It has been estimated that nearly 50% of the population will suffer from an episode of significant depression in their lifetime [35]. It is important that we attempt to address this issue with the appropriate care and referral for specialized care. Psychogenic erectile dysfunction has long been heralded as a common cause of sexual dysfunction. Many studies have attempted to propose the precise mechanism; however both erectile function and desire are controlled by the central nervous system, more specifically the cerebral cortex, limbic, and hypothalamus. Excitatory potentials as well as inhibitory potentials traveling along these pathways may facilitate inhibitory spinal and erectile reflexes. Whatever etiology may be causing this psychogenic effect – depression, social difficulties with a partner, side effects of cancer treatment – inhibitory messages may further compound sexual dysfunction [28].

Dementia is more common in older men, as are rates of schizophrenia, Parkinson's, and Alzheimer's disease. These illnesses alone are disabling and may pose significant barriers to sexual function. Outside of the burden of disease, treatment of these conditions varies widely and, similar to antidepressant medications, may also cause erectile dysfunction. Antipsychotics may cause extrapyramidal effects and an increase in serum prolactin levels, suppressing central gonadotropin release and stimulation [28]. Generalizing the side effects of antipsychotics is very difficult as the mechanism of action, targeted receptors, metabolites, and side effects vary widely with each drug. These conditions call for specialized care beyond the scope of this chapter. It is important however to be knowledgeable of the possible consequences of treatment and illness as we work to address sexual function in the aging male population.

Treating erectile and sexual dysfunction

Given the recent advances in both medical and surgical interventions for erectile and sexual dysfunction, focus on treating the disease has markedly increased. This increase has mirrored the rise in aggressively advertised –albeit unproven - supplements.

The first line of therapy in the treatment of sexual dysfunction in the aging male is always an attempt to reverse medical causes. Smoking cessation, moderation of alcohol use, daily exercise, and a healthy diet can help prevent and alleviate underlying sexual dysfunction [8, 12, 13]. These actions will decrease the rate or degree of hypertension, hyperlipidemia, atherosclerosis, diabetes, and other conditions mentioned above. Other non-medical therapies for erectile and sexual dysfunction include pelvic floor exercises and psychosexual therapy. Sexual therapy may be beneficial in identifying cognitive behaviors that are contributing to or compounding sexual dysfunction in the aging male. This may, of course, be most effective as a part of the larger treatment plan, or if the treating physician has a high suspicion for psychogenic sexual dysfunction [19, 30].

Admittedly, some of the treatments as discussed above can further compound sexual dysfunction (e.g. the use of antihypertensives to treat hypertension) but alterations and adjustments may ultimately help minimize the medical side effects while still obtaining the desired treatment goal. Changing medications should ideally occur when the side effect is first noted [35].

Medical therapies

Medical therapy may start with alleviating conditions such as treating hyperglycemia, hypogonadism, or other endocrine imbalances. Appropriate use of medications to treat reversible conditions, such as statins for hyperlipidemia, will have a positive impact regarding overall and sexual health. Generally the treatment of many of these causes will not be handled by a specialist in sexual health. They will frequently be started, or solely addressed, by a general internist or family practice physician, who may not be versed in the complex interplay between global health and sexual health in the aging male. As with many aspects of medicine a clear team approach by the physicians and the patient will be the most effective at identifying reversible causes and improving health.

As discussed earlier, low testosterone may be treated with a variety of formulations including oral, transdermal patches, topical gels, and intramuscular injections or depots. The recognition and treatment of this disorder has risen in recent years and will continue to be an important and evolving diagnosis for clinicians. Treatment may improve libido and sexual drive, as well as allow for optimal use of pharmacologic agents for ED.

The most widely employed agents in the treatment of ED are PDE-5s. Included in these agents are Viagra (sildenafil), Levitra (vardenafil), and Cialis (tadalafil). These agents do not directly cause erections. Their actions are primarily to block the conversion of cyclic guanosine monophosphate (cGMP) and thereby potentiate calcium-mediated smooth muscle relaxation in the corpus cavernosa. This allows NO-mediated vasodilation and tumescence of the corporal bodies.

PDE-5 inhibitors are recognized as a common and safe treatment of erectile dysfunction. More than 30 million doses have been consumed since the initial debut of Viagra in 1998 [9, 32]. Improvement in erectile function has been noted with large randomized studies even in difficult-to-treat populations such as post-prostatectomy and diabetics [36]. No head-to-head study has been conducted comparing these agents, but overall their efficacies are similar, with studies demonstrating improvement in erections in at least 70% of men, although certain populations (such as men with diabetes or those who have undergone prostatectomy) do not respond as well [37].

PDE-5 agents do have a number of side effects and contraindications, which must be weighed in the elderly male population. A direct contraindication for any PDE-5 inhibitor use is the use of nitrates for chest pain, severe hypotension, a history of uncontrolled arrhythmias, recent myocardial infarction, or stroke. Cardiovascular assessment may be needed for patients prior to use of these medications. Other common side effects include headaches, visual disturbances, and flushing. To date a very small percentage of patients have developed non-arteritic anterior ischemic optic neuropathy (NAION), which is a loss of vision related to ischemic damage to the optic nerve, but the relationship between NAION and PDE-5 use is controversial [38]. According to multiple recent studies, 25–30% of men attempting PDE-5 inhibitors will ultimately have an inadequate reaction. These are the patients who will benefit from the second- and third-line medical therapies [39].

Intraurethral suppository, commonly called MUSE, is a second-line medical therapy, which is administered by placing a small suppository about the size of a grain of rice within the meatus. Alprostadil, a synthetic prostaglandin E1, causes smooth muscle relaxation and vasodilation by raising the levels of cyclic AMP within the cells. This vasodilation, similar to the PDE-5 inhibitors, promotes tumescence of the erectile bodies. The medication is absorbed via urothelial tissue within the urethra, which allows diffusion of the medication into corpus spongiosal tissue. Absorption into the spongiosal tissue allows for transportation to the corpus cavernosal tissue and erectile response. The rate of successful office response to this medication is approximately 30–60% although successful home use is somewhat lower. The most common side effects of this medication are penile pain, hypotension, and syncope. The rates of penile pain are directly related to the dosing of MUSE therapy [40].

Vacuum constriction devices (VCDs) are another commonly used adjunct to treat sexual dysfunction. The device works by negative pressure, causing engorgement of the penis. The artificial erection created by this device is maintained by a ring constriction device. This ring should be left in place for 30 minutes or less. The portion of the penis proximal to the ring does not engorge, and therefore there may be a "pivoting" effect with erectile instability. The erection obtained with this device does engorge the glans as well and may be used with other supplemental devices such as PDE-5 inhibitors or urethral suppositories. Side effects of this therapy include penile pain, ecchymosis, and numbness. Care should be taken by men on anticoagulant therapy. Barriers to VCD use include penile hinging, pain, discoloration, and the lack of spontaneity accompanying the need to place the device. As a result, long-term acceptance rates are disappointing. In a retrospective study 20% of people rejected the device primarily after an initial trial, 30% after a period of 16 weeks, with an additional 7% rejecting the device within the first year [41].

Another line of medical therapy is intracavernous injection therapy. This therapy was first introduced in 1983. Injections have been carried out with a variety of agents. The injections may consist of monotherapy (such as papaverine or PGE-1) or in combination (such as "trimix," a combination of papaverine, phentolamine, and PGE-1). Papaverine acts to inhibit phosphodiesterase. This increases the levels of cyclic GMP causing relaxation of the cavernosal smooth muscle. Phentolamine is an alpha-adrenoreceptor antagonist. Phentolamine works by blocking adrenoreceptors; this prevents sinusoidal relaxation and thus prolongs engorgement and erections. Alprostadil, described above in the section on urethral suppositories, is also commonly used.

Table 11.1 Common treatments and dosing for the aging male.

Medical therapy	Agent	Dosing	Notes
Testosterone	Intramuscular; transdermal gel; buccal; subQ implant patch	50–400 mg every 1–4 weeks 5–10 mg every 24 hours 30 mg every 12 hours 150–750 mg every 3–6 months 2.5–10 mg (depending on manufacturer)	Injected into large muscle; apply to dry skin, do not shower for 6 hours, do not apply to genitals; alternate side of mouth used; generally implanted in gluteal region, alternate site of patch daily, may cause rash
PDE-5 inhibitors	Viagra (sildenafil) Levitra (vardenafil) Cialis (tadalafil)	50 mg (range 25–100 mg) 10 mg (5–20 mg) 10 mg (5–20 mg)	Generally recommended to be taken on empty stomach, absorption unaffected by food
Intraurethral suppository	alprostadil (MUSE)	125, 250, 500, 1,000 µg	First dose should be administered under supervision Do NOT use if female partner may be pregnant unless condom is used
Intracavernosal injection therapy	papaverine alprostadil bimix (papaverine + phentolamine) trimix (papaverine + phentolamine + alprostadil)	7.5–60 mg 1–60 µg 0.1–1.0 mL 0.1–1.0 mL	May cause fibrous and priapism, common complaint of painful erection, requires refrigeration May cause fibrous and priapism, requires refrigeration

Common combinations are termed bimix (papaverine and phentolamine) as well as trimix (papaverine, phentolamine, and alprostadil) for intracavernosal injections (Table 11.1). Combination medications have been found to be as or more effective than monotherapy with alprostadil, with success rates in greater than 70% of patients and lower rates of penile pain, a common side effect in higher doses required for using a single agent. The ultimate goal of therapy is to obtain an erection sufficient for sexual activity while avoiding major side effects [39, 42].

The primary side effects of injection therapy include fibrosis, pain at the injection site, hematoma, fibrosis, and priapism. Fibrosis may occur as a solitary nodule, plaque, or ultimate curvature of the penis [19, 42]. Priapism rates vary depending on which treatment is being used. Initial injections should be carried out in the doctor's office, to appropriately assess dosing, while also ensuring detumescence and hopefully decreasing the rate or frequency of priapism. Despite injection therapy's efficacy, it has been estimated that the compliance rate with continued injection therapy is only approximately 50% or lower [43]. Respondents discontinued therapy because they felt it was unnatural, dissatisfaction with the process, or they were not having an appropriate erectile response [42].

However, satisfaction is high in those who continue to use injection therapy and should still be considered a very viable second-line option [43]. Contraindications for this therapy include blood dyscrasias, like hemophilia. Anticoagulants are not a contraindication to injection therapy, however this should be taken into consideration and these patients should be advised to hold pressure on the injection site.

Surgical therapy

The above therapies are all effective. However when they fail, either secondary to poor erectile response or discontinuation of therapy, there are surgical options for the repair and treatment of erectile dysfunction. Considering surgical options should not be taken lightly, and should be for patients who have failed other interventions. There are multiple devices that are currently used for penile prosthetic surgery. They come in the form of self-contained inflatable devices or semi-rigid malleable devices (Figure 11.1). The basic design of these devices is that inflatable cylinders occupy the corporal cavernosal spaces, thus replacing the role of the non-functional corpus cavernosal tissue. A pump in the scrotum is used to transfer saline from a reservoir, typically located in the pelvis, adjacent to the

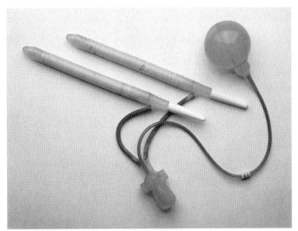

A. AMS 700, 3 piece device

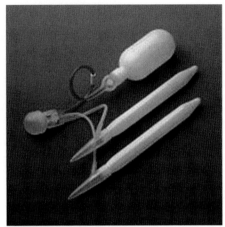

B. Coloplast Titan, 3 piece device

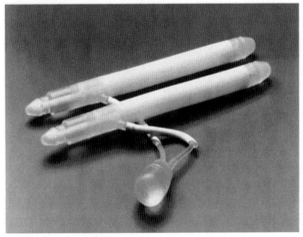

C. AMS Ambicor, 2 piece device

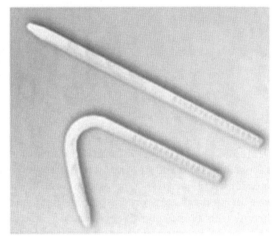

D. AMS Spectra, malleable device

Figure 11.1. IMAGES of Coloplast and AMS penile prosthetics. (A) AMS 700, 3 piece device. Image courtesy of American Medical Systems. (B) Coloplast Titan, 3 piece device. Image courtesy of Coloplast. (C) AMS Ambicor, 2 piece device. Image courtesy of American Medical Systems. (D) AMS Spectra, malleable device. Image courtesy of American Medical Systems.

bladder, into the cylinders. A deflation mechanism reverses the process. Rare risks of implantation include urethral injury during implantation, erosion of the device, improper sizing, pump complications, or auto-inflation. The most serious concerns are perioperative risks associated with a general anesthetic as well as infection of the implanted device. Infections may cause removal and loss of the implanted device as well as severe systemic illness [44]. These devices have continued to evolve over the years, as research has continued with efforts attempting to prevent device infection. The devices may now be impregnated with an antibiotic coating, helping to prevent the

formation of bacterial biofilms. With these antibiotic treatments, the infection rates have dropped to 1–2% for first-time patients, with slightly higher rates closer to 3% for diabetics [44].

These devices are implanted via either a suprapubic approach, or an incision at the penile scrotal junction. The procedure is generally well tolerated. Recovery is generally 2–6 weeks in uncomplicated scenarios. The device allows more spontaneity then many of the medical therapies. Patient satisfaction rates are over 90% in most studies [45]. In 2009 22,420 implantable devices were placed in the USA alone, an increase from 17,540 in 2000 [46].

Erectile dysfunction in the aging male may be thought of as analogous to medical renal disease, where disease may be treated medically at less advanced stages and may require organ replacement or substitution when there is end-stage organ dysfunction. A PDE-5 inhibitor may work if there is mild to moderate erectile dysfunction, but many patients will go on to require more aggressive treatments as their underlying condition worsens. Tissue engineering and gene therapy technology offers the eventual goal of regeneration or recreation of functional erectile tissue, whether done on a tissue, cellular, or gene level. In the foreseeable future, vectors may be introduced into corporal tissue containing specialized growth factors that regenerate or create endothelial and smooth muscular tissue as well as the necessary nervous input. Tissues or stem cells may be implanted and coerced to differentiate into erectile tissue. Even corporal replacement may be an option, given the advances of tissue engineering.

Conclusions

Sexual health in the aging male is a reflection of mental, physical, and social health. As the world population over 45 years of age continues to climb the rates of sexual health-related issues will continue to climb. With the projected population of men and women older than 45 being 2 billion in 2050, and the incidence of sexual dysfunction nearing 50%, we can project that there may be up to 500 million men who will need treatment and care for sexual and erectile dysfunction.

The treatment of sexual and erectile dysfunction is a multi-billion dollar industry in healthcare and pharmacotherapy. The goal of our treatment should be to pursue a safe medical or surgical option allowing for satisfying sexual intimacy.

Causes of sexual dysfunction may include medical comorbidities such as diabetes, hypertension, hyperlipidemia, or endocrine dysfunction, which should also be treated in conjunction with sexual and erectile function [18]. The identification of these causes may be through basic health screenings, laboratory examination, or patient self-referral. The treatments of erectile and sexual dysfunctions are as varied as the causes. Psychogenic erectile dysfunction or underlying sexual issues may be addressed effectively via psychological therapy. Heart disease, hypertension, hyperlipidemia,

and diabetes, all common place in Western society, may cause vascular atherosclerotic plaques and vascular dysfunction. Treatment of these conditions should focus on the primary cause as well as the end-organ effects [8].

As we have tried to emphasize, the treatment of sexual function in the aging male is an attempt to address the patient's global health. Erectile dysfunction may in fact serve as the harbinger of other underlying diseases. While our treatments seek to improve, they can at times cause dysfunction in their own right. It is important that general caregivers and subspecialists work together to address sexual dysfunction and health.

Beyond our methods to treat underlying medical comorbidities through diet, exercise, or primary medical care, there are a wide variety of medical aides to supplement, improve, or simply replace erectile function. Phosphodiesterase inhibitors, intraurethral suppositories, vacuum devices, and intracavernosal injections are common, proven erectile dysfunction therapies currently on the market. Surgical interventions may also be employed with excellent functional results and high patient satisfaction. The demand will continue to rise and will generate newer generations of medical and surgical therapy. The horizon likely includes improvements in gene therapy and tissue engineering.

As the market and demand for sexual health "fixes" continues to rise, we must approach the treatment of this condition with hopes to improve aging males' health and life.

References

1. Feldman HA, Goldstein I, Hatzichristou DG *et al.* Impotence and its medical and psychosocial correlates: results of the Massachusetts Male Aging Study. *J Urol.* 1994;**151**(1):54–61.

2. Bacon CG, Mittleman MA, Kawachi I *et al.* Sexual function in men older than 50 years of age: results from the health professionals follow-up study. *Ann Intern Med.* 2003;**139**(3):161–8.

3. Hyde Z, Flicker L, Hankey GJ *et al.* Prevalence and predictors of sexual problems in men aged 75–95 years: a population-based study. *J Sex Med.* 2012;**9** (2):442–53.

4. Egan BM, Zhao Y, Axon RN. US trends in prevalence, awareness, treatment, and control of hypertension, 1988–2008. *J Am Med Assoc.* 2010;**303**(20):2043–50.

5. Reffelmann T, Kloner RA. Sexual function in hypertensive patients receiving treatment. *Vasc Health Risk Manag*. 2006;**2**(4):447–55.

6. Srilatha B, Adaikan PG, Arulkumaran S *et al*. Sexual dysfunction related to antihypertensive agents: results from the animal model. *Int J Impot Res*. 1999;**11**(2):107–13.

7. Parazzini F, Ricci E, Chiaffarino F *et al*. Diabetes, cardiovascular diseases and risk of erectile dysfunction: a brief narrative review of the literature. *Arch Ital Urol Androl*. 2009;**81**(1):24–31.

8. Meldrum DR, Gambone JC, Morris MA *et al*. The link between erectile and cardiovascular health: the canary in the coal mine. *Am J Cardiol*. 2011;**108**(4):599–606.

9. Napoli C, Ignarro LJ. Nitric oxide and pathogenic mechanisms involved in the development of vascular diseases. *Arch Pharm Res*. 2009;**32**(8):1103–8.

10. Lewis RW, Fugl-Meyer KS, Bosch R *et al*. Epidemiology/risk factors of sexual dysfunction. *J Sex Med*. 2004;**1**(1):35–9.

11. Cheng JY, Ng EM, Chen RY *et al*. Alcohol consumption and erectile dysfunction: meta-analysis of population-based studies. *Int J Impot Res*. 2007;**19**(4):343–52.

12. Boddi V, Corona G, Monami M *et al*. Priapus is happier with venus than with bacchus. *J Sex Med*. 2010;**7**(8):2831–41.

13. Yusuf S, Hawken S, Ounpuu S *et al*. Effect of potentially modifiable risk factors associated with myocardial infarction in 52 countries (the Interheart Study): case-control study. *Lancet*. 2004;**364**(9438):937–52.

14. Brant WO, Bella AJ, Lue TF. Erectile and sexual dysfunction in the aging diabetic male. *Aging Health*. 2006;**2**(6):1025–34.

15. Matfin G, Jawa A, Fonseca VA. Erectile dysfunction: interrelationship with the metabolic syndrome. *Curr Diab Rep*. 2005;**5**(1):64–9.

16. Laumann EO, Paik A, Rosen RC. Sexual dysfunction in the United States: prevalence and predictors. *J Am Med Assoc*. 1999;**281**(6):537–44.

17. Broderick GA, Arger P. Duplex doppler ultrasonography: noninvasive assessment of penile anatomy and function. *Semin Roentgenol*. 1993;**28**(1):43–56.

18. Lue TF. Erectile dysfunction. *N Engl J Med*. 2000;**342**(24):1802–13.

19. Wein AJ, Kavoussi LR, Novick AC *et al*., editors. *Campbell-Walsh Urology*. 9th edn. Philadelphia, PA: Saunders/Elsevier; 2007.

20. Mulligan T, Frick MF, Zuraw QC *et al*. Prevalence of hypogonadism in males aged at least 45 years: the HIM study. *Int J Clin Pract*. 2006;**60**(7):762–9.

21. Kilminster S, Muller S, Menon M *et al*. Predicting erectile function outcome in men after radical prostatectomy for prostate cancer. *BJU Int*. 2012;**110**(3):422–6.

22. Mulhall JP, Rojaz-Cruz C, Muller A. An analysis of sexual health information on radical prostatectomy websites. *BJU Int*. 2010;**105**(1):68–72.

23. Choi WW, Freire MP, Soukup JR *et al*. Nerve-sparing technique and urinary control after robot-assisted laparoscopic prostatectomy. *World J Urol*. 2011;**29**(1):21–7.

24. Munding MD, Wessells HB, Dalkin BL. Pilot study of changes in stretched penile length 3 months after radical retropubic prostatectomy. *Urology*. 2001;**58**(4):567–9.

25. McVary K. Lower urinary tract symptoms and sexual dysfunction: epidemiology and pathophysiology. *Br J Urol*. 2006;**97**(Suppl. 2):23–8.

26. Barqawi AB, Myers JB, O'Donnell C *et al*. The effect of alpha-blocker and 5alpha-reductase inhibitor intake on sexual health in men with lower urinary tract symptoms. *BJU Int*. 2007;**100**(4):853–7.

27. McVary KT, Roehrborn CG, Kaminetsky JC *et al*. Tadalafil relieves lower urinary tract symptoms secondary to benign prostatic hyperplasia. *J Urol*. 2007;**177**(4):1401–7.

28. Traish AM, Hassani J, Guay AT *et al*. Adverse side effects of 5alpha-reductase inhibitors therapy: persistent diminished libido and erectile dysfunction and depression in a subset of patients. *J Sex Med*. 2011;**8**(3):872–84.

29. Chung SD, Keller JJ, Lin HC. A case-control study on the association between chronic prostatitis/chronic pelvic pain syndrome and erectile dysfunction. *Br J Urol*. 2012;**110**(5):726–30.

30. Araujo AB, O'Donnell AB, Brambilla DJ *et al*. Prevalence and incidence of androgen deficiency in middle-aged and older men: estimates from the Massachusetts Male Aging Study. *J Clin Endocrinol Metab*. 2004;**89**(12):5920–6.

31. Kapoor D, Goodwin E, Channer KS *et al*. Testosterone replacement therapy improves insulin resistance, glycaemic control, visceral adiposity and hypercholesterolaemia in hypogonadal men with type 2 diabetes. *Eur J Endocrinol*. 2006;**154**(6):899–906.

32. Greco EA, Spera G, Aversa A. Combining testosterone and PDE5 inhibitors in erectile dysfunction: basic rationale and clinical evidences. *Eur Urol*. 2006;**50**(5):940–7.

33. Basaria S, Coviello AD, Travison TG *et al*. Adverse events associated with testosterone administration. *N Engl J Med*. 2010;**363**(2):109–22.

34. Kantor J, Bilker WB, Glasser DB *et al.* Prevalence of erectile dysfunction and active depression: an analytic cross-sectional study of general medical patients. *Am J Epidemiol.* 2002;**156**(11):1035–42.

35. Clayton AH, Pradko JF, Croft HA *et al.* Prevalence of sexual dysfunction among newer antidepressants. *J Clin Psychiatry.* 2002;**63**(4):357–66.

36. Latini DM, Penson DF, Lubeck DP *et al.* Longitudinal differences in disease specific quality of life in men with erectile dysfunction: results from the exploratory comprehensive evaluation of erectile dysfunction study. *J Urol.* 2003;**169**(4):1437–42.

37. Briganti A, Salonia A, Gallina A *et al.* Drug insight: oral phosphodiesterase type 5 inhibitors for erectile dysfunction. *Nat Clin Pract Urol.* 2005;**2**(5):239–47.

38. Bella AJ, Brant WO, Lue TF *et al.* Non-arteritic anterior ischemic optic neuropathy (NAION) and phosphodiesterase type-5 inhibitors. *Can J Urol.* 2006;**13**(5):3233–8.

39. Eardley I, Donatucci C, Corbin J *et al.* Pharmacotherapy for erectile dysfunction. *J Sex Med.* 2010;**7**(1 Pt 2):524–40.

40. Mulhall JP, Jahoda AE, Ahmed A *et al.* Analysis of the consistency of intraurethral prostaglandin e(1) (MUSE) during at-home use. *Urology.* 2001;**58**(2):262–6.

41. Derouet H, Caspari D, Rohde V *et al.* Treatment of erectile dysfunction with external vacuum devices. *Andrologia.* 1999;**31**(Suppl. 1):89–94.

42. de la Taille A, Delmas V, Amar E *et al.* Reasons of dropout from short- and long-term self-injection therapy for impotence. *Eur Urol.* 1999;**35**(4):312–17.

43. Hsiao W, Bennett N, Guhring P *et al.* Satisfaction profiles in men using intracavernosal injection therapy. *J Sex Med.* 2011;**8**(2):512–17.

44. Wilson SK, Salem EA, Costerton W. Anti-infection dip suggestions for the coloplast titan inflatable penile prosthesis in the era of the infection retardant coated implant. *J Sex Med.* 2011;**8**(9):2647–54.

45. Akin-Olugbade O, Parker M, Guhring P *et al.* Determinants of patient satisfaction following penile prosthesis surgery. *J Sex Med.* 2006;**3**(4):743–8.

46. Montague DK. Penile prosthesis implantation in the era of medical treatment for erectile dysfunction. *Urol Clin North Am.* 2011;**38**(2):217–25.

Chapter 12

Supplements and replacement therapies for the aging male and their effects on reproductive fitness

Armand Zini and Naif Al-Hathal

Introduction

Aging represents a series of universal biological changes that occur with time. The process of aging, like any biological process, is affected by environmental and genetic factors. It is noteworthy that worldwide the population is aging, with the proportion of the population over 65 years of age expected to more than double by the year 2050 [1]. This longevity is attributed to biomedical progress in healthcare and increased self-awareness of disease-preventive strategies, like improved diet and regular exercise. The term "aging" has many definitions, but is perhaps best defined as "progressive, generalized impairment of bodily functions resulting in a loss of adaptive response to stress and a growing risk of age associated disease" [2]. However, there is no global consensus on the exact definition of "old age." Some indicators that are commonly used to define old age are the retirement age, reproductive pause, becoming a grandparent, or poor health that limits a person's capacity to work. The World Health Organization (WHO) uses 65 and 80 years of age to categorize elderly (old persons), and oldest-old, respectively [1]. As the incidence of disability increases with age, an increasing number of social and health-related conditions arise, including nutritional and hormone deficiencies.

Old age is a risk factor for malnutrition. Chronic diseases, polypharmacy, living alone, and limited physical activity contribute to inadequate food intake in the elderly. A national survey of 5000 elderly people (over 60 years) in the USA indicated that the median intake of total energy in the elderly was lower than the recommended daily intake for men (2300 kcal) and women (1900 kcal) [3]. Moreover, in the elderly, the intake of essential micronutrients (e.g. vitamin E and calcium) is lower than the recommended daily levels.

The inadequate food intake and malnutrition has been attributed to factors such as income limitations, disability, inability to chew food, and presence of multiple diseases with several drugs usage [4]. Since the functional deterioration associated with aging is believed to result, at least in part, from free radical reactions with biomolecules (e.g. proteins and lipids), restoring physiological body levels of vitamins and antioxidants is of paramount importance for general and reproductive health particularly in old age.

The term "male reproductive aging" refers to the gradual decline in male sexual and fertility potential during or after midlife, suggesting that only a minority of men will retain normal reproductive function throughout the lifespan. Unlike women during menopause, men do not experience an abrupt decline in gonadal function. Hence, the insidious reproductive impairment in males provides a good model to study age-related changes. The Massachusetts Male Aging Study has clearly shown an increasing prevalence of male sexual dysfunction with increasing age [5]. Similarly, a gradual decline in male reproductive potential (decreasing semen parameters and reduced pregnancy rates independent of maternal age) is reported in most studies although much of the age-related decline in fertility is attributed to female aging [6–9]. Hence, this chapter will focus on reproductive aging in men as well as the common supplements and replacement therapies used to treat age-related sexual dysfunction and infertility.

Reproductive changes in aging men

Late-onset hypogonadism

Testosterone has a number of physiological functions in the male (Table 12.1) [10]. Testosterone is responsible for

Paternal Influences on Human Reproductive Success, ed. Douglas T. Carrell. Published by Cambridge University Press.
© Cambridge University Press 2013.

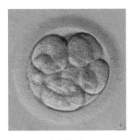 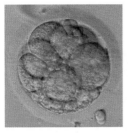 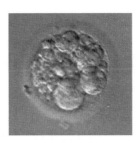

Level 1 Embryo   **Level 2 Embryo**   **Level 3 Embryo**

Figure 1.2. Examples of normal embryotic cleavage at the 8 cell stage (level 1), moderately abnormal cleavage with some blastomere fragmentation (level 2), and poor cleavage with extreme fragmentation (level 3).

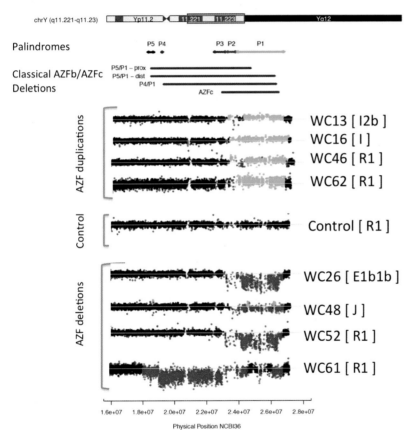

Figure 2.1. Copy number variation on the Y chromosome in men with azoospermia. We used the Affymetrix 6.0 oligonucleotide array to screen a small group of azoospermic individuals ascertained at a tertiary care clinic, and identified a number of classical AZF deletions, as well as duplications of AZFc. Next to each CNV is listed the sample ID and Y haplogroup of the sample. These data demonstrate that existing array platforms can cleanly identify Y chromosome rearrangements involving both gain and loss of sequence, and will facilitate investigation of the full spectrum of Y chromosome variation in future studies of male infertility. In both panels, for each individual, deviations of probe $\log_2$ ratios from 0 are depicted by gray lines or black dots, and probes spanning CNV calls are colored as either red (losses) or green (gains). The location of the region plotted is highlighted by a red box on the Y karyogram at top, followed by horizontal lines depicting the location of DNA sequence features that facilitate the formation of recurrent CNVs in the region ("palindromes"), and the location of the "classical" AZFb/c deletions described in the literature.

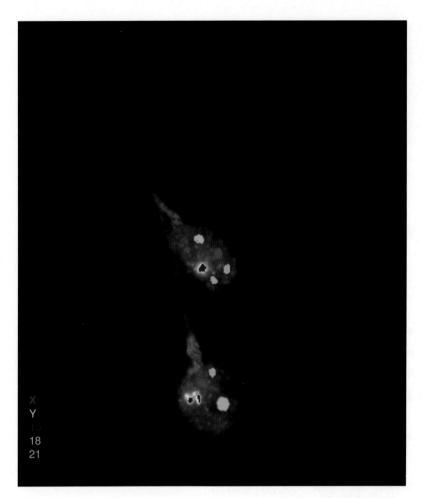

Figure 2.2. A chromosomally normal sperm (upper) and aneuploid sperm aneuploid for chromosome 13 (lower) identified by 5-color chromosome FISH. Sperm were probed for chromosomes X, Y, 13, 18, and 21 (photo courtesy of Benjamin Emery, University of Utah Andrology and IVF Laboratories).

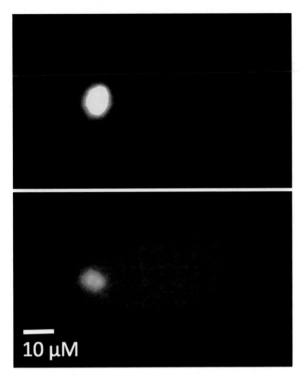

Figure 2.3. Photomicrographs of spermatozoa analyzed for DNA damage using the Comet assay. The top panel displays a cell with minimal DNA damage, and the bottom panel displays a cell with extensive DNA fragmentation, resulting in a pronounced comet-like tail (photos courtesy of Luke Simon, University of Utah Andrology and IVF Laboratories).

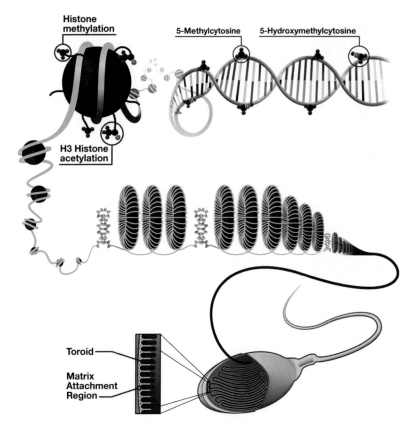

Histone methylation

H3 Histone acetylation

5-Methylcytosine   5-Hydroxymethylcytosine

Toroid

Matrix Attachment Region

Figure 3.1. Chromatin and epigenetic modifications to sperm. Epigenetic modifications consist of DNA methylation of 5 position of cytosine including 5-methylcytosine and 5-hydroxymethylcytosine. Histone tail modifications confer structural and spatial confirmations that influence the binding of transcription factors and enzymes to the chromatin. Chromatin modifications result from the extensive, but not complete, removal of most histones and replacement with protamines. Protamines facilitate a higher order of chromatin packaging consisting of toroidal units with interspersed histone regions.

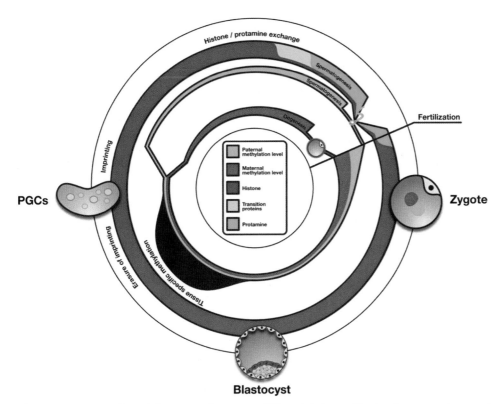

PGCs

Zygote

Blastocyst

Figure 3.2. Summary of critical chromatin and concurrent DNA methylation modifications in sperm, embryos, and primordial germ cells. Key events include the protamination of sperm during spermiogenesis, followed by replacement of protamines with histones at the pronuclear stage of embryogenesis. After fertilization, sperm-derived DNA is actively demethylated in contrast with passive demethylation of maternally derived DNA. Resetting of imprinting occurs in the primordial germ cells and tissue-specific methylation changes occur throughout development.

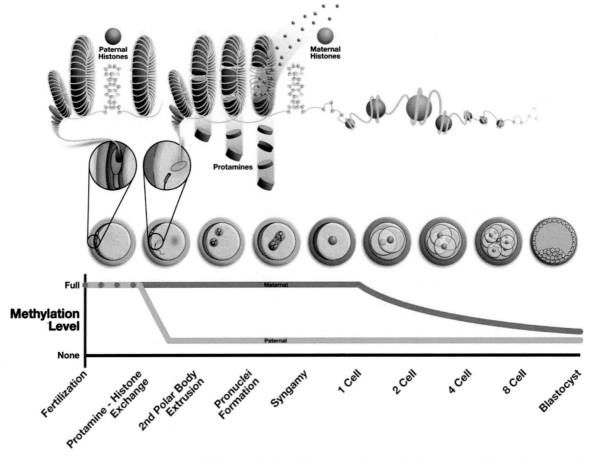

Paternal Histones

Maternal Histones

Protamines

Full

Methylation Level

None

Maternal

Paternal

Fertilization

Protamine - Histone Exchange

2nd Polar Body Extrusion

Pronuclei Formation

Syngamy

1 Cell

2 Cell

4 Cell

8 Cell

Blastocyst

Figure 3.3. Alterations to the epigenome post-fertilization. This figure demonstrates the removal of protamines and their replacement with maternal histones during the very early stages post-fertilization, as well as DNA methylation changes to the paternal and maternal DNA throughout embryogenesis.

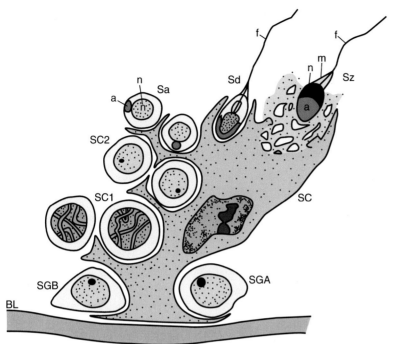

Figure 4.1. Schematic representation of human spermatogenesis in the germinal epithelium. Basal Lamina (BL); Sertoli cell (SC); Spermatogonia A (SGA) and B (SGB); Primary spermatocytes (SC1); Secondary spermatocytes (SC2); Round spermatids (Sa) with round nucleus (n) and acrosomic vesicle (a); Elongated spermatids (Sd) with a flagellum (f); Spermatozoa (Sz) with mitochondria (m) in the mid piece.

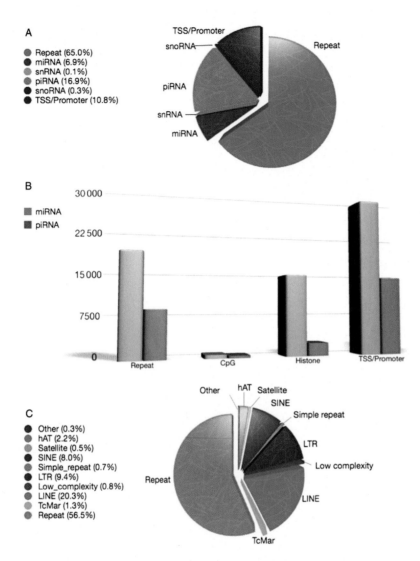

A

- Repeat (65.0%)
- miRNA (6.9%)
- snRNA (0.1%)
- piRNA (16.9%)
- snoRNA (0.3%)
- TSS/Promoter (10.8%)

B

- miRNA
- piRNA

C

- Other (0.3%)
- hAT (2.2%)
- Satellite (0.5%)
- SINE (8.0%)
- Simple_repeat (0.7%)
- LTR (9.4%)
- Low_complexity (0.8%)
- LINE (20.3%)
- TcMar (1.3%)
- Repeat (56.5%)

Figure 5.2. Small non-coding (snc) RNAs in human spermatozoa (three donors). (A) Sequences mapping to known genomic elements, Transcription Start Sites (TSS) and promoters. The distribution of sequences mapping to miRNA, piRNA, snoRNA, snRNA, and repeats are shown here. In addition, those sequences that did not map to known genomic elements were analyzed for TSS and promoter association. (B) Sequences mapping to miRNA or piRNA as well as repeats, CpG islands, histones, and TSS or promoters. All sequences associated with miRNA (blue) or piRNA (red) were further analyzed to determine if they also map to repeats, CpG islands, histones, or TSS/promoters. (C) Sequences mapping to known repeat classes. This figure shows the majority of sequences associated with an undefined repeat category. Of the remaining categories, LINE, LTR, and SINE are highly represented. From Krawetz *et al.* (2011) [24] with permission.

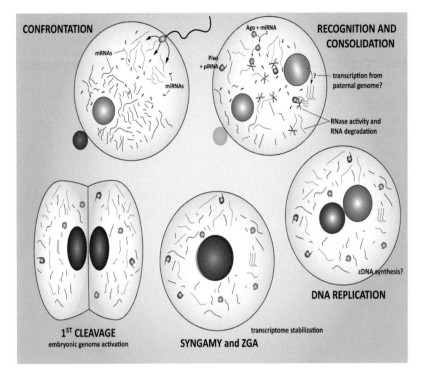

Figure 5.3. Introduction of sperm RNA to the egg leads to possible cytoplasmic confrontation mediated through miRNAs and other RNA types (including piRNAs). This serves mainly as protection against the proliferation of sperm-borne LTR and non-LTR retrotransposons. Assuming that this threat is neutralized, confrontation is defused following compatibility "checking" and the sperm is recognized and consolidated into the early zygote. The compatibility check itself may be driven by oocyte Ago and Piwi proteins using sperm miRNAs as downregulators of key maternal mRNAs. These may be required prior to syngamy and before the first round of DNA replication can commence. DNA replication may offer a window for cDNA synthesis from unknown RNA templates using an endogenous reverse transcriptase present in the ooplasm. The role of RT in the process is implied by the prevention of ZGA in the presence of RT inhibitors.

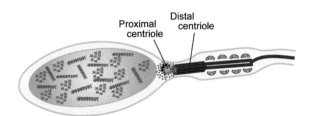

Figure 6.1. Schematic representation of non-rodent sperm showing sperm head with DNA and nuclear matrix proteins and the centriole complex consisting of two centrioles that are in perpendicular orientation to each other. The centriole close to the nucleus (proximal centriole) will become important for microtubule nucleation of sperm aster, zygote aster, and mitotic apparatus in the fertilized oocyte while the centriole associated with the sperm tail (distal centriole) will be destroyed along with the sperm tail after fertilization.

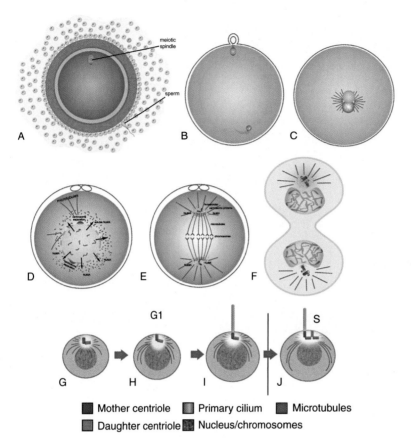

Figure 6.2. Fertilization takes place at the MII stage in most mammalian systems (A); shortly after fertilization a sperm aster becomes nucleated and organized by the sperm's centriole-centrosome complex, indicating successful sperm incorporation and centrosome functions (B). Duplication and subsequent separation of the centriole-centrosome complex occurs at the pronuclear stage (C) followed by nuclear envelope breakdown and dispersion of nuclear proteins including NuMA (D) and maturation of centrosomes into division-competent centrosomes in mitosis (E). The distribution of centrosomal material to the dividing daughter cells may be symmetric or asymmetric (F). During later stages of embryo development there is a close relationship between the older (mother) centriole of the centrosome complex and the formation of the primary cilium (G–J). The assembly of the primary cilium is initiated during G1 (G–H) when the distal end of the mother centriole becomes associated with a membrane vesicle. An axoneme assembles (I) and centrioles duplicate and lengthen during the subsequent S phase (J). Please see text for more detailed description.

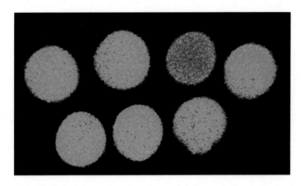

Figure 15.1. The injection of a caged-IP3 into mouse oocytes to determine its ability to trigger calcium oscillation compared with normal fertilization events. Calcium oscillations are shown below the micrograph.

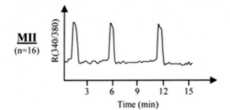

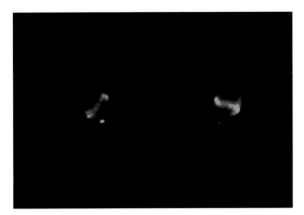

Figure 15.2. Fluorescent micrograph of spermatozoa evaluated for the presence of PLCζ, utilizing a polyclonal antibody.

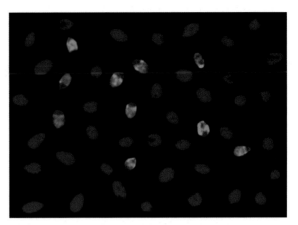

Figure 15.3. Evaluation of sperm DNA integrity using the TUNEL assay.

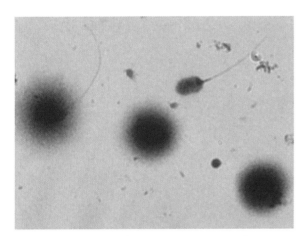

Figure 15.4. Evaluation of sperm DNA integrity using the sperm chromatin dispersion (SCD) assay.

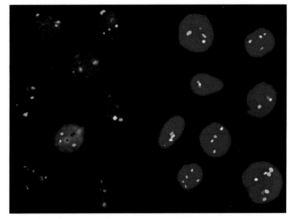

Figure 15.5. Sperm aneuploidy analysis using probes for multiple chromosomes. Each color reflects a specific chromosome probe. Sperm are shown without and with DAPI staining.

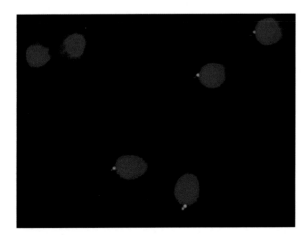

Figure 15.6. Fluorescent micrographic assessment of the presence and integrity of the centriole axis (green dot) of the sperm centrosome in sperm of infertile men.

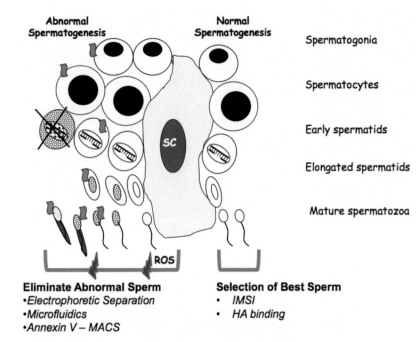

Abnormal
Spermatogenesis

Normal
Spermatogenesis

Spermatogonia

Spermatocytes

Early spermatids

Elongated spermatids

Mature spermatozoa

SC

ROS

Eliminate Abnormal Sperm
•*Electrophoretic Separation*
•*Microfluidics*
•*Annexin V – MACS*

Selection of Best Sperm
•   *IMSI*
•   *HA binding*

Figure 16.1. Spermatogenesis can lead to the production of spermatozoa (left side) with persistence of apoptotic marker proteins on the membrane (green flags), retention of cytoplasm and membrane abnormalities (purple shading), and possession of nuclear DNA damage (black shading). Both the normal and abnormal spermatozoa can then be damaged by Reactive Oxygen Species (ROS). These sperm can be eliminated from a sperm preparation using techniques that are designed to eliminate them from the final preparation. Normal spermatogenesis (right side) produces sperm carrying none of these traits. Individual normal sperm can be selected using high magnification intracytoplasmic morphologically selected sperm injection (IMSI) or by selecting sperm whose membranes possess the Hyaluronan receptor (HA binding).

Table 12.1 Clinical effects of testosterone (see references [10, 11]).

Organ	Effect of physiologic doses	Potential effect(s) of deficiency
Genital organs	Growth, masculinization	Testis atrophy
Bone	Growth, improved mineralization	Osteoporosis
Larynx	Growth at puberty with deep voice	No deepening of voice at puberty
Skin	Growth of facial/body/axillary hair Loss of scalp hair Enlargement of sebaceous glands	Alopecia, skin dryness
Kidney	Improved erythropoietin production	Lowered erythropoietin levels
Lipid metabolism	Favorable lipid profile	Adverse lipid profile
Cardiovascular system	Improved cardiovascular health	Increased cardiovascular risk
Fatty tissue	Decrease in visceral fat	Reduced lean body mass
Bone marrow	Stimulation of erythropoiesis	Anemia
Muscle	Increase in muscle strength/mass	Sarcopenia
Testis	Maintenance of spermatogenesis	Infertility
Prostate	Improved growth and function	Prostate carcinoma (?)
Mammary gland	Growth inhibition	Gynecomastia
Psychosexual functions	Sexual stimulation	Decreased libido
Cognition	Improved cognition	Decreased cognition/spatial memory
Mood	Stable mood	Depression/mood disorder

the development of secondary sexual characteristics in the adolescent and for the maintenance of reproductive (e.g. testicular) and sexual function (libido, as well as quality and frequency of morning erections) in adults [11]. Moreover, testosterone is important for bone health, fat distribution, and cardiovascular health [12]. The gradual decline in testosterone level that is observed in some men with advancing age has led to new and inexact terminology. While the term "menopause" represents an abrupt hormonal pause that occurs in all women during aging, applying counterpart terms for men like "male menopause" or "andropause" does not precisely describe the insidious testosterone deficiency syndrome that occurs in a subset of men with aging [13]. More recently, the term late-onset hypogonadism (LOH) was adopted by many international andrology societies. Late-onset hypogonadism is defined as "a clinical and biochemical syndrome" associated with advancing age and characterized by a complex of signs and symptoms, and, a low

serum testosterone level [14]. This condition may result in significant loss of quality of life and can adversely affect the function of multiple organs [14].

The reported prevalence of LOH in longitudinal population studies varies according to the definition used. In one study, the prevalence of hypogonadism was 4.2% between 30 and 50 years and 8.4% between 50 and 79 years [15], while other studies have reported a much higher prevalence [13]. In an attempt to define LOH, Wu *et al.* used complex statistical analysis in a population-based study to define whether any cluster of sexual symptoms was strongly associated with testosterone levels below a threshold concentration [16]. Using Wu's diagnostic criteria, the overall prevalence of late-onset hypogonadism was reported to be 3% between 60 and 69 years and 5% between 70 and 79 years, which is lower than the reported prevalence of LOH by other authors. The sexual symptoms most strongly associated with a low serum T level were (1) reduced early morning erections, (2) reduced sexual desire, and (3) erectile dysfunction.

The diagnosis of late-onset hypogonadism is challenging as it is confounded by the non-specificity of LOH-associated symptoms that are commonly related to advancing age. These symptoms include fatigability, irritability, and loss of motivation and energy. Nonetheless, several societies agree that loss of libido is the most common symptom associated with LOH, although other manifestations of hypogonadism include erectile dysfunction, decreased muscle mass and strength, increased body fat, decreased bone mineral density with osteoporosis, decreased vitality, and depressed mood [14]. In addition to the aforementioned signs and symptoms, LOH must be accompanied by a low, morning total serum testosterone level. The general consensus is that serum total testosterone levels above 12 nmol/L (350 ng/dL) do not require replacement whereas patients with serum total testosterone levels below 8 nmol/L (230 ng/dL) usually benefit from testosterone substitution [14, 17]. However, for serum total testosterone between 8 and 12 nmol/l, repeating total testosterone levels and determination of free testosterone may be helpful [15, 17].

Aging is a known risk factor for multiple health issues, including hypogonadism. Other risk factors for LOH include obesity, chronic diseases (diabetes, chronic obstructive lung disease, renal disease, inflammatory arthritic disease), metabolic syndrome, and hemochromatosis [18]. Late-onset hypogonadism may be due to a testicular insult (primary testicular failure) or to a central (pituitary or hypothalamic) insult (secondary testicular failure) or a combination of both. Primary testicular failure results in low circulating testosterone, impaired spermatogenesis, and elevated gonadotropin levels (hypergonadotropic hypogonadism). In contrast, secondary testicular failure, or hypogonadotropic hypogonadism, is associated with impaired spermatogenesis, low or low normal gonadotropin levels, and low testosterone levels.

Fertility decline with aging

Studies have shown that paternal age is independently associated with natural fertility and time to pregnancy, and, moreover, paternal age may compound the adverse effect of advanced maternal age on natural pregnancy rates [6, 19, 20]. Several studies have also suggested that paternal age may be associated with an increased risk of miscarriage [21–24]. However, to date, paternal age has

not been shown to have a consistent adverse impact on pregnancy rates with assisted reproduction (intrauterine insemination (IUI), in vitro fertilization (IVF) or intracytoplasmic sperm injection (ICSI)) [25–27].

A number of studies have reported an age-related decline in semen quality and spermatogenic potential. Experimental studies have shown specific characteristics of aging testes that include multinucleated and multilayered spermatogonia, megalospermatocyte, giant spermatids, diverticula of seminiferous tubules and reduced type-A spermatogonia [28]. In addition, the number of Sertoli cells and Leydig cells decreases with aging [29]. Kidd *et al.* conducted a systematic review on semen quality in aging men. In their report, a 50-year-old man would on average have a 3–20% decrease in semen volume, a 3–37% decrease in sperm motility, and a 4–18% decrease in sperm concentration when compared with a 30-year-old man [19, 30]. When controlled for sexual abstinence, the expected annual decrease of semen volume was reported to be 0.5% per year, and there was a yearly decrease of sperm motility of 0.17–0.7% [6]. More recently, several studies have shown that sperm DNA integrity may also deteriorate with advancing age, although most studies have examined populations of infertile men [31–35].

Studies suggest that paternal age may also be associated with an increased risk of genetic and chromosomal abnormalities in the offspring [36]. Studies have shown that advanced paternal age is associated with an increased risk of sperm bearing fibroblast growth factor receptor 2 (FGFR2) and fibroblast growth factor receptor 3 (FGFR3) mutations [37–39]. Fibroblast growth factor receptor 2 and FGFR3 mutations have been associated with an increased risk of achondroplasia and Apert syndrome, respectively [37–39]. Paternal age has also been associated with an increasing risk of neurocognitive disorders (e.g. autism, schizophrenia) in the offspring [40, 41].

Supplements and replacement therapies for the aging male

Testosterone replacement therapy

The body of literature on testosterone replacement therapy (TRT) stresses the importance of an accurate diagnosis of LOH prior to initiating TRT. Once a patient is deemed eligible for treatment, the goals of testosterone therapy are to: (1) restore serum testosterone levels to the physiological range; (2) restore metabolic parameters to eugonadal state; (3) increase muscle mass, strength, and function; (4) maintain bone mineral density (BMD) and reduce fracture risk; (5) improve neuropsychological function (cognition and mood); (6) improve libido and sexual function; (7) enhance quality of life [42].

Before commencing treatment for LOH, the treating physician should be aware of the absolute contraindications of TRT. Testosterone administration is absolutely contraindicated in men with suspected or documented carcinoma of the prostate or breast. Relative contraindications of TRT include the following: polycythemia, untreated sleep apnea, severe heart failure, severe symptoms of lower urinary tract obstruction based on high scores on the IPSS (International Prostate Symptom Score), or clinical findings of bladder outflow obstruction (increased post-micturition residual volume, decreased peak urinary flow, pathological pressure flow-studies) due to an enlarged, clinically benign prostate. Moderate obstruction represents a partial contraindication. After successful treatment of the obstruction, TRT can be initiated [43]. Age per se is not a contraindication to initiating testosterone therapy.

Testosterone exerts its effects on multiple target sites in the body:

1. In men (as well as women) the incidence of hip fractures increases with age due to the gradual decline in bone mineral density. This devastating problem is believed to result, at least partly, from testosterone deficiency. Retrospective studies have reported a 48–66% prevalence of hypogonadism in older men who have sustained a hip fracture [44, 45]. The association between low testosterone and osteoporosis may be explained by several putative mechanisms, the most likely being the fact that low serum T levels leads to reduced aromatization of T to estrogens.

2. Aging is associated with muscle weakness and increased adipose tissue in the central and upper body. Older people tend to have more chronic morbidities, malnutrition, immobilization, and polypharmacy that might predispose them to generalized muscle weakness. Cross-sectional studies have shown an inverse relationship between serum testosterone levels and visceral fat accumulation with weaker muscle strength parameters of the upper and lower extremities [46, 47].

3. The relationship between sex hormone levels and cardiovascular mortality has been controversial. However, recent cross-sectional studies suggest a beneficial effect of androgens on cardiovascular mortality, demonstrating a positive correlation between free testosterone level and HDL (good) cholesterol, and a negative correlation between free testosterone and coronary heart disease [48].

4. It is well established that endogenous androgens stimulate erythropoiesis and hypogonadal men tend to have lower hemoglobin levels than age-matched controls [49]. The main mechanism of testosterone-induced erythropoiesis is believed to be through a direct effect of androgens on the kidney to produce erythropoietin.

5. Low testosterone has been linked to depressed mood, memory loss, and impaired cognitive function in older men [50, 51].

6. Low testosterone levels have been associated with sexual dysfunction. While erectile function and libido tend to decline with advancing age, these symptoms are only partly attributable to decreasing testosterone levels (with age) because sexual dysfunction in older men is multifactorial. The effect of testosterone replacement therapy on male sexual dysfunction will be discussed in greater detail in subsequent sections.

Antioxidants

Oxidative stress (OS) is a pathologic state that is caused by an imbalance between the production and scavenging of reactive oxygen species (ROS). Reactive oxygen species refers to a number of chemically reactive molecules derived from oxygen which include superoxide, hydroxyl radical, and hydrogen peroxide [52]. Oxidative stress leads to an increased oxidation of biomolecules (e.g. proteins, lipid membranes) and is one of the proposed mechanisms responsible for the functional deterioration of cells and tissues related to aging in mammals. Indeed, lipid peroxidation, protein oxidation, and oxidation of nuclear DNA have been associated with aging [53]. In addition, factors that reduce oxidative stress and enhance antioxidant capacity were shown to be associated with longer lifespan in animals [54].

Antioxidants protect cells against free radical-induced damage. Antioxidants may be enzymatic (e.g. superoxide dismutase, catalase, and glutathione peroxidase) and small, non-enzymatic molecules (e.g. vitamin E, vitamin C, carotenoids, and ubiquinone) [55]. In the elderly, the lack of natural antioxidant defense mechanisms (due to prevalent vitamin and mineral deficiency) can compound the oxidative stress associated with aging. This is particularly true in frail and institutionalized individuals, and, is often accompanied by cognitive impairment, poor wound healing, anemia, and increased propensity for developing infections [56]. Therefore, there is a growing interest in treating elderly men with multivitamin supplements, particularly, those with a poor dietary intake of vitamin-rich nutrients.

Despite the lack of strong evidence in support for the routine use of antioxidant supplementation in the elderly, oral vitamin and mineral supplements are being prescribed frequently. The national health and nutrition examination survey (NHANES 1999–2000) reported that over 50% of the 4,862 adults surveyed were taking supplements (47% of the men, 57% of the women). The most commonly utilized supplements were multivitamin/multimineral supplements (35%). Female gender, white race, older age, and higher level of education were some of the factors associated with greater use of supplement intake [57]. In addition, the sales of vitamins and dietary supplements has increased dramatically over the last 20 years and it is estimated that in the USA alone, about $8 billion was spent on these products in 2006 [58].

Studies have shown that the use of vitamins and antioxidants may reduce overall mortality and age-related disease morbidity. Vitamin C is known to promote vascular health and an intake that maintains blood levels above 60 mmol per day was associated with a 4-fold decrease in overall mortality in a group of European men and women aged 40–79 years old [59]. Vitamin C was also associated with a reduced risk of atherosclerosis in 4,000 Chinese aged 65 years and older after adjusting for common risk factors like age, gender, smoking habit, and alcohol intake [60]. Vitamin C is an essential nutrient that functions as a cofactor in several enzymatic reactions (including those involved in the formation of collagen) and as a protective antioxidant. However, in randomized controlled studies, vitamin C (in combination with other antioxidants) showed no benefit in the prevention of cancer and cardiovascular diseases [61, 62].

Vitamin E (alpha tocopherol) has also been studied for its potential role in modulating oxidative stress associated with aging and age-related chronic diseases but the results have been disappointing. Experimental, observational, and clinical studies have specifically focused on the relationship between cardiovascular disease and vitamin E intake. Diets high in alpha tocopherol are associated with reduced risk of coronary artery disease, and reduced formation of atherosclerotic plaque in mouse models [63]. An observational study of 90,000 women, the Nurses Health Study, demonstrated a 30–40% lower incidence rate of heart disease in those with the highest intakes of vitamin E supplements [64]. In addition, a longitudinal Finnish study involving 5,133 men and women showed decreased mortality from congestive heart failure (CHF) among those with higher intakes of vitamin E-rich foods [65]. However, the role of vitamin E in reducing the overall mortality and/or prevention of CHF has been challenged. A large study with long follow-up, The Heart Outcomes Prevention Evaluation study demonstrated no benefit of daily 400 IU vitamin E in the prevention of cardiovascular events or overall mortality but those taking vitamin E were 21% more likely to be hospitalized with heart failure [66]. Vitamin E has also been studied in cancer prevention trials. The alpha-tocopherol, beta-carotene cancer prevention study demonstrated a 32% reduction in the incidence of prostate cancer with alpha-tocopherol, but a 23% increase in the incidence of the same cancer with beta-carotene [67]. The authors of a 2005 meta-analysis on 139,967 participants concluded that high-dose vitamin E may increase all-cause mortality and should be avoided [64, 68].

Vitamin B complex and folic acid were studied in older men for the prevention of dementia, cancer, and cardiovascular-related events, based on the premise that these vitamins may lower homocysteine levels. However, randomized controlled trials (RCTs) have failed to show a beneficial effect of vitamin B complex and/or folic acid supplementation in the prevention of vascular, neurological, or cancer-related events in the elderly [69–71]. Likewise, selenium (Se – a known antioxidant and cofactor of glutathione peroxidase) has been studied extensively. In a meta-analysis of 68 RCTs that included 232,606 participants, supplementation with Se was not associated with an overall survival benefit [72].

Other supplements (vitamin D, calcium)

Vitamin D is involved in several physiological functions including the regulation of bone metabolism and bone health, muscle function, cardiovascular, and mental health. Vitamin D deficiency is relatively common and the elderly are especially prone due to poor oral intake, and, the lack of exposure to sun and outdoor activities. Oral vitamin D supplementation has been shown to reduce the risk of fractures and falls, and to increase physical performance [73]. Furthermore, vitamin D was studied in cancer prevention trials, especially colorectal cancer. A meta-analysis of studies examining high-dose vitamin D supplementation (1,000–2,000 IU) suggests that this vitamin may reduce the risk of colorectal cancer. However, additional RCTs are needed to establish the effectiveness of vitamin D in the prevention of cancer in general, and colorectal cancer specifically [74]. Although there was a higher risk of cardiovascular events among participants who had low serum vitamin D levels (in the Framingham offspring study), there is no strong evidence supporting a role of vitamin D supplementation on cardiovascular events [75].

Adequate intake of calcium is important to decrease the risk of osteoporosis. The recommended daily intake of calcium in the elderly is at least 800 mg, with higher values (> 900 mg) required to reduce bone loss [76]. Calcium supplementation in high doses has been associated with lower risks of hypertension and colonic cancer [77]. However, clinical trials have not shown an association between calcium intake and cardiovascular events. One has to balance the preventive role of calcium supplementation in elderly and the risk of kidney stones [64].

Effects of testosterone replacement on male sexual dysfunction

Experimental studies have shown that testosterone deficiency is associated with a marked decline in nitric oxide synthase (NOS) activity and protein expression [78, 79]. Moreover, testosterone treatment restores erectile response and NOS activity in castrated rats [80–82]. Furthermore, testosterone supplementation restores cavernosal phosphodiesterase-5 (PDE-5) gene and protein expression in a rabbit model with hypogonadotropic hypogonadism [83–85]. On an ultrastructural scale, castrated animals have a thinner and less elastic tunica albuginea [86], a reduced trabecular smooth muscle content, increased connective tissue deposition in the corpora cavernosa [87, 88] and deleterious changes in the penile dorsal nerve [86]. Testosterone replacement restored the majority of these penile changes [89]. Hence, the clinical implication of testosterone replacement in the treatment of patients with sexual dysfunction, especially erectile dysfunction, has gained great interest.

The National Institute of Health consensus defined ED as the persistent inability to achieve or maintain an erection sufficient for satisfactory sexual performance. Population-based studies have derived an estimated prevalence of combined mild, moderate, and severe ED to be 52%. Across age groups, ED prevalence has been reported at 7% in men aged 18–29, 40% at age of 40, and 70% at age of 70 [5]. From an etiological perspective, ED can be stratified into three groups: organic, psychogenic, or most commonly a combination of both.

It is unclear whether the age-related decline in testosterone levels plays a role in the prevalence of erectile dysfunction in aging men. This debate stems from the fact that sexual function declines with advancing age in healthy (endocrinologically normal) men [90]. Moreover, testosterone replacement trials have not clearly demonstrated that testosterone replacement improves erectile function in aging eugonadal men. Indeed, a meta-analysis of 17 RCTs (656 subjects) has shown that testosterone treatment improves the number of nocturnal erections, sexual thoughts and motivation, number of successful intercourse, scores of erectile function, and overall sexual satisfaction in men with a low testosterone level (average baseline testosterone below 12 nmol/l), whereas testosterone treatment had no effect on erectile function in eugonadal men [91]. Due to the heterogeneity of the evaluable studies and short-term testosterone treatment (median 3 months), no major conclusions can be drawn from such a review and large-scale, long-term, randomized controlled trials are needed to investigate the effect of testosterone replacement in the treatment of symptomatic elderly men with erectile dysfunction.

Most studies on hypogonadal men have shown that androgen administration improves penile rigidity, the number of successful erections, orgasmic function and sexual satisfaction [92, 93]. Many authors have reported positive effects of testosterone replacement on sexual interest and libido, symptoms that are frequently present in older men [94, 95]. Several international andrology societies (ISA, ASA, ISSAM, EAU, EAA) recommend initiation of testosterone therapy in older men with symptoms of erectile dysfunction and/or poor libido, and, unequivocally low serum testosterone. Moreover, men with symptoms of sexual dysfunction and borderline testosterone levels warrant short-term (e.g. 3 months) testosterone treatment [43]. More recently, testosterone treatment was shown to have a synergistic effect when used in combination with phosphodiesterase type 5 inhibitors (PDE-5i)) [96], improving erectile function in men who have failed PDE-5i treatment initially. The currently available intramuscular (IM), subdermal, transdermal, oral, and buccal testosterone preparations are safe and effective and the selection of any preparation should be a joint decision by the treating physician and the patient [43].

Deleterious effects of exogenous testosterone on male germline

Spermatogenesis is regulated by pituitary gonadotropins (follicle-stimulating hormone (FSH) and luteinizing hormone (LH)). Follicle-stimulating hormone is required for Sertoli cell support of the mitotic and meiotic processes during spermatogenesis, and testosterone synthesis (by Leydig cells) occurs in response to LH stimulation of Leydig cells. Both FSH and high concentrations of intra-testicular testosterone (50–100 × serum T concentration) play a principal role for the quantitative maintenance of spermatogenesis. When administered in eugonadal men with normal sperm parameters, testosterone functions as a contraceptive by suppressing pituitary gonadotropins. Low levels of FSH and LH are detrimental for normal spermatogenesis and exogenous testosterone, not endogenous, will cause markedly reduced sperm counts and reversible infertility in most cases [97]. Thus, testosterone treatment causes a state of hypogonadotropic hypogonadism with variable degrees of oligospermia, and virtual azoospermia. Indeed, there has been growing interest in the use of testosterone as a male contraceptive, to be used singly or in combination with other agents (i.e. progestins and GNRH analogues) [98].

The WHO-sponsored multinational studies on the use of androgens as male contraceptives have demonstrated the potent adverse effects of androgens on spermatogenesis. In these studies, healthy fertile men were given high-dose testosterone enanthate (200 mg) IM, weekly. After 6 months of treatment, 70% of the participants became azoospermic and the remainder became severely oligozoospermic with a mean sperm concentration of 3 million/mL [98, 99]. The effect of testosterone-induced hypogonadotropic hypogonadism tends to be reversible and sperm quality usually recovers within 4–12 months after discontinuation [100]. Occasionally, the negative effects on sperm quality may persist and patients need to be treated

actively with gonadotropins, like human chorionic gonadotropin (hCG), human menopausal gonadotropin (hMG), or FSH [101].

Vitamin and antioxidant supplements in male sexual dysfunction

The most common cause of erectile dysfunction (ED) in the aging male is organic vasculogenic ED. This is due to atherosclerotic disease of the vascular endothelium, a condition that is mediated, at least in part, by oxidative stress (OS) [102]. As such, oxidative stress may have an important role in the development of ED (vasculogenic) in the aging male yet, to date, very few studies have explored the potential role of oxidative stress in the context of ED and the potential benefit of vitamin and antioxidant supplements in the treatment of this condition. Indeed, oxidants such as superoxide, hydrogen peroxide, and hydroxyl radicals, can impair the formation and/or activity of several mediators of penile tumescence (e.g. nitric oxide, prostacyclin) [103]. The only widely studied antioxidant in the context of ED is vitamin E for Peyronie's disease. Although the beneficial effect of vitamin E in the treatment of Peyronie's disease is unproven, the second meeting of the International Consultation On Erectile Dysfunction reported that vitamin E, in combination with other modalities, might help to improve disease progression in Peyronie's disease [104].

Several natural products have been used in the treatment of ED, however, none has been subjected to randomized trials. Of greater concern is the fact that regulatory agencies in North America have found that a significant proportion of marketed herbal products for erectile dysfunction contain PDE-5i and carry the risk of fatal interaction with nitrates [105].

Vitamin and antioxidant supplements for sperm health and fertility

Oxidative stress (OS) represents one of the main factors in the pathogenesis of sperm dysfunction and sperm DNA damage [106–108]. Although low levels of semen oxidants or ROS are required for sperm physiology (sperm hyperactivation, capacitation) and sperm fertilizing capacity, the uncontrolled release of ROS (by immature germ cells and leukocytes) causes lipid peroxidation, loss of motility, and sperm DNA damage [109–111]. Spermatozoa are particularly susceptible to oxidative injury due to the abundance of polyunsaturated fatty acids on the plasma membrane. Seminal plasma is a rich source of antioxidants and this is believed to protect spermatozoa from oxidative stress [108].

The rationale for antioxidant therapy for infertile men with sperm abnormalities (e.g. poor motility, DNA damage) comes from the observed inherent susceptibility of human spermatozoa to oxidative injury and the fact that over 25% of infertile men have high levels of semen ROS (fertile men do not have high levels of semen oxidants) [108]. Furthermore, some studies suggest that infertile men have a poor seminal oxidant scavenging capacity. As previously discussed in this chapter, oxidative stress is one of the proposed theories to explain the process of aging in mammalian species, especially in humans. In view of the expected increase in oxidative stress with aging, we suspect that older men are more likely to experience ROS-induced sperm dysfunction [112–114].

Several studies have shown that men will generally experience a significant improvement in semen parameters after oral intake of antioxidants. Although there are no studies specifically aimed at the aging male population, there are now a number of RCTs demonstrating a beneficial effect of oral vitamins and antioxidants (with improvement in semen parameters and pregnancy outcomes) in men with infertility. However, it is hard to arrive at a clear consensus regarding the role of antioxidant supplements due to the heterogeneity of the study designs, the short duration of treatment (3–6 months only) and the variable treatment regimens (combination and dosage of antioxidants) [115].

A single RCT has evaluated the effects of vitamin C alone and reported a significant improvement in sperm parameters in the treatment arm only [116]. Six RCTs evaluated the effects of vitamin E alone or in combination with vitamin C or selenium. Two of these studies reported a significant improvement in sperm motility [117, 118] and one reported a significant improvement in sperm DNA integrity [119] in the treatment arm only. In contrast, three RCTs reported no significant improvement in sperm parameters after vitamin E ± C treatment [120–122] although sperm–zona binding improved in one of these studies [120]. Five RCTs evaluated the effects of zinc alone or in combination with folic acid and all five reported a significant improvement in sperm parameters in the treatment arm only. Three RCTs evaluated the effects of selenium alone or in combination with N-acetyl cysteine and two of the three studies reported a significant

improvement in sperm parameters in the treatment arm only [123–125]. Four RCTs evaluated the effects of L-carnitine alone or in combination with L-acetyl carnitine and three of the four reported a significant improvement in sperm parameters in the treatment arm only [126–129]. Three RCTs evaluated the effects of coenzyme Q10 and all three reported a significant improvement in sperm parameters in the treatment arm only [124, 130, 131].

Conclusions

In summary, male aging is associated with a gradual decline in sexual function and reproductive potential. The pathophysiology of male reproductive aging is multifactorial and the proposed underlying mechanisms include age-associated oxidative stress, chronic disease, and late-onset hypogonadism. Testosterone replacement is recommended in those men with LOH and sexual dysfunction although testosterone replacement will have an adverse effect on male reproductive fitness. The role of antioxidants and vitamins in the maintenance of overall health in the aging male remains to be fully elucidated but some vitamins (e.g. vitamins C and D) appear to be beneficial in this regard. The potential effects of vitamin supplements on sexual and reproductive function in the aging male have not been studied extensively but a number of small studies suggest a potential beneficial effect on reproductive function in men with infertility.

References

1. World Health Organization. Men, ageing and health: ageing and health programme, social change and mental health cluster. *Aging Male*. 2000;**3**(1):3–36.

2. Kirkwood T. Mechanisms of ageing. In Ebrahim S, Kalache A, editors. *Epidemiology in Old Age*. London: BMJ; 1996.

3. Burt VL, Harris T. The third national health and nutrition examination survey: Contributing data on aging and health. *Gerontologist*. 1994;**34**(4):486–90.

4. Meydani M. The Boyd Orr lecture. Nutrition interventions in aging and age-associated disease. *Proc Nutrition Soc*. 2002;**61**(2):165–71.

5. Feldman HA, Goldstein I, Hatzichristou DG *et al.* Impotence and its medical and psychosocial correlates: results of the Massachusetts Male Aging Study. *J Urol*. 1994;**151**(1):54–61.

6. Kuhnert B, Nieschlag E. Reproductive functions of the ageing male. *Hum Reprod Update*. 2004;**10**(4):327–39.

7. Stewart AF, Kim ED. Fertility concerns for the aging male. *Urology.* 2011;**78**(3):496–9.

8. Hammiche F, Laven JS, Boxmeer JC *et al.* Sperm quality decline among men below 60 years of age undergoing IVF or ICSI treatment. *J Androl.* 2011;**32**(1):70–6.

9. Cardona Maya W, Berdugo J, Cadavid Jaramillo A. The effects of male age on semen parameters: analysis of 1364 men attending an andrology center. *Aging Male: Official J Int Soc Study Aging Male.* 2009;**12**(4):100–3.

10. Oddens BJ, Vermeulen A, editors. *Androgens in the Aging Male: The Proceedings of a Workshop Organized by the International Health Foundation, Geneva, Switzerland, December 1995.* New York, NY: The Parthenon Publishing Group, Inc.; 1996.

11. Krause W, Mueller U, Mazur A. Testosterone supplementation in the aging male: which questions have been answered? *Aging Male: Official J Int Soc Study Aging Male.* 2005;**8**(1):31–8.

12. Gooren LJ. Late-onset hypogonadism. *Frontiers Hormone Res.* 2009;**37**:62–73.

13. Jones TH. Late onset hypogonadism. *Br Med J.* 2009;**338**:b352.

14. Nieschlag E, Swerdloff R, Behre HM *et al.* Investigation, treatment and monitoring of late-onset hypogonadism in males. ISA, ISSAM, and EAU recommendations. *Eur Urol.* 2005;**48**(1):1–4.

15. Araujo AB, Esche GR, Kupelian V *et al.* Prevalence of symptomatic androgen deficiency in men. *J Clin Endocrinol Metabol.* 2007;**92**(11):4241–7.

16. Wu FC, Tajar A, Beynon JM *et al.* Identification of late-onset hypogonadism in middle-aged and elderly men. *New Engl J Med.* 2010;**363**(2):123–35.

17. Wang C, Nieschlag E, Swerdloff R *et al.* Investigation, treatment, and monitoring of late-onset hypogonadism in males: ISA, ISSAM, EAU, EAA, and ASA recommendations. *Eur Urol.* 2009;**55**(1):121–30.

18. Bhasin S, Cunningham GR, Hayes FJ *et al.* Testosterone therapy in adult men with androgen deficiency syndromes: an endocrine society clinical practice guideline. *J Clin Endocrinol Metabol.* 2006;**91**(6):1995–2010.

19. Kidd SA, Eskenazi B, Wyrobek AJ. Effects of male age on semen quality and fertility: a review of the literature. *Fertil Steril.* 2001;**75**(2):237–48.

20. Hassan MA, Killick SR. Effect of male age on fertility: evidence for the decline in male fertility with increasing age. *Fertil Steril.* 2003;**79**(Suppl. 3):1520–7.

21. Belloc S, Cohen-Bacrie P, Benkhalifa M *et al.* Effect of maternal and paternal age on pregnancy and miscarriage rates after intrauterine insemination. *Reprod Biomed Online.* 2008;**17**(3):392–7.

22. Slama R, Bouyer J, Windham G *et al.* Influence of paternal age on the risk of spontaneous abortion. *Am J Epidemiol.* 2005;**161**(9):816–23.

23. de La Rochebrochard E, Thonneau P. Paternal age: are the risks of infecundity and miscarriage higher when the man is aged 40 years or over? *Rev d'epidemiol sante publique.* 2005;**53** Spec No 2:2S47–55.

24. de la Rochebrochard E, Thonneau P. Paternal age and maternal age are risk factors for miscarriage; results of a multicentre European study. *Hum Reprod.* 2002;**17**(6):1649–56.

25. Wiener-Megnazi Z, Auslender R, Dirnfeld M. Advanced paternal age and reproductive outcome. *Asian J Androl.* 2012;**14**(1):69–76.

26. Dain L, Auslander R, Dirnfeld M. The effect of paternal age on assisted reproduction outcome. *Fert Steril.* 2011;**95**(1):1–8.

27. Bellver J, Garrido N, Remohi J *et al.* Influence of paternal age on assisted reproduction outcome. *Reprod Biomed Online.* 2008;**17**(5):595–604.

28. Holstein AF, Voigt K-D, Grässlin D *et al. Reproductive Biology and Medicine.* Berlin: Diesback; 1989.

29. Johnson L. Spermatogenesis and aging in the human. *J Androl.* 1986;**7**(6):331–54.

30. Eskenazi B, Wyrobek AJ, Sloter E *et al.* The association of age and semen quality in healthy men. *Hum Reprod.* 2003;**18**(2):447–54.

31. Belloc S, Benkhalifa M, Junca AM *et al.* Paternal age and sperm DNA decay: discrepancy between chromomycin and aniline blue staining. *Reprod Biomed Online.* 2009;**19**(2):264–9.

32. Brahem S, Mehdi M, Elghezal H *et al.* The effects of male aging on semen quality, sperm DNA fragmentation and chromosomal abnormalities in an infertile population. *J Assist Reprod Genet.* 2011;**28**(5):425–32.

33. Singh R, Artaza JN, Taylor WE *et al.* Androgens stimulate myogenic differentiation and inhibit adipogenesis in C3H 10T1/2 pluripotent cells through an androgen receptor-mediated pathway. *Endocrinology.* 2003;**144**(11):5081–8.

34. Vagnini L, Baruffi RL, Mauri AL *et al.* The effects of male age on sperm DNA damage in an infertile population. *Reprod Biomed Online.* 2007;**15**(5):514–19.

35. Wyrobek AJ, Eskenazi B, Young S *et al.* Advancing age has differential effects on DNA damage, chromatin integrity, gene mutations, and aneuploidies in sperm. *Proc Natl Acad Sci USA.* 2006;**103**(25):9601–6.

36. Schmid TE, Eskenazi B, Baumgartner A *et al.* The effects of male age on sperm DNA damage in healthy non-smokers. *Hum Reprod.* 2007;**22**(1):180–7.

37. Yoon SR, Qin J, Glaser RL et al. The ups and downs of mutation frequencies during aging can account for the Apert syndrome paternal age effect. *PLoS Genet.* 2009;**5**(7):e1000558.

38. Glaser RL, Broman KW, Schulman RL et al. The paternal-age effect in Apert syndrome is due, in part, to the increased frequency of mutations in sperm. *Am J Hum Genet.* 2003;**73**(4):939–47.

39. Tiemann-Boege I, Navidi W, Grewal R et al. The observed human sperm mutation frequency cannot explain the achondroplasia paternal age effect. *Proc Natl Acad Sci USA.* 2002;**99**(23):14,952–7.

40. Buizer-Voskamp JE, Laan W, Staal WG et al. Paternal age and psychiatric disorders: findings from a Dutch population registry. *Schizophr Res.* 2011;**129** (2–3):128–32.

41. Petersen L, Mortensen PB, Pedersen CB. Paternal age at birth of first child and risk of schizophrenia. *Am J Psych.* 2011;**168**(1):82–8.

42. Lunenfeld B, Nieschlag E. Testosterone therapy in the aging male. *Aging Male: Official J Int Soc Study Aging Male.* 2007;**10**(3):139–53.

43. Nieschlag E, Swerdloff R, Behre HM et al. Investigation, treatment and monitoring of late-onset hypogonadism in males: ISA, ISSAM, and EAU recommendations. *Int J Androl.* 2005;**28**(3):125–7.

44. Stanley HL, Schmitt BP, Poses RM et al. Does hypogonadism contribute to the occurrence of a minimal trauma hip fracture in elderly men? *J Am Geriatr Soc.* 1991;**39**(8):766–71.

45. Abbasi AA, Rudman D, Wilson CR et al. Observations on nursing home residents with a history of hip fracture. *Am J Med Sci.* 1995;**310**(6):229–34.

46. Couillard C, Gagnon J, Bergeron J et al. Contribution of body fatness and adipose tissue distribution to the age variation in plasma steroid hormone concentrations in men: the Heritage Family Study. *J Clin Endocrinol Metabol.* 2000;**85**(3):1026–31.

47. Perry HM, 3rd, Miller DK, Patrick P et al. Testosterone and leptin in older African-American men: relationship to age, strength, function, and season. *Metabol: Clin Exp.* 2000;**49**(8):1085–91.

48. Crandall C, Palla S, Reboussin B et al. Cross-sectional association between markers of inflammation and serum sex steroid levels in the postmenopausal estrogen/progestin interventions trial. *J Women's Health.* 2006;**15**(1):14–23.

49. Spivak JL. The blood in systemic disorders. *Lancet.* 2000;**355**(9216):1707–12.

50. Barrett-Connor E, Von Muhlen DG, Kritz-Silverstein D. Bioavailable testosterone and depressed mood in older men: the Rancho Bernardo study. *J Clin Endocrinol Metabol.* 1999;**84**(2):573–7.

51. Flood JF, Farr SA, Kaiser FE et al. Age-related decrease of plasma testosterone in samp8 mice: replacement improves age-related impairment of learning and memory. *Physiol Behav.* 1995;**57**(4):669–73.

52. Nordberg J, Arner ES. Reactive oxygen species, antioxidants, and the mammalian thioredoxin system. *Free Radical Biol Med.* 2001;**31**(11):1287–312.

53. Harman D. Free radical theory of aging. *Mutat Res.* 1992;**275**(3–6):257–66.

54. Yu BP. Aging and oxidative stress: modulation by dietary restriction. *Free Radical Biol Med.* 1996;**21** (5):651–68.

55. Morley JE, Armbrecht HJ, Coe RM. The free radical theory of aging. In *The Science of Geriatrics. Facts, Research, and Intervention in Geriatrics Series.* Paris and New York, NY: Serdi Publisher/Springer; 2000.

56. Fairfield KM, Fletcher RH. Vitamins for chronic disease prevention in adults: scientific review. *J Am Med Assoc.* 2002;**287**(23):3116–26.

57. Radimer K, Bindewald B, Hughes J et al. Dietary supplement use by US adults: data from the National Health and Nutrition Examination Survey, 1999–2000. *American J Epidemiol.* 2004;**160**(4):339–49.

58. Lowe FC, Patel T. Complementary and alternative medicine in urology: what we need to know in 2008. *BJU International.* 2008;**102**(4):422–4.

59. Khaw KT, Wareham N, Bingham S et al. Combined impact of health behaviours and mortality in men and women: the EPIC-Norfolk Prospective Population Study. *PLoS Med.* 2008;**5**(1):e12.

60. Woo J, Lynn H, Wong SY et al. Correlates for a low ankle-brachial index in elderly Chinese. *Atherosclerosis.* 2006;**186**(2):360–6.

61. Lin J, Cook NR, Albert C et al. Vitamins C and E and beta carotene supplementation and cancer risk: a randomized controlled trial. *J Natl Cancer Inst.* 2009;**101**(1):14–23.

62. Gaziano JM, Glynn RJ, Christen WG et al. Vitamins E and C in the prevention of prostate and total cancer in men: the Physicians' Health Study II randomized controlled trial. *J Am Med Assoc.* 2009;**301** (1):52–62.

63. Cyrus T, Yao Y, Rokach J et al. Vitamin E reduces progression of atherosclerosis in low-density lipoprotein receptor-deficient mice with established vascular lesions. *Circulation.* 2003;**107**(4):521–3.

64. Skully R, Saleh AS. Aging and the effects of vitamins and supplements. *Clin Geriatr Med.* 2011;**27** (4):591–607.

65. Knekt P, Reunanen A, Jarvinen R *et al.* Antioxidant vitamin intake and coronary mortality in a longitudinal population study. *Am J Epidemiol.* 1994;**139**(12):1180–9.

66. Lonn E, Bosch J, Yusuf S *et al.* Effects of long-term vitamin E supplementation on cardiovascular events and cancer: a randomized controlled trial. *J Am Med Assoc.* 2005;**293**(11):1338–47.

67. The Alpha-Tocopherol, Beta Carotene Cancer Prevention Study Group. The effect of vitamin E and beta carotene on the incidence of lung cancer and other cancers in male smokers. *New Engl J Med.* 1994;**330** (15):1029–35.

68. Miller ER, 3rd, Pastor-Barriuso R, Dalal D *et al.* Meta-analysis: high-dosage vitamin E supplementation may increase all-cause mortality. *Annals Internal Med.* 2005;**142**(1):37–46.

69. Toole JF, Malinow MR, Chambless LE *et al.* Lowering homocysteine in patients with ischemic stroke to prevent recurrent stroke, myocardial infarction, and death: the Vitamin Intervention for Stroke Prevention (VISP) randomized controlled trial. *J Am Med Assoc.* 2004;**291**(5):565–75.

70. Seshadri S, Beiser A, Selhub J *et al.* Plasma homocysteine as a risk factor for dementia and Alzheimer's disease. *New Engl J Med.* 2002;**346**(7):476–83.

71. Ebbing M, Bonaa KH, Nygard O *et al.* Cancer incidence and mortality after treatment with folic acid and vitamin B12. *J Am Med Assoc.* 2009;**302**(19):2119–26.

72. Bjelakovic G, Nikolova D, Gluud LL *et al.* Mortality in randomized trials of antioxidant supplements for primary and secondary prevention: systematic review and meta-analysis. *J Am Med Assoc.* 2007;**297** (8):842–57.

73. Bischoff-Ferrari HA, Willett WC, Wong JB *et al.* Prevention of nonvertebral fractures with oral vitamin D and dose dependency: a meta-analysis of randomized controlled trials. *Arch Intern Med.* 2009;**169**(6):551–61.

74. Gorham ED, Garland CF, Garland FC *et al.* Optimal vitamin D status for colorectal cancer prevention: a quantitative meta analysis. *American J Prevent Med.* 2007;**32**(3):210–16.

75. Wang TJ, Pencina MJ, Booth SL *et al.* Vitamin D deficiency and risk of cardiovascular disease. *Circulation.* 2008;**117**(4):503–11.

76. Woo J. Nutritional strategies for successful aging. *Med Clin North Am.* 2011;**95**(3):477–93, ix–x.

77. Wu K, Willett WC, Fuchs CS *et al.* Calcium intake and risk of colon cancer in women and men. *J Natl Cancer Inst.* 2002;**94**(6):437–46.

78. Penson DF, Ng C, Rajfer J *et al.* Adrenal control of erectile function and nitric oxide synthase in the rat penis. *Endocrinology.* 1997;**138**(9):3925–32.

79. Mills TM, Stopper VS, Wiedmeier VT. Effects of castration and androgen replacement on the hemodynamics of penile erection in the rat. *Biol Reprod.* 1994;**51**(2):234–8.

80. Lugg JA, Rajfer J, Gonzalez-Cadavid NF. Dihydrotestosterone is the active androgen in the maintenance of nitric oxide-mediated penile erection in the rat. *Endocrinology.* 1995;**136**(4):1495–501.

81. Baba K, Yajima M, Carrier S *et al.* Delayed testosterone replacement restores nitric oxide synthase-containing nerve fibres and the erectile response in rat penis. *BJU Int.* 2000;**85**(7):953–8.

82. Park KH, Kim SW, Kim KD *et al.* Effects of androgens on the expression of nitric oxide synthase mRNAs in rat corpus cavernosum. *BJU Int.* 1999;**83**(3):327–33.

83. Morelli A, Filippi S, Mancina R *et al.* Androgens regulate phosphodiesterase type 5 expression and functional activity in corpora cavernosa. *Endocrinology.* 2004;**145**(5):2253–63.

84. Traish AM, Munarriz R, O'Connell L *et al.* Effects of medical or surgical castration on erectile function in an animal model. *J Androl.* 2003;**24**(3):381–7.

85. Zhang XH, Morelli A, Luconi M *et al.* Testosterone regulates PDE5 expression and in vivo responsiveness to tadalafil in rat corpus cavernosum. *Eur Urol.* 2005;**47** (3):409–16; discussion 16.

86. Shen ZJ, Zhou XL, Lu YL *et al.* Effect of androgen deprivation on penile ultrastructure. *Asian J Androl.* 2003;**5**(1):33–6.

87. Traish AM, Park K, Dhir V *et al.* Effects of castration and androgen replacement on erectile function in a rabbit model. *Endocrinology.* 1999;**140**(4):1861–8.

88. Rogers RS, Graziottin TM, Lin CS *et al.* Intracavernosal vascular endothelial growth factor (VEGF) injection and adeno-associated virus-mediated VEGF gene therapy prevent and reverse venogenic erectile dysfunction in rats. *Int J Impotence Res.* 2003;**15** (1):26–37.

89. Shabsigh R, Rajfer J, Aversa A *et al.* The evolving role of testosterone in the treatment of erectile dysfunction. *Int J Clin Pract.* 2006;**60**(9):1087–92.

90. Martin CE. Factors affecting sexual functioning in 60–79-year-old married males. *Arch Sex Behav.* 1981;**10** (5):399–420.

91. Isidori AM, Giannetta E, Gianfrilli D *et al.* Effects of testosterone on sexual function in men: results of a meta-analysis. *Clin Endocrinol.* 2005;**63**(4):381–94.

92. Arver S, Dobs AS, Meikle AW *et al.* Improvement of sexual function in testosterone deficient men treated for 1 year with a permeation enhanced testosterone transdermal system. *J Urol.* 1996;**155** (5):1604–8.

93. Morales A, Johnston B, Heaton JP *et al*. Testosterone supplementation for hypogonadal impotence: assessment of biochemical measures and therapeutic outcomes. *J Urol*. 1997;**157**(3):849–54.

94. Carani C, Zini D, Baldini A *et al*. Effects of androgen treatment in impotent men with normal and low levels of free testosterone. *Arch Sex Behav*. 1990;**19** (3):223–34.

95. Boyanov MA, Boneva Z, Christov VG. Testosterone supplementation in men with type 2 diabetes, visceral obesity and partial androgen deficiency. *Aging Male: Official J Int Soc Study Aging Male*. 2003;**6**(1):1–7.

96. Shabsigh R, Kaufman JM, Steidle C *et al*. Randomized study of testosterone gel as adjunctive therapy to sildenafil in hypogonadal men with erectile dysfunction who do not respond to sildenafil alone. *J Urol*. 2004;**172**(2):658–63.

97. Wu FC. Hormonal approaches to male contraception: approaching reality. *Mol Cell Endocrinol*. 2006;**250** (1–2):2–7.

98. Nieschlag E. The struggle for male hormonal contraception. *Best Pract Res Clin Endocrinol Metabol*. 2011;**25**(2):369–75.

99. World Health Organization Task Force on methods for the regulation of male fertility. Contraceptive efficacy of testosterone-induced azoospermia in normal men. *Lancet*. 1990;**336** (8721):955–9.

100. Turek PJ, Williams RH, Gilbaugh JH, 3rd *et al*. The reversibility of anabolic steroid-induced azoospermia. *J Urol*. 1995;**153**(5):1628–30.

101. de Souza GL, Hallak J. Anabolic steroids and male infertility: a comprehensive review. *BJU Int*. 2011;**108** (11):1860–5.

102. Lloyd-Jones DM, Bloch KD. The vascular biology of nitric oxide and its role in atherogenesis. *Ann Rev Med*. 1996;**47**:365–75.

103. Jeremy JY, Angelini GD, Khan M *et al*. Platelets, oxidant stress and erectile dysfunction: an hypothesis. *Cardiovasc Res*. 2000;**46**(1):50–4.

104. Chiao TB, Lee AJ. Role of pentoxifylline and vitamin E in attenuation of radiation-induced fibrosis. *Annals Pharmacother*. 2005;**39**(3):516–22.

105. Fleshner N, Harvey M, Adomat H *et al*. Evidence for contamination of herbal erectile dysfunction products with phosphodiesterase type 5 inhibitors. *J Urol*. 2005;**174**(2):636–41; discussion 41; quiz 801.

106. Aitken RJ. The role of free oxygen radicals and sperm function. *Int J Androl*. 1989;**12**(2):95–7.

107. Aitken RJ, Clarkson JS. Cellular basis of defective sperm function and its association with the genesis of

108. Zini A, de Lamirande E, Gagnon C. Reactive oxygen species in semen of infertile patients: levels of superoxide dismutase- and catalase-like activities in seminal plasma and spermatozoa. *Int J Androl*. 1993;**16**(3):183–8.

reactive oxygen species by human spermatozoa. *J Reprod Fertil*. 1987;**81**(2):459–69.

109. Aitken RJ. Molecular mechanisms regulating human sperm function. *Mol Hum Reprod*. 1997;**3**(3):169–73.

110. Aitken RJ, Paterson M, Fisher H *et al*. Redox regulation of tyrosine phosphorylation in human spermatozoa and its role in the control of human sperm function. *J Cell Sci*. 1995;**108** (Pt 5):2017–25.

111. de Lamirande E, Jiang H, Zini A *et al*. Reactive oxygen species and sperm physiology. *Rev Reprod*. 1997;**2** (1):48–54.

112. Zubkova EV, Robaire B. Effects of ageing on spermatozoal chromatin and its sensitivity to in vivo and in vitro oxidative challenge in the Brown Norway rat. *Hum Reprod*. 2006;**21**(11):2901–10.

113. Zubkova EV, Wade M, Robaire B. Changes in spermatozoal chromatin packaging and susceptibility to oxidative challenge during aging. *Fertil Steril*. 2005;**84**(Suppl. 2):1191–8.

114. Weir CP, Robaire B. Spermatozoa have decreased antioxidant enzymatic capacity and increased reactive oxygen species production during aging in the Brown Norway rat. *J Androl*. 2007;**28**(2):229–40.

115. Showell MG, Brown J, Yazdani A *et al*. Antioxidants for male subfertility. *Cochrane Database System Rev*. 2011(1):CD007411.

116. Dawson EB, Harris WA, Teter MC *et al*. Effect of ascorbic acid supplementation on the sperm quality of smokers. *Fertil Steril*. 1992;**58**(5):1034–9.

117. Suleiman SA, Ali ME, Zaki ZM *et al*. Lipid peroxidation and human sperm motility: protective role of vitamin E. *J Androl*. 1996;**17**(5):530–7.

118. Keskes-Ammar L, Feki-Chakroun N, Rebai T *et al*. Sperm oxidative stress and the effect of an oral vitamin E and selenium supplement on semen quality in infertile men. *Arch Androl*. 2003;**49**(2):83–94.

119. Greco E, Iacobelli M, Rienzi L *et al*. Reduction of the incidence of sperm DNA fragmentation by oral antioxidant treatment. *J Androl*. 2005;**26**(3):349–53.

120. Kessopoulou E, Powers HJ, Sharma KK *et al*. A double-blind randomized placebo cross-over controlled trial using the antioxidant vitamin E to treat reactive oxygen species associated male infertility. *Fertil Steril*. 1995;**64**(4):825–31.

121. Moilanen J, Hovatta O, Lindroth L. Vitamin E levels in seminal plasma can be elevated by oral administration

of vitamin E in infertile men. *Int J Androl.* 1993;**16**(2):165–6.

122. Rolf C, Cooper TG, Yeung CH *et al.* Antioxidant treatment of patients with asthenozoospermia or moderate oligoasthenozoospermia with high-dose vitamin C and vitamin E: a randomized, placebo-controlled, double-blind study. *Hum Reprod.* 1999;**14**(4):1028–33.

123. Hawkes WC, Alkan Z, Wong K. Selenium supplementation does not affect testicular selenium status or semen quality in North American men. *J Andrology.* 2009;**30**(5):525–33.

124. Safarinejad MR, Safarinejad S. Efficacy of selenium and/or n-acetyl-cysteine for improving semen parameters in infertile men: a double-blind, placebo controlled, randomized study. *J Urol.* 2009;**181**(2):741–51.

125. Scott R, MacPherson A, Yates RW *et al.* The effect of oral selenium supplementation on human sperm motility. *Br J Urol.* 1998;**82**(1):76–80.

126. Cavallini G, Ferraretti AP, Gianaroli L *et al.* Cinnoxicam and l-carnitine/acetyl-l-carnitine treatment for idiopathic and varicocele-associated oligoasthenospermia. *J Androl.* 2004;**25**(5):761–70; discussion 771–2.

127. Lenzi A, Lombardo F, Sgro P *et al.* Use of carnitine therapy in selected cases of male factor infertility: a double-blind crossover trial. *Fertil Steril.* 2003;**79**(2):292–300.

128. Sigman M, Glass S, Campagnone J *et al.* Carnitine for the treatment of idiopathic asthenospermia: a randomized, double-blind, placebo-controlled trial. *Fertil Steril.* 2006;**85**(5):1409–14.

129. Balercia G, Regoli F, Armeni T *et al.* Placebo-controlled double-blind randomized trial on the use of l-carnitine, l-acetylcarnitine, or combined l-carnitine and l-acetylcarnitine in men with idiopathic asthenozoospermia. *Fertil Steril.* 2005;**84**(3):662–71.

130. Ciftci H, Verit A, Savas M *et al.* Effects of n-acetylcysteine on semen parameters and oxidative/antioxidant status. *Urology.* 2009;**74**(1):73–6.

131. Paradiso Galatioto G, Gravina GL, Angelozzi G *et al.* May antioxidant therapy improve sperm parameters of men with persistent oligospermia after retrograde embolization for varicocele? *World J Urol.* 2008;**26**(1):97–102.

Environment and lifestyle effects on fertility

Marc A. Beal and Christopher M. Somers

Introduction

The male reproductive system is complex and can be very sensitive to perturbations. The environment and lifestyle of individuals can interfere with spermatogenesis, disrupting healthy sperm production and potentially leading to sub- or infertility. Proper function of the male reproductive system, and thereby fertility, requires intricate interactions between individual components within and outside of the testes. Hormone and sperm production are determined by a complex feedback loop involving the hypothalamus, pituitary gland, and testes, which make up the hypo-thalamic–gonadal–pituitary (HGP) axis. Each component plays a critical role in male fertility, and each may be sensitive to different environmental influences. It is therefore very important for clinicians to be aware of which environmental and lifestyle factors alter male fertility, and what potential risk they pose to particular individuals or populations.

Rather than attempt to deal with the whole HGP, this chapter focuses on environmental and lifestyle factors that have a direct effect on sperm quantity or quality, affecting measures of sperm count, concentration, density, motility, or morphology, or reducing capacity to fertilize the egg. Environmental factors are known to affect other components of male reproduction that are independent of spermatogenesis such as libido, impotence, orgasm, and ejaculation, but these etiologies are not discussed. The purpose of the chapter is to inform clinicians about exogenous factors, either independent of, or in conjunction with, genetic or developmental disorders in patients that could contribute to reduced fertility. Also, the chapter is meant to inform researchers about the current state of the field and where more studies are needed. The field is large enough that each subsection presented

here could be a chapter in its own right; therefore, the studies we have chosen are those best suited to illustrate the general concepts discussed. For additional information, other reviews are available on the subject matter and should be consulted to expand perspective in this important area of male reproductive health [1, 2]. Figure 13.1 summarizes all of the different environmental and lifestyle factors we discuss here. The epidemiological/etiological evidence for some of the factors presented is not yet fully convincing or is still controversial; however, the studies are still discussed here because of their potential relevance to male fertility. Furthermore, some of the factors discussed may only exert mild effects on semen quality, but either affect very large numbers of men, or have the potential to interact with other conditions or exposures in an additive or synergistic way that may impair fertility. By the end of the chapter it should be apparent that some proportion of men may have reduced fertility due to environmental or lifestyle effects that could be reversible. A thorough assessment of environmental and lifestyle factors should be part of considering assisted reproductive technology (ART) to help these patients; men should be made aware of how lifestyle choices might affect their fertility.

Tobacco smoking and chewing

It is estimated that one-third of adults of reproductive age in the world smoke tobacco [3]; as a result, there is ongoing research investigating how tobacco smoke affects male fertility. A recent review of published articles on male fertility and smoking by Mostafa is a good resource for a compiled list of relevant studies and discussion of evidence [4]. In this review, Mostafa lists 10 studies in which smoking was correlated with reduced sperm count/concentration/density, 15 studies

Paternal Influences on Human Reproductive Success, ed. Douglas T. Carrell. Published by Cambridge University Press.
© Cambridge University Press 2013.

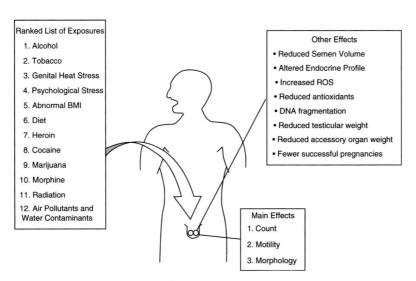

Figure 13.1. Exogenous factors that are deleterious to male fertility. Exposure or lifestyle factors have been ranked in relative order of importance by the authors based on the magnitude of effect on male fertility, and/or the size of the population potentially affected. The main effects identified have clear links to human fertility problems, whereas the other effects are more variable.

in which smokers had impaired sperm motility, 10 studies showing an increase in teratozoospermia in smokers, and nine studies showing no differences between smokers and controls [4]. In a good example of a clinically relevant study, Künzle *et al.* found that male smokers attending an infertility clinic had significantly lower sperm density (67.7 million/mL compared with 79.9 million/mL), total motility (105.6 million compared with 126.6 million), and percent of normal forms (21.2% compared with 23.7%) relative to controls [5]. The review by Mostafa also covers other parameters affected by tobacco smoke such as reduced acrosin activity, which may reduce zona pellucida penetration by spermatozoa [4, 6]. Although some of the evidence requires further corroboration, smoking tobacco should be considered a male infertility risk factor because of its clearly negative effects on sperm functional parameters. Heavy-smoking subfertile men in particular may benefit from quitting tobacco use.

Smoking is not the only way that tobacco can impair male fertility; evidence also suggests that chewing tobacco can have negative effects on sperm quality. Said *et al.* divided men with a history of chewing tobacco into mild, medium, and severe chewers and evaluated their sperm parameters [7]. A significant dose–response was observed among the three categories. The percent of azoospermic men was 1%, 3%, and 14% among mild, medium, and severe chewers, respectively, while the percent of men with oligoasthenoteratozoospermia (OAT) was 2%, 8%, and 29% in the same categories. Although none of the subjects participating in the study were non-chewers, background rates of

oligozoospermia and azoospermia are likely comparable to those of the mild chewers. Comparisons of semen samples between medium and severe chewers characterized by OAT showed significant reductions in the numbers of motile or morphologically normal sperm in the severe group. Thus, chewing tobacco made an existing fertility issue worse. Among the normozoospermic men, all sperm parameters (count, motility, morphology, viability) got significantly worse from a mild to severe chewing habit. The average sperm count dropped 48% from 79.69 million/mL in the mild chewing group to 36.51 million/mL in the severe group. Consequently, men with an existing propensity for low sperm counts may be more severely affected by chewing tobacco. This study demonstrates that it does not necessarily matter how the tobacco is consumed, it can still negatively affect male sperm quality. More research is needed to determine the mechanisms by which chewing tobacco affects sperm quality and how it compares with smoking tobacco.

One of the main ingredients of tobacco is nicotine, and it is therefore important to determine how male fertility is potentially affected by nicotine exposure. Oyeyipo *et al.* treated male rats with nicotine at two different doses: a low dose of 0.5 mg/kg (equivalent dose to an 80 kg man smoking one pack of cigarettes a day) and a high dose of 1.0 mg/kg [8]. Some of the rats were allowed a 30-day period to recover before analysis (recovery group). A significant decrease in sperm motility and concentration was observed in the treated rats compared with the control. Sperm counts in the control, 0.5 mg/kg, and 1.0 mg/kg groups were 103.60,

71.80, and 51.40 million/mL respectively. The decrease of ~50% in the high-dose group was similar in magnitude to that observed in the chewing tobacco study described above, suggesting a potentially important role for nicotine in tobacco-related effects [7]. The recovery group also had reduced sperm motility and concentration, but it was improved compared with non-recovery treatment groups. The sperm counts for the 0.5 mg/kg and 1.0 mg/kg recovery groups were 93.40 and 70.80 million/mL respectively. All treatment groups showed a dose-dependent relationship with the number of abnormal sperm, mostly due to the appearance of curved tails. Litter size was significantly decreased in both treatment groups and in the high-dose recovery group. A key implication of this study is that nicotine itself may impair fertility, so men considering quitting tobacco products in order to improve their fertility need to be made aware that nicotine patches may also be detrimental.

Another way tobacco products may affect fertility is through altering the levels of metals and antioxidants in the seminal plasma, leading to an increase in oxidative stress to sperm cells. Kiziler *et al.* demonstrated that smokers have elevated levels of Pb and Cd (shown to negatively affect male fertility) in seminal fluids [9, 10]. They also found that levels of malondialdehyde, protein carbonyls, and reactive oxygen species, markers for oxidative stress, were increased in the seminal fluid of smokers. The same study found smokers to have a reduction in glutathione levels and glutathione *S*-transferase activity, both of which are proteins involved in antioxidant defense against free radical production. It has been observed that levels of the antioxidant superoxide dismutase and its cofactors, Zn and Cu, are also reduced in smokers [11]. Therefore, smoking may be causing oxidative stress while inhibiting natural defenses against it. Interestingly, supplementation with the antioxidant ascorbic acid has been shown to improve sperm quality in heavy smokers [12]. Thus, subfertile men, especially those that smoke, should consider taking antioxidant supplements to reduce oxidative damage in sperm.

The oxidative stress caused by smoking is likely leading to increased DNA damage in the sperm of smokers. Sun *et al.* found that the percentage of sperm with DNA fragmentation, or DNA fragmentation index (DFI), increased on average from 1.1% in non-smokers to 4.7% in smokers [13]. They also found that DFI was negatively correlated with sperm concentration, morphology, motility, in vitro fertilization rate, and embryo cleavage rate. A DFI of 4.7% is still well below the benchmark for infertility (>30%) [14]; however some of the individuals had DFIs as high as 40% [13]. Thus, individuals predisposed to DNA fragmentation due to underlying genetic factors or other exposures, may be more severely impacted by cigarette smoke, leading to higher DFI values. Other types of DNA damage or alterations caused by smoking have been discussed by Mostafa [4]. DNA damage in early cell types may disrupt spermatogenesis by preventing proliferation and differentiation at cell cycle checkpoints, thereby reducing the total count of viable sperm. Based on the evidence discussed here, DNA damage is likely an important component of tobacco-induced subfertility.

Based on the studies discussed above, the spermatozoa of tobacco users are likely to be compromised compared with non-users. This is due in large part to the harmful chemicals in tobacco products entering the testes and seminal plasma. To better understand how the seminal plasma of smokers influenced sperm quality, Zavos *et al.* transferred isolated spermatozoa from the seminal plasma of smokers to that of non-smokers, and vice-versa [15]. Exposure of smoker spermatozoa to non-smoker plasma increased sperm quality, viability, and longevity. For example, after 48 hours of incubation, the unprocessed smoker sperm motility declined 50.0% while in the non-smoker seminal plasma the sperm motility only declined 43.6%. Transferring the non-smoker spermatozoa to the smoker seminal plasma had the opposite effect. These results show that quality of the seminal plasma is reduced in smokers, and that the reduced quality has a negative impact on sperm functional parameters. Smokers using assisted reproductive technology may benefit from having their seminal plasma replaced with a physiological media that increases sperm quality. Based on the research discussed in this section it is clear that using tobacco products decreases the likelihood of successful pregnancies simply by decreasing the number of normal sperm. Therefore, subfertile men should be strongly advised against smoking, both for their fertility and for their general health.

Alcohol

Alcohol is one of the most highly addictive substances next to nicotine. Alcohol consumption can range from rare/casual drinking to alcoholism, and severe drinking can have many adverse health consequences, one of which is impaired fertility. Consumption of alcohol can disrupt the HPG axis and result in reduced sperm functional parameters. Comparisons of serum hormonal levels between alcoholics and non-alcoholics shows that in alcoholics FSH, LH, and estradiol are elevated, testosterone and progesterone are both diminished, but no significant changes in prolactin levels were detected [16]. Based on the results of Muthusami and Chinnaswamy, alcohol causes a reduction in progesterone, leading to reduced testosterone synthesis [16]. Increased estradiol also provides evidence for increased metabolic clearance of testosterone through aromatase conversion. The reduction of testosterone then results in increased LH and FSH. Muthusami and Chinnaswamy measured sperm parameters in addition to hormone levels and found that the changes in the HPG axis were correlated with reduced semen quality [16]. They found that sperm count in alcoholics was reduced to 51.99 million/mL compared with 132.97 million/mL in healthy controls. The percent of morphologically normal sperm (head, neck, or tail) in alcoholics was also reduced to 67.17% from 82.00% in the control. The percent of immotile sperm increased to 35.91% in alcoholics from 20.17% in the control. Other etiologies found were reductions in semen volume, live sperm, and progressively motile sperm.

Similar results were obtained by Brzek [17]: semen volume, sperm density, sperm count, and sperm motility were reduced in alcohol abusers compared with non-abusers. However, the authors found that after 10 weeks of abstaining from alcohol, following a regimen of proper nutrition and exercise, and taking disulfiram, a chemical that causes hangover-like symptoms when alcohol is consumed, certain sperm parameters improved. Sperm density, count, and velocity all improved significantly in some men undergoing treatment, whereas volume improved non-significantly. Among nine of the men that had azoospermia, after 3 months of treatment seven had motile sperm, four had sperm density over 40 million/mL, and two had sperm with normal motility. By simply stopping alcohol abuse some azoospermic men in the study were able to recover normal fertility parameters. Thus, there is evidence that a healthy lifestyle free of alcohol may cause recrudescence of fertility in heavy drinkers.

It is important to emphasize that the effects of alcohol may be experienced in moderate drinkers as well as heavy abusers. In an autopsy study done by Pajarinen

et al., a dose response was observed between daily alcohol consumption and spermatogenic arrest [18]. In the study, autopsies of 195 men aged 35–69 that had died from cardiac causes, violent death, poisoning, or undetermined causes were used. The control group consisted of individuals that consumed less than 10 g of alcohol per day (40 g per day could be achieved by drinking ~1.1 liters of beer or 112 mL of spirits). The authors found that normal spermatogenesis occurred equally in control individuals and those that had between 10–40 g of alcohol per day. Relative to the controls, the proportion of normal spermatogenesis was 10.7% lower for men who consumed 40–80 g, 28.4% lower for 80–160 g, and 37.3% lower at >160 g of alcohol consumed per day. Partial or complete spermatogenic arrest (SA) increased with higher alcohol consumption rates; 42% of men that consumed 40–80 g had SA, 54% consuming 80–160 g had SA, and 64% consuming >160 g had SA. Men who drank high levels (>80 g) of alcohol had significantly reduced testicular weight and significantly smaller seminiferous tubular diameter. A few individuals displayed Sertoli-cell only (SCO) syndrome and they were all in the higher alcohol consumption range. One man had SCO (3%) in the 40–80 g group, three in 80–160 (9%), and three in >160 (8%). Although consumption of lower doses (10–40 g) of alcohol is safe in regards to testicular function, patients should still be aware of the potential consequences of drinking, particularly when combined with other factors (e.g. underlying genetics, smoking).

Recreational drugs

There has been a longstanding belief that recreational drugs can affect the health and fertility of users. However, a limited amount of information is available on how use of recreational drugs alters the male reproductive system and sperm quality. This is most likely due to the illegality of the drugs and the difficulty of finding cohorts to study. Therefore, most of our knowledge on the relationships between drug use and fertility comes from work done in animal models. This section focuses specifically on three common recreational drugs: cocaine, opioids, and marijuana. However, other recreational drugs, prescription medications, or over-the-counter drugs may have negative effects on male fertility as well.

Cocaine use may be a significant factor affecting male fertility. Bracken et al. found that a history of cocaine use was more common in men with lower sperm motility, concentration, and a higher proportion of abnormal-shaped sperm [19]. They also found that men who were oligozoospermic were twice as likely to have used cocaine within 2 years of semen analysis. Rats receiving a daily and weekend exposure to cocaine had reduced seminiferous tubule diameter, germinal epithelium thickness, and spermatid count (daily and weekend treatments reduced germ cell counts by 19.40% and 15.90%, respectively) [20]. In rats administered cocaine daily there was also a decrease in the number of successful pregnancies with untreated females, and reduced birth weight in progeny. No changes in FSH, LH, or testosterone levels were observed after exposure [20]. Thus, there is strong evidence that chronic cocaine exposure can be detrimental to the fertility of rodents, but only limited information on the effects of cocaine use in humans. Given the uncertainties, we suggest that the use of cocaine should be assessed during diagnostic interviews, and considered when developing a treatment plan.

A few studies have investigated the effects of opioids, such as heroin and morphine, on male reproduction. Mice administered a high dose of 5 mg/kg of heroin had reduced sperm viability, fertility, and serum testosterone levels compared with controls, but no differences in testicular weight were detected [21]. Humans taking either heroin alone, or heroin while undergoing methadone treatment were also shown to have impaired sperm parameters [22]. All of the humans taking either heroin or both heroin and methadone had sperm abnormalities. All of the heroin/dual users had asthenospermia, 24% showed teratospermia, 17% showed oligospermia, and 24% showed hypospermia, providing evidence that heroin is toxic to the male reproductive system in humans. There is contradictory evidence in terms of hormonal changes attributed to heroin use. For example, Ragni et al. [22] found that heroin subjects had normal FSH, LH, and testosterone, but elevated prolactin, while Malik et al. [23] found that heroin users had reduced FSH and testosterone, but normal LH. Therefore, heroin is likely affecting hormones but the mechanisms are not yet fully understood. Hormone levels in rats are also altered through the administration of morphine, which is a product of heroin metabolism. Male rats injected twice daily with a high dose of 5 mg/kg morphine had reduced testosterone and LH but not FSH [24]. In addition to disrupting the endocrine system, morphine also exerts detrimental effects on fertility. Female rats mated with males chronically exposed to morphine had a marked decrease in the number of pregnancies (33%) compared with controls (74.5%) [25]. This is most likely due to defective sperm with an impaired ability to fertilize the egg or increased preimplantation fetal loss. Overall there is still a lack of knowledge regarding the degree to which opioids impair fertility, especially in humans. However, it appears that heroin use may be a factor to consider when assessing all possible influences on male fertility.

Studies have been conducted that determine how marijuana, its major psychoactive drug delta-9-tetrahydrocannabinol (THC), and other cannabinoids affect male fertility. The effects have been most widely studied in animals [26]. The results of some of the animal studies (mostly done in rodents) show that THC may block gonadotropin-releasing hormone release by the hypothalamus, resulting in a reduction of LH and FSH levels, and a subsequent depression of testosterone production by Leydig cells. Some of the results also showed reduced mass in testes and accessory reproductive organs, lower levels of sperm in the epididymis, increased numbers of abnormal sperm, and fewer pregnancies. It was not determined whether the decrease in the quality and quantity of sperm was due to changes in hormone levels or direct action of cannibinoids on spermatogenesis. All of the effects marijuana had on the fertility of animals appeared to be reversible. In humans evidence showing reduced fertility by marijuana is either limited or has not been reproduced. Hembree et al. showed that fertile men who smoked between 6–20 cigarettes with 2% THC per day (average 8) had around a 30% decrease in sperm concentration in the first 2 weeks post-smoking [27]. A significant decrease due to the marijuana smoke was also observed in sperm motility and the percent of sperm with normal morphology. Despite a large body of evidence linking marijuana with impaired fertility in animals, more research is needed to determine the effects in humans. However, given that marijuana does impair fertility in animals and a few studies have shown some effect in humans, clinicians should still consider marijuana use when developing a treatment plan.

Body mass index and diet

The prevalence of obesity in the Western world is rising to the point where it is becoming an epidemic. In 2008 it was estimated that 1.5 billion adults were overweight and more than 200 million men were obese [28]. Obesity is one of the most preventable causes of death worldwide and it is associated with many disorders such as heart disease and type II diabetes. A body mass index (BMI) that is above normal levels (20–25 kg/m^2) is also associated with a decrease in male fertility independent of erectile dysfunction or changes to libido. Jensen *et al.* showed that men with a higher than normal BMI had reduced sperm concentrations and sperm counts (39.0 million/mL and 116.0 million, respectively) relative to men with a normal BMI (46.0 million/mL and 138.0 million, respectively) [29]. Furthermore, 24.4% of men with a higher BMI were oligozoospermic compared with only 21.7% of normal men. When examining the percentage of motile sperm, morphologically normal sperm, semen volume, and testis size, there was no effect associated with high BMI. Hormonal profiles were different between overweight and normal individuals, and this difference may be responsible for the decrease in sperm count. Total serum testosterone, sex hormone-binding globulin, and inhibin B all decreased significantly, while free androgen index and estradiol increased significantly with increasing BMI. Having an above-average BMI may therefore be detrimental in men with marginal fertility.

In contrast to the Western world, in less developed countries malnutrition and starvation are major concerns rather than obesity. In 2000 it was estimated that malnutrition affected 800 million people worldwide [30]. Similar to high BMI, a below-normal BMI (<20 kg/m^2) has also been associated with decreased fertility in men. Jensen *et al.* showed that underweight men also had lower sperm concentrations and total sperm counts (40.0 million/mL and 105 million, respectively) relative to normal weight men (46.0 million/mL and 138.0 million, respectively) [29]. Similar to overweight men, there were more slender men with oligozoospermia (29.0%) compared with normal weight men (21.7%). In contrast to observations in overweight men, testis size, semen volume, and percentage of motile sperm were all reduced in slim men. Hormonal changes are likely responsible for the decrease in sperm count but the mechanisms are probably different between overweight and underweight men. In underweight men, sex hormone-binding globulin levels were higher, while free androgen index and levels of estradiol decreased significantly. The only other significant hormonal change in slim men was that serum FSH was higher. Unlike overweight men,

no changes in total serum testosterone or inhibin B were observed in underweight men. It is apparent that having a BMI outside the normal range can cause decrements in sperm count. However, studies need to be done to determine whether losing or gaining weight improves semen quality; if so, some cases of subfertility caused by BMI may be preventable. Men attending an infertility clinic with BMIs outside the healthy range should therefore be made aware of the potential importance of maintaining a healthy weight.

There is evidence that diet can play a major role in fertility. For example, it was found that men with a high intake of soy (0.3 servings per day) had a ~33% reduced sperm concentration (72 million/mL) compared with men that did not consume soy (106 million/mL) [31]. After adjusting for confounding variables, the same men had 41 million sperm/mL less than men that do not eat soy products [31]. The inverse relationship between soy intake and sperm concentration was more pronounced in overweight men compared with men of normal weight, again reiterating the importance of a healthy lifestyle for fertility. Other foods that have estrogenic activity may also impair fertility and should be avoided. Caffeine, a stimulant drug prevalent in most people's diet (coffee, tea, soda, chocolate) has not been shown to affect male fertility [32]. However, cola, which does have a relatively small amount of caffeine, has been shown to affect sperm parameters, while the other sources of caffeine did not [32]. After controlling for confounding variables, Jensen *et al.* showed that semen volume, sperm concentration, total sperm count, and the percentage of morphological normal sperm decreased in men who consume cola compared with non-drinkers [32]. Men that drink excessive amounts of cola (>1 liter per day) had an adjusted total sperm count and sperm concentration of 121 million and 40 million/mL, respectively, compared with 181 million and 56 million/mL in non-cola-drinkers. Unlike many of the other lifestyle factors that affect male fertility, no differences in serum hormone levels were observed. It is important to emphasize that the men in the study that drank the excessive amounts of cola tended to live an unhealthier lifestyle in other ways as well. Whether or not the impaired sperm parameters were due to the cola or a generally unhealthy lifestyle (including other factors), it is clear that different lifestyle choices are important for fertility. Thus, changing unhealthy eating habits, as part of a series of lifestyle changes, could improve fertility in some males.

Improving fertility is not just a matter of limiting unhealthy dietary factors; it also requires maximizing healthy nutrition. Eating a balanced, moderate diet may be beneficial to some subfertile men. In addition, evidence has shown that dietary supplementation with certain compounds may improve fertility. For example, supplementation with l-cartinine and its acyl derivative l-acetyl-cartinine, which are important for cellular energy production, may improve fertility in subfertile men. Lenzi *et al.* conducted a 6-month double-blind placebo-controlled study that analyzed how men with varying degrees of OAT responded to l-cartinine + l-acetyl-cartinine treatment [33]. Subjects that underwent the cartinine treatment had an improvement in total and forward sperm motility relative to the placebo group. Following treatment, total sperm motility went from 23.17% to 31.11% and forward sperm motility from 14.83% to 25.00%. Only minor increases in other sperm parameters (semen volume, sperm concentration) were observed after the combined treatment. During the observation period, four spontaneous pregnancies occurred, all of which were in the treatment group (two pregnancies after 4 months of treatment, one after 5 months, and one after 6 months). The patients that had successful fertilizations were in a subgroup with the highest initial motility percentages and after treatment they had no significant increase in motility. This may suggest that treatment of carnitine over the long term can improve fertility in ways that are not apparent by microscopic analyses. Future studies investigating how different dietary factors influence fertility will aid to help clinicians recommend a diet plan tailored to subfertile individuals.

Psychological stress

Stress can be responsible for various disorders and is seen as an important medical and social problem. Psychological stress could have an indirect effect on male fertility by leading men to make unhealthy decisions such as drinking alcohol or taking drugs (shown to impair male fertility) to try and cope with the stress. Furthermore, there is evidence that stress is related to male fertility directly. Mental stress has been associated with a decline in testosterone levels, which impairs spermatogenesis, and many studies have examined how stress affects semen parameters in infertile and fertile men [34]. The mechanisms linking stress to male fertility are most likely complex, but

there are studies that have explored how stress might affect semen quality at the cellular level. For example, Eskiocak *et al.* examined 27 healthy, non-smoking, normozoospermic medical students before and after their final exams (high and low stress respectively) [35]. Sperm parameters and the levels of two antioxidants important in the seminal plasma, superoxide dismutase (SOD) and catalase, were measured in the subjects. Perceived stress scores and SOD levels increased during the stress period (before exam), while no changes in catalase levels were observed. Significant decreases in sperm density (78.00 million/mL to 41.93 million/mL) and the number of motile sperm (42.51 million/mL to 21.14 million/mL) were detected during the stress period. Stress also increased the percent of abnormal sperm (45.56% to 52.59%) but non-significantly. Data suggest that SOD is responding to the psychological stress but is not sufficient enough to protect the sperm from damage. In a similar study, Eskiocak *et al.* assessed the effect of exam stress on the semen quality of healthy medical students, as well as the content of glutathione and free sulphydryl in semen [36]. During the period of stress, glutathione and free sulphydryl levels in the seminal plasma were significantly lower compared with the non-stress period. Sperm motility index decreased while the percent of morphologically abnormal sperm increased significantly. The results show that stress may reduce the levels of glutathione and free sulphydryl in the seminal plasma, causing a reduction in sperm quality.

There is evidence to suggest that types of stress impair semen quality differently. For example, Fenster *et al.* assessed psychological job stress and life-event stress in parallel with sperm parameters in 157 volunteers representative of the general population [37]. Work stress and life-event stress were not related to any changes in semen quality; however, recent death of a close family member significantly reduced straight-line velocity from 39.0 μm/s to 32.5 μm/s, and the percent of progressively motile sperm from 66.3% to 58.1%. The sperm from this high-stress group also had significantly longer sperm-head measurements and a slight increase in sperm with larger and more tapered nuclei. These results suggest that bereavement stress may temporarily lessen male fertility. Efforts to reduce the amount of psychological stress in male infertility patients will help to improve their semen quality and possibly fertility. Providing patients with a sense of hope that they can be partly in charge of their fertility by living a healthy lifestyle may help their fertility by reducing psychological stress. For example, in the study described above regarding l-cartinine supplementation, the authors observed a positive effect in the placebo group [33]. The pressure of trying to conceive while undergoing infertility treatment may be very stressful for individuals; anything that can be done to minimize stress will be beneficial to the health and fertility of patients.

Genital heat stress

It is commonly accepted that scrotal heat near or above body temperature is harmful to male fertility, and several studies have shown that genital heat stress directly impairs semen quality [38]. Stage-specific apoptosis of male germ cells, resulting in a reduction of the number of viable sperm is one of the main processes through which genital hyperthermia alters semen quality [39]. Increased heat in the genital area should therefore be avoided in subfertile men. Examples of factors that have been shown to increase scrotal temperature include sleeping posture, sitting, laptop use, tight-fitting underwear, external heat exposure, fever, and history of varicocele [38]. In some of the studies data pertaining to semen quality was not available. In those that did measure semen quality, heat was associated with a reduction in sperm count, percent of motile sperm and normal forms. Some studies were limited by design (i.e. had confounding variables) and others had convincing results that need to be further validated in larger cohort studies. However, any potential factors that may increase testicular temperatures should be avoided.

Studies have shown that semen quality can be improved by reducing the temperature of the scrotum, suggesting that genital heat stress may be reversible. For example, 11 infertile men with a history of wet heat exposure in hot tubs or baths were evaluated during heat exposure periods and 3–6 months after cessation [40]. Five of the 11 patients responded beneficially and the mean increase in total motile sperm count (TMC = ejaculate volume × sperm concentration × fraction of motile sperm) was 491% (excluding one individual that had a TMC increase from zero to 200,000). This increase was not statistically significant and was mostly due to the increase in sperm motility from 12% to 34%. The largest improvement in TMC (excluding the individual with an initial TMC of 0) was from 1.1 million to 10.7 million motile sperm. Another individual actually went from having 3.2

million to 21.1 million motile sperm, putting that individual in the normal range for fertility. A smoking history of 5.6 pack-years was observed in five of the six men that had no post-intervention changes in sperm quality, compared with only 0.11 pack-years in three of the five men who responded to avoidance of wet heat. This finding reiterates the potentially harmful effects of smoking on male fertility, and also demonstrates how combinations of lifestyle factors can impair fertility. Based on the results of this study, it is apparent that the fertility of some men can be improved through the avoidance of testicular wet heat exposure.

The type of undergarments worn by men may also play a significant role in producing unwanted genital heat stress. Tiemessen *et al.* conducted semen analysis biweekly for a year to determine how the type of underpants worn affected semen parameters in 11 fertile men [41]. Men wore tight and loose-fitting underwear for half a year each. A significant increase in concentration from 46.0 million to 89.5 million sperm per mL was observed when men switched from wearing tight-fitting underwear to loose-fitting boxer shorts. Additionally, the number of motile sperm improved significantly from 17.4 million to 53.1 million sperm per mL, and the number of progressively motile sperm improved significantly from 6.9 million to 17.4 million sperm per mL. Therefore, changing the type of underwear worn may improve fertility in men.

A study conducted by Jung *et al.* determined that direct cooling of the testicles during sleeping hours improved semen quality in 20 men with idiopathic or varicocele-induced OAT [42]. The volunteers in the study were found to have high scrotal heat stress compared with normozoospermic men. A scrotal temperature profile of an individual showed that temperatures were maximal during periods of rest, and higher during sitting compared with doing physical activity. The men with OAT were given an air stream cooling device to facilitate nocturnal cooling of the testicles. The device resulted in a decrease of scrotal temperature by approximately 1 °C (median change from 35.8 °C to 34.9 °C). The men undergoing the nocturnal cooling experiment also had a significant increase in sperm count and sperm density (median change from ~7.3 million/mL before to ~17.7 million/mL after cooling). Significant improvements were also seen in sperm motility (median change from ~21% to ~28.5%) and the percent of sperm with normal morphology (median change from ~3% to ~9%), but the increase was small compared with the improvement in sperm count/concentration. A significant increase in LH was detected at the end of cooling, but there were no changes for testosterone or FSH. The results of the studies described in this section show that cooling the temperature of the testicles (in moderation) may be suitable for increasing sperm quality parameters in males. However, studies have only evaluated how reduction in testicle temperature increases semen quality. Evidence regarding whether or not reduced heat increases the number of spontaneous pregnancies, such as in the case with carnitine treatment, needs to be investigated further [33].

Radiation

It is well known that ionizing radiation causes damage to sperm and results in a decline in sperm count. The most controlled and long-term study on the effects of ionizing radiation on male fertility was done by Rowley et al. [43]. This study determined how sperm was affected in normal healthy male volunteers, between the ages of 25 and 52, receiving different acute gonadal doses of X-rays. Radiation exposure was followed by a marked decrease in sperm concentration. Sixty-seven days after irradiation exposure the sperm concentrations dropped to azoospermia at all doses above 78 rads. Complete recovery of sperm concentrations following exposure to <100 rads occurred within 9–18 months, 30 months for 200–300 rads, and at least five years for 400–600 rads. Only one subject in the high-dose group completely recovered, indicating that high doses of radiation have the potential to cause permanent damage. Hormonal changes in the plasma were also associated with the radiation exposure. Levels of FSH did not change at the 8 rad exposure, but there was a slight increase following 20 rad, and a highly significant increase between 75 and 600 rad (as high as four-fold). Increases in LH levels were seen at higher doses between 75 and 600 rad. At 600 rad LH levels were twice as high compared with pre-irradiation levels. No effect of radiation on plasma testosterone was observed. Seven subjects were irradiated a second or third time and the results did not change. The radiation doses used in this study are exceptionally high (up to 640 rads) compared with background (between several micro- and millirads) and the radiation is directly targeted at the testicles; however chronic low dose exposures could potentially have an impact. The

primary group of individuals that would be exposed to high doses of radiation are cancer patients. The results of this study show how important it is for men receiving radiotherapy to preserve sperm samples prior to treatment because of the potential of sterility as well as the possibility of genomic damage. Clinicians should be aware that men who had been recently exposed to high doses of ionizing radiation may have temporary infertility.

Non-ionizing radiation, which is any type of electromagnetic radiation such as ultraviolet light, visible light, infrared light, microwaves, radio waves, and static fields, may also affect semen quality. This type of exposure is potentially much more relevant to human health because people are exposed on a daily basis. Sources of non-ionizing radiation include sunlight, microwave ovens, wi-fi, television, power lines, and cellular phones. There is major concern over the effects of cell phone use on fertility because many of the several million men who use cell phones, which emit electromagnetic waves (EMW), either keep their phones in their pocket or on their belt, near the scrotum. Gutschi et al. compared sperm parameters of 991 cell phone users to 1119 non cell phone users; all of the subjects were infertility patients, but those with a history of smoking, alcohol abuse, or systematic disease were excluded [44]. All sperm parameters assessed (count, morphology, motility) were lower in the cell phone users. However, the only significant differences were that the cell phone users had a higher proportion of sperm with abnormal morphology (68.0% compared with 58.1%) and a lower percentage of rapid progressive motile sperm (23.98% compared with 25.19%). Teratozoospermia was found in 45.3% of cell phone users compared with only 27.7% in the control group. The altered sperm quality caused by cell phones could be due to the emission of electromagnetic waves, thermal effects, or both. Cell phone use was also associated with an altered endocrine profile. Cell phone users had higher serum testosterone and lower LH, while no changes in prolactin or FSH were observed. The increased levels of testosterone suggests that electromagnetic waves may be inhibiting or altering the activities of enzymes responsible for testosterone conversion, thereby disrupting maintenance of normal epididymal functions associated with sperm maturation. Although there is limited evidence to evaluate how electromagnetic waves may affect male reproduction, it is clear that cell phone use has a negative impact on sperm quality. The study described here did not determine the effects of having phones on stand-by-mode, the effect of cell phone proximity to the scrotum, or other factors surrounding cell phone use. However, it may be beneficial for patients to think of alternative ways to use and carry their cell phones to ensure they are well removed from the scrotum. More research is required to better understand how cell phones, and other types of non-ionizing radiation, may impair male fertility.

Air pollution and water contamination

Air pollution, both natural and anthropogenic, can be in the form of solid particles, liquid droplets, or gases. Several studies have been published that show negative associations between ambient air pollution and semen quality [45, 46]. Areas with high air pollution levels have been associated with a reduction in sperm concentration, fewer morphologically normal sperm, reduced motility in sperm, and increased DNA fragmentation. There is also growing evidence that air pollution can be both aneugenic and mutagenic in the male germline [45, 46]. Studies addressing the effects of air pollution have not been able to determine a direct impact of air pollution on fertility. Furthermore, the magnitude of the sperm quality effects measured in these studies was small and unlikely to be of any clinical relevance [46]. However, air pollution studies demonstrate that the male reproductive system is negatively affected by poor air quality [46], which could be one of the many contributing factors associated with male subfertility. Because air pollution occurs as complex mixtures, it is difficult to determine the causal agents that could be impairing semen quality; therefore, more effort is required to identify agents that are harmful to reproductive health. Unfortunately, human studies are limited by control of confounding variables, accurate assessment of exposures, and inability to link exposures and clinical outcomes. Thus, controlled studies with model species may be a more suitable experimental approach for understanding the relationship between air pollution and fertility [46].

Chlorine used to disinfect drinking water reacts with natural organic contaminants to produce unwanted disinfection byproducts (DBPs). Recently, there has been a focus on the reproductive effects of DBPs, but information is either unavailable or minimal in regards to the effects on male fertility [47, 48].

Studies in which rodents were exposed to different doses and types of DBPs have shown a reduction in epididymal sperm count, sperm motility, and sperm morphology [47, 48]. For example, Toth *et al.* found that there was a negative relationship between sodium dichloroacetate dose and epididymal sperm count [49]. Rats administered 0, 31.25, 62.5, and 125 mg/kg had sperm counts of 630.3, 582.5, 502.6, and 367.8 million/g cauda respectively. The doses administered would be considered high for a typical human exposure, so the effects observed in rats may not be clinically relevant. Similar to studies addressing the effects of air pollution, studies that attempt to determine the relationship between male fertility and DBP exposure in humans are limited by exposure assessment and confounding variables. More epidemiological studies with large cohorts are needed to determine how individual DBPs and byproduct mixtures found commonly in drinking water affect semen quality in male humans. Understanding the harmful effects of the different DBPs at different doses will aid regulatory bodies in determining the maximal levels at which different DBPs need to be maintained to protect the fertility of individuals in the population.

Conclusions

Despite ongoing research associating male infertility with environmental and lifestyle factors, knowledge gained from the available literature is still limited. There is very little information available on how adjusting lifestyle habits (removing bad habits and initiating good ones) can improve fertility. Evaluations of other potentially harmful factors, such as home cleaning products, prescription drugs, food additives, etc., and their influences on male fertility are also needed. Furthermore, most studies examine extreme cases, such as high-dose exposures to environmental factors or very unhealthy lifestyles. Studies using large cohorts are needed to examine environmental and lifestyle effects in men that more accurately represent the general population. In addition, men are exposed to complex mixtures in the environment and may make a series of poor lifestyle choices, the combined effect of which could be a significant impairment of fertility. For example, many men worldwide simultaneously smoke tobacco, abuse alcohol, are overweight with poor diets, wear briefs instead of boxer shorts, are psychologically stressed, and live in polluted urban areas. More studies investigating multiple factors simultaneously are needed, as well as studies evaluating the efficacy of interventions. Considering that additive or synergistic effects could be occurring, cessation of all harmful exposures and negative lifestyles may in some cases improve fertility, particularly for males that are predisposed to having poor sperm quality (e.g. because of genetic factors). Moreover, a large percent of male infertility is idiopathic; adjusting for environmental and lifestyle effects may improve fertility in some of these men with no other apparent underlying genetic or developmental etiology. Changes in lifestyle should therefore be considered before, or in conjunction with, invasive and expensive ART procedures.

References

1. Mendiola J, Torres-Cantero AM, Agarwal A. Lifestyle factors and male infertility: an evidence-based review. *Arch Med Sci.* 2009;**5**:S3–S12.

2. Kumar DP, Sangeetha N. Mitochondrial DNA mutations and male infertility. *Indian J Hum Genet.* 2009;**15**(3):93–7.

3. World Health Organization. *Tobacco or Health : A Global Status Report.* Geneva: WHO; 1997.

4. Mostafa T. Cigarette smoking and male infertility. *J Adv Res.* 2010;**1**:179–86.

5. Künzle R, Mueller MD, Hänggi W *et al.* Semen quality of male smokers and nonsmokers in infertile couples. *Fertil Steril.* 2003;**79**(2):287–91.

6. Gerhard I, Frohlich E, Eggert-Kruse W *et al.* Relationship of sperm acrosin activity to semen and clinical parameters in infertile patients. *Andrologia.* 1989;**21**(2):146–54.

7. Said TM, Ranga G, Agarwal A. Relationship between semen quality and tobacco chewing in men undergoing infertility evaluation. *Fertil Steril.* 2005;**84**(3):649–53.

8. Oyeyipo, Yinusa R, Emikpe BO *et al.* Effects of nicotine on sperm characteristics and fertility profile in adult male rats: a possible role of cessation. *J Reprod Infertil.* 2011;**12**(3):201–8.

9. Kiziler AR, Aydemir B, Onaran I *et al.* High levels of cadmium and lead in seminal fluid and blood of smoking men are associated with high oxidative stress and damage in infertile subjects. *Biol Trace Elem Res.* 2007;**120**(1–3):82–91.

10. Telisman S, Cvitkovic P, Jurasovic J *et al.* Semen quality and reproductive endocrine function in relation to biomarkers of lead, cadmium, zinc, and copper in men. *Environ Health Perspect.* 2000;**108**(1):45–53.

11. Zhang JP, Meng QY, Wang Q *et al.* Effect of smoking on semen quality of infertile men in Shandong, China. *Asian J Androl.* 2000;**2**(2):143–6.

12. Dawson EB, Harris WA, Teter MC *et al.* Effect of ascorbic acid supplementation on the sperm quality of smokers. *Fertil Steril.* 1992;**58**(5):1034–9.

13. Sun JG, Jurisicova A, Casper RF. Detection of deoxyribonucleic acid fragmentation in human sperm: correlation with fertilization in vitro. *Biol Reprod.* 1997;**56**(3):602–7.

14. Evenson DP, Larson KL, Jost LK. Sperm chromatin structure assay: its clinical use for detecting sperm DNA fragmentation in male infertility and comparisons with other techniques. *J Androl.* 2002;**23**(1):25–43.

15. Zavos PM, Correa JR, Antypas S *et al.* Effects of seminal plasma from cigarette smokers on sperm viability and longevity. *Fertil Steril.* 1998;**69**(3):425–9.

16. Muthusami KR, Chinnaswamy P. Effect of chronic alcoholism on male fertility hormones and semen quality. *Fertil Steril.* 2005;**84**(4):919–24.

17. Brzek A. Alcohol and male fertility (preliminary report). *Andrologia.* 1987;**19**(1):32–6.

18. Pajarinen J, Karhunen PJ, Savolainen V *et al.* Moderate alcohol consumption and disorders of human spermatogenesis. *Alcohol Clin Exp Res.* 1996;**20**(2):332–7.

19. Bracken MB, Eskenazi B, Sachse K *et al.* Association of cocaine use with sperm concentration, motility, and morphology. *Fertil Steril.* 1990;**53**(2):315–22.

20. George VK, Li H, Teloken C *et al.* Effects of long-term cocaine exposure on spermatogenesis and fertility in peripubertal male rats. *J Urol.* 1996;**155**(1):327–31.

21. Fazelipour S, Kiaei S, Tootian Z. Adverse effect of heroin hydrochloride on selected male reproductive parameters in mice. *Comp Clin Pathol.* 2010;**19**(6):565–9.

22. Ragni G, De Lauretis L, Bestetti O *et al.* Gonadal function in male heroin and methadone addicts. *Int J Androl.* 1988;**11**(2):93–100.

23. Malik SA, Khan C, Jabbar A *et al.* Heroin addiction and sex hormones in males. *J Pak Med Assoc.* 1992;**42**(9):210–12.

24. Yilmaz B, Konar V, Kutlu S *et al.* Influence of chronic morphine exposure on serum LH, FSH, testosterone levels, and body and testicular weights in the developing male rat. *Arch Androl.* 1999;**43**(3):189–96.

25. Cicero TJ, Davis LA, LaRegina MC *et al.* Chronic opiate exposure in the male rat adversely affects fertility. *Pharmacol Biochem Behav.* 2002;**72**(1–2):157–63.

26. Harclerode J. Endocrine effects of marijuana in the male: preclinical studies. *NIDA Res Monogr.* 1984;**44**:46–64.

27. Hembree WC, III, Nahas GG, Zeidenberg P *et al.* Changes in human spermatozoa associated with high

dose of marihuana smoking. In Nahas GG, Paton W D M, editors. *Advances in the Biosciences. Vol. 22 & 23. Marihuana: Biological Effects; Analysis, Metabolism, Cellular Responses, Reproduction and Brain.* Oxford: Pergamon Press, 1979; 429–39.

28. World Health Organization. Obesity and overweight. 2012; Available from: http://www.who.int/mediacentre/factsheets/fs311/en/.

29. Jensen TK, Andersson AM, Jorgensen N *et al.* Body mass index in relation to semen quality and reproductive hormones among 1,558 Danish men. *Fertil Steril.* 2004;**82**(4):863–70.

30. World Health Organization, Mach A. Turning the tide of malnutrition: responding to the challenge of the 21st century. Geneva: WHO; 2000; Available from: http://books.google.com/books?id=VeHVGwAACAAJ.

31. Chavarro JE, Toth TL, Sadio SM *et al.* Soy food and isoflavone intake in relation to semen quality parameters among men from an infertility clinic. *Hum Reprod.* 2008;**23**(11):2584–90.

32. Jensen TK, Swan SH, Skakkebaek NE *et al.* Caffeine intake and semen quality in a population of 2,554 young Danish men. *Am J Epidemiol.* 2010;**171**(8):883–91.

33. Lenzi A, Sgro P, Salacone P *et al.* A placebo-controlled double-blind randomized trial of the use of combined l-carnitine and l-acetyl-carnitine treatment in men with asthenozoospermia. *Fertil Steril.* 2004;**81**(6):1578–84.

34. McGrady AV. Effects of psychological stress on male reproduction: a review. *Arch Androl.* 1984;**13**(1):1–7.

35. Eskiocak S, Gozen AS, Kilic AS *et al.* Association between mental stress & some antioxidant enzymes of seminal plasma. *Indian J Med Res.* 2005;**122**(6):491–6.

36. Eskiocak S, Gozen AS, Yapar SB *et al.* Glutathione and free sulphydryl content of seminal plasma in healthy medical students during and after exam stress. *Hum Reprod.* 2005;**20**(9):2595–600.

37. Fenster L, Katz DF, Wyrobek AJ *et al.* Effects of psychological stress on human semen quality. *J Androl.* 1997;**18**(2):194–202.

38. Jung A, Schuppe HC. Influence of genital heat stress on semen quality in humans. *Andrologia.* 2007;**39**(6):203–15.

39. Lue YH, Hikim AP, Swerdloff RS *et al.* Single exposure to heat induces stage-specific germ cell apoptosis in rats: role of intratesticular testosterone on stage specificity. *Endocrinology.* 1999;**140**(4):1709–17.

40. Shefi S, Tarapore PE, Walsh TJ *et al.* Wet heat exposure: a potentially reversible cause of low semen quality in infertile men. *Int Braz J Urol.* 2007;**33**(1):50–6; discussion 56–7.

41. Tiemessen CH, Evers JL, Bots RS. Tight-fitting underwear and sperm quality. *Lancet.* 1996;**347**(9018):1844–5.

42. Jung A, Eberl M, Schill WB. Improvement of semen quality by nocturnal scrotal cooling and moderate behavioural change to reduce genital heat stress in men with oligoasthenoteratozoospermia. *Reproduction.* 2001;**121**(4):595–603.

43. Rowley MJ, Leach DR, Warner GA *et al.* Effect of graded doses of ionizing radiation on the human testis. *Radiat Res.* 1974;**59**(3):665–78.

44. Gutschi T, Mohamad Al-Ali B, Shamloul R *et al.* Impact of cell phone use on men's semen parameters. *Andrologia.* 2011;**43**(5):312–16.

45. Jurewicz J, Hanke W, Radwan M *et al.* Environmental factors and semen quality. *Int J Occup Med Environ Health.* 2009;**22**(4):305–29.

46. Somers CM. Ambient air pollution exposure and damage to male gametes: human studies and in situ 'sentinel' animal experiments. *Syst Biol Reprod Med.* 2011;**57**(1–2):63–71.

47. Nieuwenhuijsen MJ, Toledano MB, Eaton NE *et al.* Chlorination disinfection byproducts in water and their association with adverse reproductive outcomes: A review. *Occup Environ Med.* 2000;**57**(2):73–85.

48. Tardiff RG, Carson ML, Ginevan ME. Updated weight of evidence for an association between adverse reproductive and developmental effects and exposure to disinfection by-products. *Regul Toxicol Pharmacol.* 2006;**45**(2):185–205.

49. Toth GP, Kelty KC, George EL *et al.* Adverse male reproductive effects following subchronic exposure of rats to sodium dichloroacetate. *Fundam Appl Toxicol.* 1992;**19**(1):57–63.

Obesity and male infertility: is there an effect on embryogenesis?

Oumar Kuzbari and Ahmad O. Hammoud

Introduction

The relationship between obesity and male infertility is gaining wider attention with an influx of recent articles exploring this association both in animal models and humans. This new research covers all aspects of this relationship, including the association of obesity to the hormonal profile, semen parameters, semen DNA fragmentation, and embryo quality (Table 14.1). A recent meta-analysis done by Sermondade et al. showed that male obesity is associated with alterations in semen parameters [1]. This study came to oppose a previously published meta-analysis that could not find this relation

in the articles analyzed and reopened a debate expected to only get wider in the coming years [2].

Obesity, among other factors, was suggested as a causal agent in the decline of semen quality in the industrialized world. During the past decades, several reports have suggested that the quality of semen in men is declining. Carlsen et al. showed, in a meta-analysis of 61 studies including 14,947 men, a significant global decline in the mean sperm count from 113 million/mL in 1940 to 66 million/mL in 1990 ($P < 0.0001$) and mean seminal volume from 3.40 mL to 2.75 mL ($P = 0.027$) among men without a history of infertility [3]. Auger et al. also found a decline in the

Table 14.1 The effects of male obesity on human reproduction.

Parameter and effects		References
Fertility in the general population	Increase the risk of infertility	Sallmen et al. [10], Nguyen et al. [11], Ramlau-Hansen et al. [12], Jokela et al. [13]
Serum reproductive hormone levels	Decrease the levels of total testosterone, SHBG, and inhibin B. Decreased or normal FSH and LH levels Increase serum estrogen levels	Hammoud et al. [9], Chavarro et al. [14], Isidori et al. [15], Tchernof et al. [16], Pauli et al. [17], Kasturi et al. [18], Winters et al. [19]
Sperm parameters	Decrease in total sperm count, concentration, and motility	Sermondade et al. [1], Hammoud et al. [8, 9, 21], Jensen et al. [22], Kort et al. [23]
Sperm functions	Increase DNA fragmentation index and seminal oxidative stress	Kort et al. [23], Chavarro et al. [14], Tunc et al. [29], Tremellen [30]
Preimplantation embryo development	Decrease in expanded blastocyst development rates per two pro-nuclei (2PN)	Bakos et al. [41]
Pregnancy rate and live birth outcomes after ART	Decrease in implantation rate, clinical pregnancy rate, and live birth rates Increase in pregnancy loss	Bakos et al. [41], Keltz et al. [42]

SHBG, sex hormone-binding globulin; FSH, follicle-stimulating hormone; LH, luteinizing hormone; ART, assisted reproduction technology.

Paternal Influences on Human Reproductive Success, ed. Douglas T. Carrell. Published by Cambridge University Press.
© Cambridge University Press 2013.

concentration, motility, and percentage of morphologically normal sperm in Parisian, fertile men studied over 20 years. In that study, the mean concentration of sperm decreased by 2.1% per year, from 89 million/mL in 1973 to 60 million/mL in 1992 ($P < 0.001$) and the percentages of motile and normal spermatozoa decreased by 0.6% and 0.5% per year, respectively ($P < 0.001$) [4]. These findings led to the estimation that sperm count is falling by as much as 1.5% each year in the USA and other western nations [5]. Several hypotheses explaining the observed decline in male fertility have been postulated and these include exposure to environmental pollution and estrogen-mimicking chemicals during fetal or adult life, and/or changes in diet and lifestyle factors such as stress, smoking, and obesity. Obesity is now a major public health concern. During the past three decades, the USA has experienced a dramatic increase in the prevalence of obesity among men and women aged 20 years or older, approximately 66.3% are overweight, 32.42% are obese, and 4.8% are extremely obese [6]. At the same rate, the percentage of overweight and obese adults is estimated to be 86.3% and 51.1% by 2030 [7].

Obesity and male infertility

Multiple reports have described the effect of obesity on male fertility [2, 8, 9]. This effect is thought to be multifactorial and is modulated by genetic and environmental influences.

Effect of male obesity on fertility in the general population

Population-based studies on the effect of men's body mass on couples' fertility suggested an adverse effect. In a secondary analysis of the Agricultural Health Study that included 52,395 certified pesticide applicators and 32,347 of their spouses, 1,329 couples met the inclusion criteria, including data available regarding body mass index (BMI) for both partners. Male BMI was associated with infertility with an odds ratio (OR) of 1.12 (95% confidence interval: 1.01–1.25), after correction for female BMI, male and female age, smoking status, alcohol use, and exposure to solvents and pesticides. The categorization of male BMI into groups showed a dose–effect relationship, with a maximal effect in the BMI 32–43 kg/m^2 group and a plateau of effect beyond this [10]. In the Norwegian Mother and Child cohort study, overweight men (BMI: 25–29.9 kg/m^2) had an OR

for infertility of 1.20 [95% confidence interval (CI) 1.04–1.38] and obese men (BMI > 30 kg/m^2) had an OR for infertility of 1.36 (95% CI 1.13–1.63) when compared with men with normal BMI, after correcting for coital frequency, female BMI, male and female age, smoking status, and various risk factors for female infertility [11]. Similar observations were reported by Ramlau-Hansen et al. who found a dose–response relationship between increasing BMI and infertility in men after analyzing the data of 47,835 couples from the Danish National Birth Cohort [12]. While current BMI in males appears to be correlated with reduced fertility, increased weight during adolescence is also correlated with reduced fertility in adulthood. In a study by Jokela et al. on the effect of increased weight in adolescence on future fertility in 583 male participants, overweight and obese adolescents had 4% and 32% fewer children, respectively, than those with normal adolescent weight [13].

Effect of male obesity on serum reproductive hormone levels

Studies have shown an inverse association of male BMI with serum levels of total testosterone, sex hormone-binding globulin (SHBG), and inhibin B, and a positive association with serum estrogen levels. Follicle-stimulating hormone (FSH) and luteinizing hormone (LH) levels can be either normal or low in obese men suggesting a hypothalamic hypogonadic profile [9, 14–18]. The main mechanism for this hormonal profile involves increased peripheral conversion of testosterone to estrogen because of the increased activity of aromatase enzyme present in the adipose tissue. Elevated estrogens have a suppressive effect on the hypothalamus and the GnRH pulses leading to secondary hypogonadism. Sex hormone-binding globulin levels are reduced in obese men in response to the hyperinsulinemia secondary to obesity-related insulin resistance. Inhibin B levels, a surrogate marker of Sertoli cell function, and associated spermatogenic activity, were also shown to be lower in obese men [9, 14, 19]. Globerman et al. showed that among obese men who underwent gastroplasty, inhibin B levels increased following weight reduction [20].

Effect of male obesity on sperm parameters

Increasing BMI or waist/hip ratio was linked to alterations in sperm parameters in several reports [1, 8, 9,

21–23]. Jensen *et al.* examined the relationship between BMI and semen quality among 1,558 young Danish men (mean age 19 years) from the general population. They found that men with a BMI > 25 kg/m^2 had a reduction in sperm concentration and total sperm count of 21.6% (95% confidence interval (CI) 4.0–39.4%) and 23.9% (95% CI 4.7–43.2%), respectively, compared with men with BMI between 20–25 kg/m^2 after controlling for confounders [22]. We studied semen parameters in 526 patients who presented to a tertiary care center for infertility evaluation. Data collected included patient demographics, past medical, social, and surgical history, and BMI. Among the 526 patients, 10.2% (54 of 526) were excluded because of the presence of a male factor known to affect fertility. The mean age of the study population was 32.8 ± 0.3 years and the mean BMI of the population was 28.5 ± 0.26 kg/m^2. Body mass index was divided into three groups: normal (BMI < 25 kg/m^2), overweight (25 kg/m^2 ≤ BMI < 30 kg/m^2), and obese (BMI ≥ 30 kg/m^2). The incidence of oligozoospermia increased with increasing BMI: normal weight = 5.32%, overweight = 9.52%, and obese = 15.62%. The odds ratio (OR) of oligozoospermia in obese patients compared with patients with normal BMI was 3.3 (95% CI 1.19–9.14). The prevalence of a low progressively motile sperm count (defined as < 10 × 10^6 progressively motile sperm) was also greater with increasing BMI: normal weight = 4.52%, overweight = 8.93%, and obese = 13.28%. The OR of having a progressively motile sperm count < 10 × 10^6 in obese patients compared with normal weight patients was 3.4 (95% CI 1.12–10.60). When comparing obese patients with non-obese patients (normal weight and overweight), the OR of having a high percentage of abnormal morphology was 1.6 (95% CI 1.05–2.59) [21]. A recent meta-analysis of 14 studies including 9,779 men by Sermondade *et al.* showed an inverse association between obesity and abnormal sperm count. Overweight and obese men were found to be at significantly increased odds of presenting with oligozoospermia (OR 1.11; 95% CI 1.01–1.20) and (OR 1.42; 95% CI 1.12–1.79) respectively, when compared with normal weight men. Azoospermia was also higher in overweight (OR 1.39; 95% CI 0.98–1.97) and obese men (OR 1.81; 95% CI 1.23–2.66) when compared with normal weight men [1].

The effect of weight loss on semen quality has been explored. In a pilot study involving 43 men with BMI > 33 kg/m^2 followed through a 14-week residential weight loss program, Håkonsen *et al.* found that weight loss was associated with an increase in total sperm count ($P = 0.02$), semen volume ($P = 0.04$), testosterone ($P = 0.02$), SHBG ($P = 0.03$) and AMH ($P = 0.02$). In that study the median (range) age was 32 (20–59) years, the median (range) BMI was 44 (33–61) kg/m^2 and the median (range) weight loss was 22 (4–39) kg, corresponding to a median weight loss of 15%, ranging from 3.5% to 25.4% [24]. This study is in contrast to reports of men developing severe oligozoospermia or azoospermia after gastric bypass surgery [25, 26].

Effect of male obesity on sperm function

While the majority of studies conducted to date explored the effect of obesity on serum reproductive hormone levels and sperm parameters, there are some studies that described the association of obesity with sperm function and sperm DNA fragmentation. In a well-designed study, Bakos *et al.* used an animal model of diet-induced obesity to examine the direct effects of obesity on sperm function. Six-week-old male mice were fed high-fat (HFD) or control diets for 9 weeks. Mice on HFD gained significantly more weight after the nine week period compared with the mice fed the control diet (16.0 vs. 8.8 g; $P < 0.001$). The sperm motility was decreased in the HFD group compared with controls (36 ± 2% vs. 44 ± 4%; $P < 0.05$). Intracellular reactive oxygen species (ROS) production was elevated (692 ± 83 vs. 409 ± 22 units; $P < 0.01$) and sperm DNA damage was increased (1.64 ± 0.6% vs. 0.17 ± 0.06%; $P < 0.05$) in the HFD group compared with controls. Furthermore, the percentage of non-capacitated sperm was significantly lower in males fed a HFD compared with controls (12.34% vs. 21.06%; $P < 0.01$). The number of sperm bound to each oocyte was significantly lower (41.14 ± 2.5 vs. 58.39 ± 2.4; $P < 0.01$) in the HFD group compared with that in controls resulting in significantly lower fertilization rates (25.9% vs. 43.9%; $P < 0.01$) [27].

In humans, Kort *et al.* assessed the DNA fragmentation index (DFI) in 520 healthy men in different BMI groups using the flow cytometry-based sperm degree of DNA fragmentation (SCSA) and found that obese and overweight men had a significantly higher DFI (27% and 25.8%, respectively) compared with normal weight men (19.9%) ($P < 0.05$) [23]. Similarly, Chavarro *et al.* concluded that sperm with high DNA damage were significantly more numerous in obese men than in normal weight men [14]. Obesity is also associated with increased oxidative stress which occurs when the production of reactive oxygen species (ROS) overwhelms the antioxidant protective systems [28]. Tunc *et al.* found a positive correlation between BMI and sperm oxidative stress ($r = 0.23$, $P = 0.039$) in a study involving 81 men undergoing semen analysis as part of infertility work-up [29]. The increased testicular oxidative stress was proposed to play a role in obesity-related impaired spermatogenesis by two main mechanisms: damaging the sperm membrane which reduces sperm motility and ability to fuse with the oocyte and directly damaging sperm DNA, leading to a possible alteration of the paternal genomic contribution to the developing embryo [30]. The detrimental effects of paternal obesity on reproductive health can be transgenerational. In an animal model, Fullston *et al.* demonstrated that paternal obesity caused by paternal exposure to a high-fat diet in mice, in the absence of diabetes, diminishes the reproductive health of both male and female offspring, suggesting an effect of male obesity on the sperm epigenome and resulting in an alteration of developmental programming of fertility in subsequent generations [31].

Effect of male obesity on preimplantation embryo development

It has been suggested that paternal effect on embryonic development can occur as early as fertilization. During fertilization, the spermatozoon contributes genetic and epigenetic factors to the developing embryo. In humans, paternal factors can affect embryo cleavage speed and morphology, the rate of in vitro blastocyst formation and implantation rates after embryo transfer, both after conventional IVF and ICSI [32–34]. The paternal effect is postulated to be either early and/or late as follows: the early effect is associated with sperm cytoplasmic deficiencies and manifested by low cleavage speed and increased fragmentation in the cleaving embryo, the late effect is associated with increased incidence of sperm DNA fragmentation and is not detected before the 8-cell stage of embryo development, a stage when expression of sperm-derived genes begins [32, 35, 36].

The detrimental effects of paternal obesity on early embryo development were shown in a mouse model. Mitchell *et al.* demonstrated that male mice fed a standard rodent chow (lean) or a high-fat diet (obese) for 13 weeks and mated with females, resulted in a significant reduction in cleavage to the two-cell stage in relation to paternal obesity ($P < 0.001$). On days 3 and 4 of culture, a significant delay in embryo development was noted in embryos from the obese males compared with embryos from lean controls ($P < 0.001$). Moreover, at day 5 of culture, just 25.5% of embryos from obese males were developing compared with 46.0% of embryos from lean controls ($P < 0.001$). In embryos reaching the blastocyst stage, the number of cells from both the inner mass cell and the trophectoderm cell populations was significantly reduced with paternal obesity. Blastocysts from obese males had a greater proportion of apoptotic cells compared with lean controls (21.3% vs. 14.1% apoptotic cells, respectively, $P < 0.05$) [37]. Similarly, Binder *et al.* found that parental diet-induced obesity leads to delays in cell cycle progression during preimplantation in the mouse embryos noted from the second cleavage stage, and altered carbohydrate utilization by the blastocyst. Moreover, blastocyst cell numbers were significantly lower when either parent was obese [38].

Obesity is part of the metabolic syndrome and can be associated with impaired glucose metabolism. Glucose is required for successful fertilization as well as to assure maintenance of viability of the embryo throughout the preimplantation period [39]. Kim and Moley found that sperm quality, fertilization rate, and subsequent embryo development are reduced in diabetic male mice compared with non-diabetic controls, suggesting an adverse paternal effect on embryogenesis in the diabetic group [40].

In humans, there is paucity of information on the effects of paternal obesity on embryo quality and subsequent pregnancy and live birth outcomes. Bakos *et al.* studied the relationship between paternal BMI and embryo development in 305 couples undergoing fresh in vitro fertilization (IVF) cycles with or without intracytoplasmic sperm injection (ICSI). Couples were classified according to the following paternal BMI ranges: normal weight BMI 20–24.9 kg/m^2, overweight 25–29.9 kg/m^2, obese 30–34.9 kg/m^2, and morbidly obese ≥ 35 kg/m^2. In this study, there was no effect of paternal BMI on day 3 cleavage rates or the morphologic grade of embryos either in conventional IVF or ICSI. In contrast, there was a significantly linear decrease in expanded blastocyst development rates per two pro-nuclei (2PN) with increasing paternal BMI ($P < 0.05$) [41].

Paternal BMI and pregnancy and live birth outcomes after ART

A retrospective study of 290 IVF cycles by Keltz *et al.* showed that males with BMI greater than 25.0 kg/m^2 had

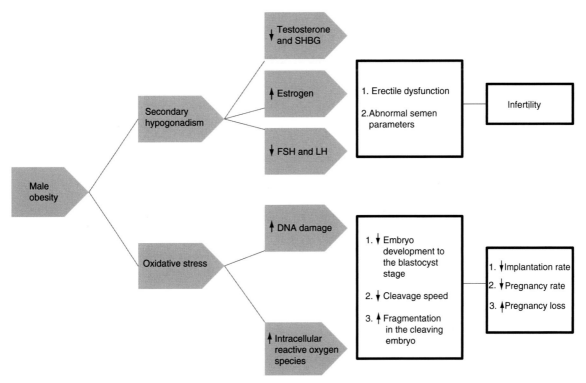

Figure 14.1. The proposed pathways in which male obesity may affect human reproduction.

a significantly lower clinical pregnancy rate compared with males with BMI of 18.5–24.9 kg/m² (53.2% vs. 33.6%). After adjustment for female age, female BMI, number of embryos transferred, and sperm concentration, male overweight status was negatively associated with pregnancy rate in IVF but not in ICSI cycles [42]. This detrimental influence of male obesity on clinical pregnancy rate after in vitro fertilization was also confirmed in a recent retrospective analysis of 305 couples undergoing fresh IVF cycles with or without ICSI. Bakos *et al.* noted linear decrease in pregnancy rates with increasing paternal BMI from normal to obese men ($P < 0.01$). Implantation rate (as measured by the presence of fetal sac) was also decreased with increased paternal BMI. Conversely, there was an overall increase in pregnancy loss with increasing paternal BMI. Similarly, viable ongoing pregnancy rates and live birth rates were decreased significantly by increasing paternal BMI ($P < 0.05$). There was no difference in gestation length or infant weight across the four groups nor any effect on sex ratios [41]. Unlike the study by Keltz *et al.*, the method of insemination did not affect these outcomes significantly. The reason for this difference may be due to the

higher number of embryos transferred in the overweight group in the study by Keltz *et al.* compared with the study by Bakos *et al.*, where the vast majority of cases were elective single-embryo transfers.

Conclusions

Obesity is associated with male infertility, and this association is more evident in extremely obese men with clear hypogonadism and altered semen parameters. Male obesity can also affect sperm function, a finding shown, in animals, to affect the developing embryo. In humans, emerging evidence suggests that male obesity can affect the developing embryo and subsequently diminish pregnancy rates in the context of IVF and ICSI (Figure 14.1).

References

1. Sermondade N, Faure C, Fezeu L *et al.* Obesity and increased risk for oligozoospermia and azoospermia. *Arch Intern Med.* 2012; **172**(5):440–2.

2. MacDonald AA, Herbison GP, Showell M *et al.* The impact of body mass index on semen parameters and

reproductive hormones in human males: a systematic review with meta-analysis. *Hum Reprod Update.* 2010;**16**(3):293–311.

3. Carlsen E, Giwercman A, Keiding N *et al.* Evidence for decreasing quality of semen during past 50 years. *Br Med J.* 1992;**305**(6854):609–13.

4. Auger J, Kunstmann JM, Czyglik F *et al.* Decline in semen quality among fertile men in Paris during the past 20 years. *New Engl J Med.* 1995;**332** (5):281–5.

5. Swan SH, Elkin EP, Fenster L. The question of declining sperm density revisited: an analysis of 101 studies published 1934–1996. *Environ Health Perspect.* 2000;**108**(10):961–6.

6. Wang Y, Beydoun MA. The obesity epidemic in the United States – gender, age, socioeconomic, racial/ethnic, and geographic characteristics: a systematic review and meta-regression analysis. *Epidemiol Rev.* 2007;**29**(1):6–28.

7. Wang Y, Beydoun MA, Liang L *et al.* Will all Americans become overweight or obese? Estimating the progression and cost of the US obesity epidemic. *Obesity.* 2008;**16**(10):2323–30.

8. Hammoud AO, Gibson M, Peterson CM *et al.* Obesity and male reproductive potential. *J Androl.* 2006;**27** (5):619–26.

9. Hammoud AO, Gibson M, Peterson CM *et al.* Impact of male obesity on infertility: a critical review of the current literature. *Fertil Steril.* 2008;**90** (4):897–904.

10. Sallmen M, Sandler DP, Hoppin JA *et al.* Reduced fertility among overweight and obese men. *Epidemiology.* 2006;**17**(5):520–3.

11. Nguyen R, Wilcox A, Skjaerven R *et al.* Men's body mass index and infertility. *Hum Reprod.* 2007;**22** (9):2488–93.

12. Ramlau-Hansen CH, Thulstrup AM, Nohr EA *et al.* Subfecundity in overweight and obese couples. *Hum Reprod.* 2007;**22**(6):1634–7.

13. Jokela M, Kivimäki M, Elovainio M *et al.* Body mass index in adolescence and number of children in adulthood. *Epidemiology.* 2007;**18**(5):599–606.

14. Chavarro JE, Toth TL, Wright DL *et al.* Body mass index in relation to semen quality, sperm DNA integrity, and serum reproductive hormone levels among men attending an infertility clinic. *Fertil Steril.* 2010;**93**(7):2222–31.

15. Isidori AM, Caprio M, Strollo F *et al.* Leptin and androgens in male obesity: evidence for leptin contribution to reduced androgen levels. *J Clin Endocrinol Metab.* 1999;**84**(10):3673–80.

16. Tchernof A, Despres JP, Belanger A *et al.* Reduced testosterone and adrenal C19 steroid levels in obese men. *Metabolism.* 1995;**44**(4):513–19.

17. Pauli EM, Legro RS, Demers LM *et al.* Diminished paternity and gonadal function with increasing obesity in men. *Fertil Steril.* 2008;**90**(2):346–51.

18. Kasturi SS, Tannir J, Brannigan RE. The metabolic syndrome and male infertility. *J Androl.* 2008;**29** (3):251–9.

19. Winters SJ, Wang C, Abdelrahaman E *et al.* Inhibin-b levels in healthy young adult men and prepubertal boys: is obesity the cause for the contemporary decline in sperm count because of fewer Sertoli cells? *J Androl.* 2006;**27**(4):560–4.

20. Globerman H, Shen-Orr Z, Karnieli E *et al.* Inhibin b in men with severe obesity and after weight reduction following gastroplasty. *Endocr Res.* 2005;**31**(1):17–26.

21. Hammoud AO, Wilde N, Gibson M *et al.* Male obesity and alteration in sperm parameters. *Fertil Steril.* 2008;**90**(6):2222–5.

22. Jensen TK, Andersson AM, Jorgensen N *et al.* Body mass index in relation to semen quality and reproductive hormones among 1,558 Danish men. *Fertil Steril.* 2004;**82**(4):863–70.

23. Kort HI, Massey JB, Elsner CW *et al.* Impact of body mass index values on sperm quantity and quality. *J Androl.* 2006;**27**(3):450–2.

24. Håkonsen L, Thulstrup A, Aggerholm A *et al.* Does weight loss improve semen quality and reproductive hormones? Results from a cohort of severely obese men. *Reprod Health.* 2011;**8**(1):24.

25. Sermondade N, Massin N, Boitrelle F *et al.* Sperm parameters and male fertility after bariatric surgery: three case series. *Reprod BioMed Online.* 2012;**24** (2):206–10.

26. Lazaros L, Hatzi E, Markoula S *et al.* Dramatic reduction in sperm parameters following bariatric surgery: report of two cases. *Andrologia.* 2012; doi: 10.1111/j.1439-0272.2012.01300.x. [Epub ahead of print].

27. Bakos HW, Mitchell M, Setchell BP *et al.* The effect of paternal diet-induced obesity on sperm function and fertilization in a mouse model. *Int J Androl.* 2011;**34** (5 pt 1):402–10.

28. Ozata M, Mergen M, Oktenli C *et al.* Increased oxidative stress and hypozincemia in male obesity. *Clin Biochem.* 2002;**35**(8):627–31.

29. Tunc O, Bakos HW, Tremellen K. Impact of body mass index on seminal oxidative stress. *Andrologia.* 2011;**43**(2):121–8.

30. Tremellen K. Oxidative stress and male infertility – a clinical perspective. *Hum Reprod Update.* 2008;**14**(3):243–58.

31. Fullston T, Palmer NO, Owens JA *et al.* Diet-induced paternal obesity in the absence of diabetes diminishes the reproductive health of two subsequent generations of mice. *Hum Reprod.* 2012; doi: 10.1093/humrep/des030 [Epub ahead of print].

32. Tesarik J, Mendoza C, Greco E. Paternal effects acting during the first cell cycle of human preimplantation development after ICSI. *Hum Reprod.* 2002;**17**(1):184–9.

33. Shoukir Y, Chardonnens D, Campana A *et al.* Blastocyst development from supernumerary embryos after intracytoplasmic sperm injection: a paternal influence? *Hum Reprod.* 1998;**13**(6):1632–7.

34. Seli E, Gardner DK, Schoolcraft WB *et al.* Extent of nuclear DNA damage in ejaculated spermatozoa impacts on blastocyst development after in vitro fertilization. *Fertil Steril.* 2004;**82**(2):378–83.

35. Ménézo YJR. Paternal and maternal factors in preimplantation embryogenesis: interaction with the biochemical environment. *Reprod BioMed Online.* 2006;**12**(5):616–21.

36. Tesarik J, Greco E, Mendoza C. Late, but not early, paternal effect on human embryo development is related to sperm DNA fragmentation. *Hum Reprod.* 2004;**19**(3):611–15.

37. Mitchell M, Bakos HW, Lane M. Paternal diet-induced obesity impairs embryo development and implantation in the mouse. *Fertil Steril.* 2011;**95**(4):1349–53.

38. Binder NK, Mitchell M, Gardner DK. Parental diet-induced obesity leads to retarded early mouse embryo development and altered carbohydrate utilisation by the blastocyst. *Reprod Fertil Dev.* 2012;**24**(6):804–12.

39. Sakkas D, Urner F, Menezo Y *et al.* Effects of glucose and fructose on fertilization, cleavage, and viability of mouse embryos in vitro. *Biol Reprod.* 1993;**49**(6):1288–92.

40. Kim ST, Moley KH. Paternal effect on embryo quality in diabetic mice is related to poor sperm quality and associated with decreased glucose transporter expression. *Reproduction.* 2008;**136**(3):313–22.

41. Bakos HW, Henshaw RC, Mitchell M *et al.* Paternal body mass index is associated with decreased blastocyst development and reduced live birth rates following assisted reproductive technology. *Fertil Steril.* 2011;**95**(5):1700–4.

42. Keltz J, Zapantis A, Jindal S *et al.* Overweight men: clinical pregnancy after ART is decreased in IVF but not in ICSI cycles. *J Assist Reprod Genet.* 2010;**27**(9):539–44.

Chapter

15

Intracytoplasmic sperm injection: does the sperm matter?

Gianpiero D. Palermo, Queenie V. Neri, and Zev Rosenwaks

Introduction

Infertility affects approximately 12–15% of couples of reproductive age [1]. Among the general population, the ability of a man to procreate appears to have progressively decreased during the past half century [2] where about half of all infertility cases are directly attributed to the male partner. Approximately 6% of males between the ages of 15 and 44 are deemed infertile or have their fecundity severely compromised [3].

Much of our understanding of the mechanisms of mammalian reproduction and advancements in this area emanated from animal husbandry and the outstanding work carried out by veterinarians [4] and reproductive biologists [5, 6]. However, it was not until the late 1970s when IVF became a reality that female infertility treatments ascended to the forefront. It was soon realized that although IVF successfully treated tubal infertility, there were great limitations in achieving predictable fertilization rates following in vitro insemination in men with suboptimal semen parameters [7].

The implementation of assisted fertilization had generated a remarkable effort in understanding the physiology of the individual spermatozoon and provided a method to bypass the limitations of a subfertile sibling cell. Assisted fertilization brought a shift from the existing in vitro approach that aimed at generating a viable embryo outside the body to target a specific step – achieving fertilization. Intracytoplasmic sperm injection (ICSI) in particular has brought down the gamete ratio one-to-one relationship where one individual spermatozoon is paired to an oocyte, paving the way to understanding the interaction between these fascinating haploid cells.

Intracytoplasmic sperm injection has proven itself as the assisted fertilization technique that grants the best results in terms of fertilization and clinical pregnancy. It is capable of providing successful fertilization almost independently of the characteristics of the semen specimens whether used fresh or after cryopreservation. Even immunological infertility with anti-sperm antibodies located on the sperm head can benefit from ICSI [8–11]. Similarly, when inconsistently mature spermatozoa are retrieved surgically from the epididymis or testis, the clinical outcome is not affected [12, 13]. Because of the dependable and versatile performance, ICSI has broadened its initial indication as a technique capable of overriding sperm dysfunction to a procedure that may partly address issues attributable to the female partner. Indeed, ICSI has allowed successful fertilization when only a few and/or abnormal oocytes are available [14] and most importantly has rendered possible the successful insemination of cryopreserved oocytes [15]. In fact, the direct sperm injection bypasses the hostile zona pellucida modified by cryo-related cortical granules extrusion [16–19]. Intracytoplasmic sperm injection is also the preferred conception method for inseminating couples undergoing preimplantation genetic diagnosis (PGD) [20]. It avoids sperm DNA zona contamination and by enhancing the number of fertilized oocytes clearly increases the number of embryos available for genetic screening [21, 22].

Finally, because a single spermatozoon is used, ICSI has allowed treatment of men who are virtually azoospermic (also defined as cryptozoospermic) and those with vasa obstruction [23]. This scenario has fueled attempts to inject oocytes with immature spermatozoa or germ cells [24–27]. However, in spite of the remarkable and consistent fertilization achieved, embryo implantation chances are similar to those observed with other assisted reproductive

Paternal Influences on Human Reproductive Success, ed. Douglas T. Carrell. Published by Cambridge University Press.
© Cambridge University Press 2013.

technologies (ART), mostly dictated by maternal age [28, 29].

The different primary and alternative indications presented have contributed to the current popular and unrestricted adoption of ICSI as the preferred insemination method in many circumstances [30–32]. In 2002, of all ART cycles reported to the International Committee Monitoring Assisted Reproductive Technologies (ICMART), ICSI represented over 50% of the cases in Australia and New Zealand (53.8%), Europe (53.9%), Latin America (76.1%), the Middle East (92.5%), and North America (60.8%) while in Asia it represented only 47.5% [33–35]. If we look at European countries insemination by ICSI started at 39.6% in 1997 and gradually increased in the ensuing years to 58.1% by 2004 [32] while in the USA, it is used in 61.4% of all cases [33]. At our center, there has been a steady and progressive increase in ICSI prevalence starting at 32% in 1993, then at 50% in 1995, and reaching 73% by 2002. The last percentage reflects the referral for male factor infertility to our unit.

The evaluation of an infertile couple calls for the screening of the male partner and according to his semen characteristics the need to carefully assess his genomic status. Thereafter, our attention needs to be focused on the spermatozoon to be used for assisted fertilization to estimate its genotype and a careful appraisal of its epigenetic phenotype. Although ICSI is capable of treating many male gamete dysfunctions, it is important to select and identify the one that has maintained its full functional capability.

Screening men

Semen analysis still provides the fundamental information on which clinicians base their initial diagnosis while gaining information on the fertility potential of a male patient. The diagnosis of male infertility is based upon the semen profile, constructed according to recognized guidelines [36–38]. This measures the volume of the ejaculate, the concentration of spermatozoa, their motility and their morphology. Marked inter-ejaculates variability is a recurrent phenomenon [39, 40], in addition many recorded parameters of the spermatogenic profile are subjective, and assessments have been inconsistent across laboratories [41–43]. Although the WHO has published a range of "normal" values, these are not evidence-based, either in terms of their diagnostic value, or in terms of their relationship to the normal ejaculate. As a consequence, many

couples with "unexplained" infertility eventually prove to have defective spermatozoa when appropriately sensitive assays (such as acrosome reaction, anti-sperm antibodies, phospholipase C zeta (PLCζ)) are used, yet some couples with subnormal semen parameters prove to have normal sperm function [44, 45]. Given this evidence, it would perhaps be most appropriate for laboratories to establish their own definition of "normal" based on their individual experience in screening ejaculates.

A number of epidemiological factors that may have a bearing on a couple's fertility include age, though the impact of male age is less certain than that of the female. Smoking by both partners is highly relevant as well, there being evidence that smokers have lower sperm concentrations than non-smokers [46–48]. Occupational, environmental, and genetic factors may also be highly relevant. In regard to the last, there is no doubt that recent advances in assisted reproduction technologies have increased our understanding of the etiology of male infertility, particularly by drawing attention to the major contribution of specific genes [49–54].

Human male germ-cell development begins in early embryogenesis, but the first mature spermatozoa appear only at puberty (c. 12 years old). Genetic disorders disrupting this male-specific cell differentiation and maturation can be reflected at the chromosomal or molecular DNA level.

In the case of chromosomal anomalies, these can be numeral, structural, or both. Aneuploidy leading to male infertility may involve the sex chromosomes (e.g. an additional X-chromosome in Klinefelter syndrome) or autosomes (e.g. trisomy 21). Structural chromosome anomalies (small deletions, translocations, inversions) can lead to male infertility and these may involve both sex and autosomal chromosomes. Chromosomal rearrangements such as reciprocal translocations can give rise to abnormal meiotic chromosome pairing, and in turn disruption of spermatogenesis. For instance, evidence has accumulated since the 1970s that disruption through meiosis and recombination follows a significant rearrangement of the Y-chromosome. In fact, deletions in the Yq region can be associated with azoospermia, suggesting a spermatogenesis locus in the region designated AZF (Azoospermia Factor) where a later study has shown three such loci (AZFa, AZFb, AZFc) in Yq [53].

While the benefits of ICSI are clear, the success of this approach may have also reinforced the perception that the sperm cell is simply a vehicle for the transport of the paternal genome. Therefore, if any motile spermatozoa are available it has become quite common to expect normal fertilization and embryogenesis, regardless of the potential intrinsic defects which may be associated with subfertile spermatozoa [55]. In addition to a haploid set of chromosomes, the human sperm cell must provide the oocyte with an activation stimulus, a functional centrosome, proper packaging and coding of the genome.

When suboptimal spermatozoa are utilized for ART procedures, claims have been made regarding a possible adverse outcome for these offspring [56–58]. Since it is not yet possible to precisely evaluate the consequences of in vitro culture procedures on imprinting, long-term, large-scale epidemiological children follow-up studies would be able to address the eventual risks posed by assisted reproduction in general and particularly the use of these gametes with dysfunction.

Choosing the male gamete

While ICSI grants the ability to utilize sperm from various forms of male infertility and extremely compromised semen parameters, it is important to consider that the individual spermatozoon chosen must carry all the different components typical of a male gamete.

The acrosome is a cap-like structure derived from the Golgi apparatus during spermiogenesis whose functional significance is believed to grant zona pellucida penetration and consequent fusion with the oolemma [59–62]. This paramount phenomenon is minimized by ICSI that apparently does not require any specific sperm pretreatment other than immobilization [12, 63, 64]. However, aggressively compressing the tail prior to injection significantly improves ICSI fertilization rates [65–69]. Although the mechanism of this beneficial effect was not immediately clear, we found indirect evidence that such immobilization triggers changes in the sperm permeability [70] and expedites membrane potential leading to sperm plasma membrane destabilization culminating in acrosomal disruption [65, 67]. This was further corroborated by the observation that epididymal spermatozoa characterized by a high lipidic content in their membrane [71] required more intense damage to trigger the induced membrane modifications [69, 72]. Therefore, proteins are added to capacitation media for partial replacement of the lipid components

rendering the sperm membrane more hydrophilic and thus, more fragile. The introduction of sequential media, formulated with limited glucose and protein, have somewhat resulted in complications in the execution of ICSI procedure requiring a more intense mechanical action on the flagellum to yield the desired membrane destabilization [73].

To achieve fertilization, spermatozoa must activate the oocyte, triggered by the increasing cytosolic free calcium concentration in mammalian ooplasms [74, 75]. One of the most important components of the male gamete is the soluble oocyte activating factor that has been recognized in rabbit, hamster, boar, and human spermatozoa [76–78]. An early form of this protein termed oscillin was claimed to exist in the equatorial segment of the sperm head and to be involved in Ca^{2+} evoking oscillation patterns similar to that seen following sperm fractions [78]. The human homolog of this hamster oscillin is glucosamine 6-phosphate isomerase (GPI, GenBank accession number D31766). The deployment of antibodies against this compound did not interfere with the sperm extract's ability to activate oocytes, nor was the injection of its recombinant form effective in inducing calcium oscillations [79]. This work helped to disprove that this compound is the specific sperm oocyte activating factor. Our work together with other investigators [79, 80] led to the identification of the sperm soluble factor that generates inositol 1,4,5-triphosphate (InsP3) and identified as phosphoinositide-specific phospholipase C (PLC) [81, 82]. Several PLC isoforms, β, γ and δ, present in the spermatozoa have been considered but were found to be absent from chromatographic fractions that specifically cause Ca^{2+} oscillations [83, 84].

The evidence of a novel PLC was first obtained on the examination of short ESTs (expressed sequence tag) from the mouse and human testis that enabled the isolation and characterization of a full-length cDNA encoding sperm protein that is now referred to as PLCζ [85]. The PLCζ triggers Ca^{2+} oscillations in the mouse indistinguishable from those at fertilization. The human PLCζ was able to elicit mouse egg activation and early embryonic development up to the blastocyst stage [86]. We attempted to inject a caged-IP3 into mouse oocytes to determine if it has the ability to trigger calcium oscillation compared with normal fertilization events (Lee and Machaca, unpublished data) (Figure 15.1).

Although ICSI results in average fertilization rates of 70% [87], complete or virtually complete fertilization

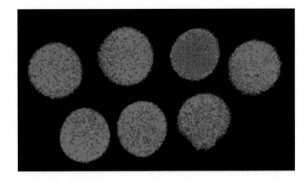

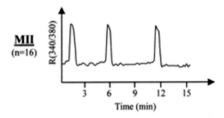

Figure 15.1. The injection of a caged-IP3 into mouse oocytes to determine its ability to trigger calcium oscillation compared with normal fertilization events. Calcium oscillations are shown below the micrograph. This figure is presented in color in the color plate section.

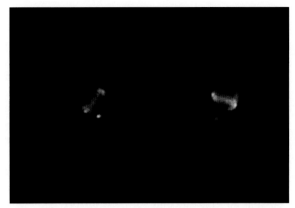

Figure 15.2. Fluorescent micrograph of spermatozoa evaluated for the presence of PLCζ utilizing a polyclonal antibody. This figure is presented in color in the color plate section.

failure still occurs in 1–5% of ICSI cycles [88, 89]. A deficiency in the level of the sperm activating factor is regarded as the principal cause of complete or partial fertilization failure after ICSI, and maintains a constant profile in repeated ART cycles [90].

At present, such cases can only be resolved using assisted oocyte activation (AOA). The most widely adopted agents for human oocytes include Ca^{2+}-ionophore and ionomycin, rarely strontium chloride, or electrical stimuli even in combination with 6-dimethylaminopurine (6-DMAP) or puromycin [90]. However, these methods are indiscriminate attempts to activate the oocyte by flooding its ooplasm with calcium ions that do not follow the physiological cascade [91]. This practice fuels concerns as to how such chemicals may be detrimental to embryo viability and future offspring well-being due to potential cytotoxic, mutagenic, and teratogenic effects [92].

A more physiologic approach would be to utilize a purified recombinant version of human PLCζ protein [93, 94]. However, the therapeutic utilization of PLCζ cRNA is not likely viable since the uncontrollable transcription of PLCζ may be detrimental to normal preimplantation development through gene expression irregularities, with eventual developmental defects observed in some embryos [94]. In addition, injected

PLCζ RNA could potentially, by reverse transcription into cDNA, be incorporated into the genome [95]. Therefore, an active, purified, and stable recombinant version of PLCζ would be the ideal alternative for therapeutic application, as it would function in a more physiologic fashion (Swann, personal communications).

In our center, we attempted to treat nine couples with histories of complete fertilization failure after ICSI. In a total of 18 cycles, we carried out assisted activation with a dual exposure of Ca^{2+}-ionophore along with a sperm membrane permeabilizing agent. Prior to their ICSI treatment, we evaluated their spermatozoa for the presence of PLCζ utilizing a polyclonal antibody. PLCζ in these men was significantly lower, ranging from 0 to no more than 14.4%, in comparison to over 37.0–80.7% in fertile individuals ($P = 0.0001$) (Figure 15.2). We were able to obtain a fertilization rate of 51.9% (41/79) with four oocytes that lysed. The cleavage rate was 87.7% with the mean number of blastomeres being 7.2 ± 1 on day 3, and a mean fragmentation rate of $8.4\% \pm 4$. Embryos were successfully transferred in all cycles with a mean of 1.7 conceptuses replaced per procedure; seven (38.9%) positive βhCG of which three (16.7%) progressed to clinical pregnancies and one couple delivered a healthy baby boy [96].

DNA damage in the male germline is considered as a major contributor to infertility, miscarriages, and birth defects in the offspring [97]. Because half of the offspring's DNA is originating from the paternal unit, it is of utmost importance to consider the detrimental effect that sperm chromatin and DNA damage may have on reproductive function.

When SCSA became available, we carried out a pilot study to understand the extent of chromatin fragmentation. We blindly assessed the DNA integrity status of sperm specimen of men that had generated ICSI children. We observed a chromatin fragmentation index ranging from 5.7% all the way up to 69.1%. When we categorized men according to DFI threshold, men with normal DFI of <30% ($n = 33$) had higher concentration and motility in comparison to those with abnormal DFI of ≥30% ($n = 27$) ($P < 0.01$). When fertilization characteristics were assessed, no differences were observed between the two groups nor in the cleavage rate of about 80%. The implantation rate was 19.8 vs 23.3%, respectively that resulted in a clinical pregnancy of 48.5% (16/33) in the normal DFI vs 66.7% (18/27) in the high DFI cohort. A total of 15 deliveries (15 singletons) were observed in the control and 14 (13 singletons and 1 set of twins) in the high DFI group. Their neonatal outcomes as well as their physical and cognitive development at 5 years of age were comparable [98, 99].

It is commonly accepted that DNA fragmentation observed in spermatozoa may play a role in embryo development and even in phenotypically normal offspring. Sperm DNA damage may become a source of epigenetic disorders later in life [100]. The fact that such fragmentation does not seem to preclude a term pregnancy [98, 99] may be attributed to a corrective role exerted by the selection of the best individual spermatozoon during the ICSI procedure [101–103] or eventually to an ability of the ooplasm to overcome and repair breaks present in the sperm DNA [104].

The sperm nucleus is very tightly packed to protect the nucleic acid during the journey that occurs prior to fertilization. Shaping of the male gamete nucleus takes place in late spermiogenesis as its chromatin is undergoing a remarkable condensation that renders the sperm transcriptionally inert and highly resistant to digestion. Following the morphological transformation of the nucleus in the testis, as sperm pass through the epididymis there occurs a stabilization of the chromatin through establishment of disulfide bonds between the thiol-rich protamines [105]. The human sperm nucleus is composed also of the DNA condensing core and linker histones that have been mostly replaced by protamines, thus changing the configuration of the sperm head to reach a more compact and hydrodynamic shape favorable for cell motility and penetration through the egg vestments [106, 107].

The vast majority of mammalian sperm chromatin is compacted into toroids that contain roughly 50 kb of DNA [108–110]. During the deployment of the sperm cells, the testicle, by the action of DNases and polymerases, induces and repairs breaks within the DNA to achieve this level of supercoiling [111]. This condensation is so complete that most of the DNA is hidden within the toroids [112]. The understanding of this unique chromatin packing has important consequences for both the development of diagnostic tests useful to screen for infertility and to understand sperm chromatin integrity, which also may have implications for the outcome of ART [101, 113–118]. It has been observed that fertile men present with some level of DNA breakage, whereas infertility presents, especially with compromised semen parameters, with an increased proportion of nicks and breaks in the chromatin [119, 120].

A systematic observation performed in our laboratory showed that when evaluating the motile fraction of the ejaculate this fraction has a remarkably lower level of fragmentation compared with the unselected portion. Even more when a motile spermatozoon was individually picked up by a microtool, the index in chromatin damage was even lower in favor of the motile cells (5.6% motile vs 71.0% immotile, respectively; $P < 0.001$) [102] (Figures 15.3 and 15.4). It is still not clear if the DNA breakage that occurs in ejaculated spermatozoa is the result of a loss of selection exerted by defects of checkpoints during spermiogenesis and to a dysfunctional epididymis or because of *de novo* occurrence due to oxygen free radicals acting during the transit through the male genital tract [121], or even,

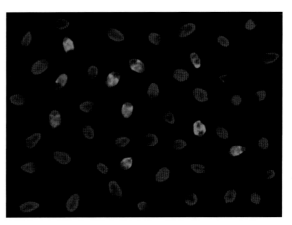

Figure 15.3. Evaluation of sperm DNA integrity using the TUNEL assay. This figure is presented in color in the color plate section.

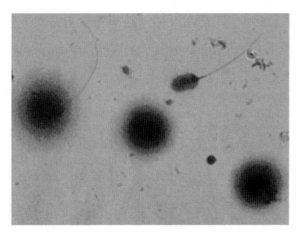

Figure 15.4. Evaluation of sperm DNA integrity using the sperm chromatin dispersion (SCD) assay. This figure is presented in color in the color plate section.

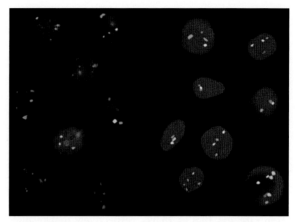

Figure 15.5. Sperm aneuploidy analysis using probes for multiple chromosomes. Each color reflects a specific chromosome probe. Sperm are shown without and with DAPI staining. This figure is presented in color in the color plate section.

according to some authors, to a cell-induced apoptic process triggered by the spermatozoon itself [104].

It appears that the etiology of sperm DNA damage is multifactorial and may be due to intrinsic and/or external factors. Intrinsic defects that may predispose spermatozoa to DNA damage include protamine deficiency and mutations that adversely affect DNA compaction [122]. An epigenetic phenomenon in the process is confirmed by the fact that advanced paternal age has been correlated with sperm DNA damage [123–126].

Although chromatin fragmentation should be completely repaired in fully developed spermatozoa, the persistence of nicks and breaks in ejaculated spermatozoa has been linked to poor embryo development and reduced implantation [127]. The converse is also true that in spite of a remarkable presence of spermatozoa with fragmented DNA, healthy offspring are still derived through ART. While this correlation may seem clear in couples attempting natural conception, artificial insemination, or in vitro fertilization, this phenomenon is less predictable of outcome where spermatozoa are selected or individually chosen such as with ICSI where only motile spermatozoa are used [102].

Concerns have been raised in the ART community regarding the possible transmission of genetic disorders and increased risk of aneuploidy offspring with the use of sperm from infertile men [128]. This is of particular concern as chromosome aneuploidy is the leading cause of pregnancy loss and mental retardation in humans, occurring in at least 4% of all clinically recognized pregnancies [129]. Most

aneuploidies are maternal in origin, nevertheless paternally derived chromosomal defects are also extraordinarily common accounting for 5–10% of autosomal aneuploidies and 50–100% of the sex chromosome aneuploidies [129].

It is also known that in subfertile men, even though they have a normal peripheral karyotype, their gametes may harbor mosaicism and thus be responsible for *de novo* gonosomal and even autosomal defects in ART offspring [130, 131]. The practice of assessing the chromosomal status of spermatozoa, although limited by the assessment of a few chromosomes (by fluorescence *in situ* hybridization (FISH)), has been correlated with some semen parameters particularly severe oligozoospermia [132–134]. The most relevant effect of sperm aneuploidy, however, has been on the compromised ability of the conceptus to retain implantation, in fact female partners of these men present with recurrent miscarriages [135–137]. Also in this situation, sperm preparation protocols or the individual selection of the male gametes may alter the outcome in a favorable manner. Currently, at our program we assess sperm aneuploidy for 10 chromosomes and in certain occasions 24 (Figure 15.5), in the spermatozoa of men with extremely dysmorphic male gametes or when their partners present with recurrent miscarriages [138].

In the 1990s, the key role of the human sperm centrosome was recognized in terms of inheritance and function [139]. The centrosome is an organelle essential for proper chromosomal migration and

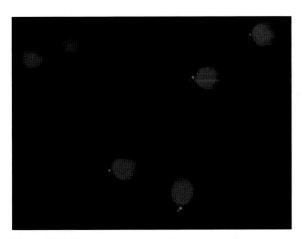

Figure 15.6. Fluorescent micrographic assessment of the presence and integrity of the centriole axis (green dot) of the sperm centrosome in sperm of infertile men. This figure is presented in color in the color plate section.

normal cell growth. In humans, the centrosome is characterized by two centrioles and the pericentriolar cytosol [140]. During fertilization, the human sperm centrosome represents the scaffold for development of an aster that later evolves into the mitotic spindle by utilizing the tubulin available in the oocyte cytosol. The centrosome's role in representing the building blocks of the mitotic spindle is paramount in embryo development by correctly segregating parental chromosomes into daughter cells. Centrosome dysfunction can result in abnormalities ranging from the inability of the zygote to cleave to embryonic aneuploidy or even mosaicism. While potential future treatments of infertility due to defective microtubule organizing centers could involve the use of donor centrosomes, such an approach would require an accurate topopgraphic assessment of this organelle for subsequent transplantation. In cases where no syngamy after ICSI or chaotic chromosomal rearrangements were observed, we assess the presence and integrity, and centriole axis, of the sperm centrosome in infertile men and compare them with fertile donors [141] (Figure 15.6).

The ability of ICSI of empowering a single spermatozoon has stimulated a trend towards the identification of the cell that would provide the best chances to generate an embryo capable of complete pre- and post-implantation development while at the same time addressing the concern of a healthy offspring. One clear example of this attempt is the selection of a spermatozoon according to its morphological characteristics in vivo.

Defined as "motile sperm organellar morphology examination" (MSOME) this approach assesses the living male gamete's phenotype [142]. The procedure referred to as "intracytoplasmic morphologically selected sperm injection" (IMSI) is claimed to yield superior clinical outcomes than conventional ICSI [143]. The promised beneficial impact of IMSI has been described in a series of small studies where the clinical outcome of patients treated by this procedure was compared with that of ICSI [144–147].

The morphological evaluation is carried out using an inverted microscope equipped with a high magnification (×100 lens under oil immersion), magnification selector (×1.5), and digital video-coupled magnification (×44) to achieve a final video monitor magnification of over ×600. The selection is restricted towards the oval shape of the spermatozoon with particular attention to the evaluation of the nuclei smooth, symmetric, oval configuration and paying attention to identifying 'vacuoles' not exceeding more than 4% of the nuclear area surface [143]. The role attributed to the putative sperm nuclear vacuole or its position within the sperm head is unclear. The rationale in identifying these structures and therefore attempting to select spermatozoa devoid of vacuoles is that it would allow identification of spermatozoa with higher DNA integrity and chromosomally normal. This may seem a little far-fetched because of the attribution to a morphologic evaluation of genetic or epigenetic screening capabilities.

Early ultrastructural studies of human sperm in the 1950s and 60s revealed that vacuoles in the sperm nucleus [148] have been seen in the large majority of human spermatozoa regardless of the fertility potential. Vacuoles in human spermatozoa have in fact been considered as a physiologic finding devoid of consequence on fertility potential [149]. Even the definition of vacuole has been challenged, in fact, they can be irrevocably identified by TEM [148] and were revealed by SEM [150, 151]. At ultrastructural evaluation they are indentations, craters, dents, or hollows observed on the sperm coat. In such cases, during sperm morphogenesis, the outer acrosomal membrane misforms and generates what appears to be a vacuole [152]. Interestingly, these presumed vacuole structures seem to disappear as the spermatozoon matures in the epididymis following in vitro maturation or at the time of the acrosome reaction [153] (Menezo, personal communications). In other circumstances, however, they seem to increase with temperature (37 °C) and incubation time (>2 hours) [154], most probably due to the plication/vacuolization of the rostral spermiolemma during capacitation. In any case, the morphological structure appears dynamic and interestingly, these appear in over 90% of spermatozoa even in obviously fertile men [150, 151].

In a joint effort to clarify the role of these sperm nuclear features, we adopted higher magnification screening for sperm surface irregularities and prospectively correlated the pre- and postimplantation development. The multicenter effort did not, however, seem to benefit the patients' clinical outcome for patients with compromised semen parameters and for those either undergoing first or repeated ART attempts [155]. Analyses of spermatozoa from different sources, ejaculated or surgically retrieved, also revealed the varying presence and size of sperm nuclear irregularities that develop during the dynamic processes of spermiogenesis and maturation. This surface irregularity did not translate to a higher incidence of DNA fragmentation or aneuploidy, nor to the ability of vacuolated spermatozoa to generate zygotes capable of developing to blastocysts [150, 151].

In addition, a link between the abnormal phenotype and the chromosomal/chromatinic integrity has also been attempted by the hyaluronic acid (HA) binding assay appearing on the surface of the mature spermatozoa [156–158]. This biochemical marker was used to identify the most viable, mature spermatozoa that has intact DNA, limited aneuploidy, restricted amount of histones, and increased spermatozoal function [156–158] to be used for ICSI. However, their concept is contradicted by the observation that immature spermatozoa such as those retrieved from epididymis and testes are capable of generating high fertilization and pregnancy rates comparable with their ejaculated counterparts [73]. In our hands, in a total of 15 men, we carried out the selection of spermatozoa that exhibit HA binding sites on which we assessed the chromosomal status and chromatinic competence. We did not find any differences in relation to the morphology, sperm compaction (aniline blue), DNA fragmentation (SCD and TUNEL), sperm aneuploidy following motility enrichment and HA selection. The selection of HA binding sites did not add any further advantage in identifying better spermatozoa than those seen after a simple method of motility enrichment [159].

Reproductive ability of suboptimal spermatozoa

In a time span of 18.5 years, we have performed 33,170 ART (IVF and ICSI) cycles consisting of 10,667 standard IVF, 20,344 ICSI with ejaculated samples and 2,159 ICSI with surgically isolated spermatozoa obtained either from the epididymis or the testis. The semen characteristics for standard in vitro insemination falls within the normal threshold of the WHO [160], having a concentration above 15 million, over 40% motility, and greater than 4% normal morphology. ICSI on the other hand, regardless of semen source, had poorer semen parameters ($P < 0.001$) (Table 15.1).

When we looked at the different semen origin such as ejaculated, electroejaculate, retrograde ejaculate and their frozen counterparts (Table 15.2), the fertilization ranged from 67.3% all the way to 83.5%. The clinical pregnancy, as determined by the presence of at least one fetal heartbeat at their seventh week ultrasound, was comparable between the different origins yielding an average of 39.8%.

At our center, we have encountered cases with severe oligozoospermia presenting with less than 1 million spermatozoa in 1,432 ICSI cycles with a mean sperm density of $0.29 \pm 0.3 \times 10^6$/mL, a motility of $17.2 \pm 21\%$, and morphology of $0.5 \pm 1\%$. Considering these severely poor parameters, zygote formation was at 66.2% (8,974/13,552) resulting in a clinical pregnancy of 43.7% ($n = 626$).

In a series of different cases when no spermatozoa were seen in the counting chamber at the initial semen analysis ($n = 160$) – formally considered to have azoospermia – we carried out high-speed centrifugation. It yielded $20.4 \pm 43 \times 10^3$/mL with $31.2 \pm 33\%$ total motility, and an acceptable fertilization of 65.3%

Table 15.1 Assisted reproduction therapies: procedure and semen origin.

Parameter	IVF	ICSI
Number of cycles	10,667	20,344
Concentration (M × 10^6/mL ± SD)	71.3 ± 21*	48.7 ± 45*
Motility (M% ± SD)	59.8 ± 4[†]	35.1 ± 22[†]
Morphology (M% ± SD)	4.2 ± 2[‡]	2.3 ± 5[‡]

*Student's t-test; [†]Semen parameters according to ART procedures and semen source; [‡]$P < 0.0001$.

Table 15.2 Intracytoplasmic sperm injection: outcome according to semen origin.

Semen origin	Cycles	Fertilization (%)	Clinical pregnancies (%)
Fresh ejaculate	18,201	113,209/150,407 (75.2)	7,280 (40.0)
Frozen ejaculate	2,023	12,354/16,691 (74.0)	767 (37.9)
Electroejaculate	59	425/556 (76.4)	30 (50.8)
Frozen electroejaculate	24	150/223 (67.3)	11 (45.8)
Retrograde ejaculate	37	263/315 (83.5)	13 (35.1)

Table 15.3 Intracytoplasmic sperm injection: outcome according to specimens retrieved through the epididymis or the testis.

	MESA	TESE
Cycles	942	1,217
Concentration (M × 10^6/mL ± SD)	28.5 ± 35	0.4 ± 2
Motility (M% ± SD)	8.9 ± 14	3.2 ± 8
Morphology (M% ± SD)	1.5 ± 2	0
Fertilization (%)	6,459/9,026 (71.6)*	6,051/10,999 (55.0)*
Clinical pregnancies (%)	482 (51.2)[†]	483 (39.7)[†]

*[†]χ^2, 2 × 2, 1 df, Effect of sperm source on fertilization and clinical pregnancy rates, $P < 0.001$.

(1,074/1,644) was attained. Moreover, in these so-called "cryptozoospermic" individuals a clinical pregnancy rate of 41.9% ($n = 67$) was achieved with an average of 3.0 conceptuses transferred.

For more severe cases of male-factor infertility, the adoption of surgical sperm retrieval techniques has made it possible for ICSI to provide children for these men. In cases of obstructive azoospermia, whether congenital, such as the case of congenital bilateral absence of the vas deferens, or acquired, as through infection or trauma, epididymal spermatozoa can produce fertilization rates of >70% and clinical pregnancy rates of 50–58%, despite severely impaired sperm motility and morphology [161]. Testicular biopsies or testicular sperm extraction (TESE) used with both obstructive and non-obstructive azoospermia, as in the case of non-mosaic Klinefelter syndrome, can retrieve sperm in even more immature stages [162]. We have retrieved 942 microsurgical epididymis sperm aspiration (MESA) and 1,217

TESE surgical samples whose female partners had an average age of 35.7 ± 5 years (Table 15.3). The epididymal cohort had better semen characteristics in comparison to those retrieved directly from the testes. When fertilization was assessed, MESA had a higher zygote formation than those from TESE ($P < 0.001$). The clinical pregnancies were also higher with MESA than in TESE ($P < 0.001$).

We also encountered men in whom, following testicular biopsy, spermatozoa are extremely scarce if not totally absent. In such cases, the extended sperm searches may take greater than 3 hours to complete, depending on the number of oocytes awaiting injection. Unsurprisingly, the level of difficulty in finding and acquiring sperm is negatively related to the clinical outcome. At our center, when extended search time is used as a parameter and categorized into 30 minutes to 1 hour, 1–2 hours, 2–3 hours, and >3 hours, both fertilization rates (54.2, 46.3, 28.0, and 25.4%, respectively; $R^2 = 0.9315$; $P < 0.001$) of the oocytes and overall pregnancy rates declined ($R^2 = 0.9812$; $P < 0.0001$) as search time increased. Although there is a pronounced decrease in pregnancy outcome as extensive search time increases, the search is still an important and valuable tool overall, as it represents the best opportunity for a male patient with non-obstructive azoospermia (NOA) to bear their own biological child. In fact, even in a search of >3 hours, the possibility of achieving pregnancy is still attainable as long as a viable spermatozoon is identified [163].

Conclusions

Male infertility represents a large component among the arrays of possible reasons for the inability of a couple to reproduce. With ICSI, we have been able to successfully treat infertile men. The ability of the direct injection in bypassing most sperm dysfunction has been confirmed for all sources of the spermatozoa and even for different maturational stages. This has resulted in the popular application of ICSI insemination with surgically retrieved spermatozoa in azoospermic men.

Infertile men, however, may carry genetic defects, therefore, it is paramount to appropriately counsel and screen them. Furthermore, spermatozoa may carry inherited genetic disorders but most importantly, they reflect the damage induced by environmental aggressors on their DNA or other important components of the male gamete such as the centrosome. In spite of all these concerns, ICSI can successfully treat male infertility by using spermatozoa from different sources, various levels of maturity, and antisperm antibody.

Despite this apparent ability to overcome all these sperm defects most of the success of the direct sperm injection comes from the fact that during ICSI it is possible to choose the sperm cell that has viability as displayed by its motility, and rule out gross morphological defects by assessing its size, shape, and dynamic progression in a viscous medium. These are aspects of the sperm integrity that are paramount to its role such as its chromosomal status, DNA integrity, centrosomal function, and most importantly the cytosolic activation factor. Without the ability to complete the first step of fertilization even gamete syngamy cannot be evaluated. These extreme cases of sperm dysfunction can be rescued by tweaking fertilization through assisted oocyte activation.

Screening for DNA fragmentation, with careful morphological assessment at high magnification, can help in better selection of the ideal spermatozoon to be injected. Other methods to study sperm genetic constitution or structural components as well as ways to permeabilize the sperm membrane or activate the oocyte will help to address gamete dysfunction.

At the present time, however, there is no individual approach or technique that will pinpoint the ideal cell to launch a thriving embryo development as it appears that different aspects need to be considered when selecting a spermatozoon for injection. The process should start at the time of consultation and with the male partner evaluation. Male partner medical history, past and present, helps to exclude or consider certain genetic aspects of the couple's infertility. Male partner evaluation should include the involvement of the urologist or geneticist according to the situation. Once the semen specimen is obtained, other genetic or epigenetic aspects can be considered ranging from chromosomal aberrations,

to the centrosomal presence and their chromatin defects. While considering the candidate spermatozoon to be injected, we can use simple morphological assessment whether carried out on the entire sperm population, when available, or individual spermatozoa. The selection for the spermatozoa expressing hyaluronic acid receptors does not grant the ideal sperm capable of producing the optimal conceptus. Every effort should be devoted to screen and select the best possible male gamete because of the obvious limitations of each individual assessment.

Current experience gained from severe forms of male factor infertility ranging from severe oligozoospermia, to cryptozoospermia, and even azoospermia support the fact that as long as we are able to identify a single viable spermatozoon, we have a fair chance of achieving a pregnancy.

Acknowledgments

We thank the clinicians, embryologists, andrologists, and scientists of The Ronald O. Perelman & Claudia Cohen Center for Reproductive Medicine and Urology Department, Weill Cornell Medical College. We are grateful to Bong Kyo Seo for their FISH and TUNEL photos.

References

1. National Center for Chronic Disease and Prevention and Health Promotion. *Assisted Reproductive Technology Success Rates. National Summary and Fertility Clinic Reports.* National Center for Chronic Disease and Prevention and Health Promotion; 2008.

2. Stefankiewicz J, Kurzawa R, Drozdzik M. [Environmental factors disturbing fertility of men]. *Ginekologia polska.* 2006;77(2):163–9.

3. Wright VC, Chang J, Jeng G et al. Assisted reproductive technology surveillance – United States, 2003. *MMWR Surveill Summ /CDC.* 2006;**55**(4):1–22.

4. Wales RG, Whittingham DG. Development of eight-cell mouse embryos in substrate-free medium. *J Reprod Fertil.* 1973;**32**(2):316–17.

5. Edwards RG. Immunological control of fertility in female mice. *Nature.* 1964;**203**:50–3.

6. McLaren A, Biggers JD. Successful development and birth of mice cultivated in vitro as early embryos. *Nature.* 1958;**182**(4639):877–8.

7. Cohen J, Edwards RG, Fehilly CB et al. Treatment of male infertility by in vitro fertilization: factors affecting fertilization and pregnancy. *Acta Eur Fertil.* 1984;**15**(6):455–65.

8. Mansour RT, Aboulghar MA, Serour GI *et al.* The effect of sperm parameters on the outcome of intracytoplasmic sperm injection. *Fertil Steril.* 1995;**64**(5):982–6.

9. Nagy ZP, Liu J, Joris H *et al.* The result of intracytoplasmic sperm injection is not related to any of the three basic sperm parameters. *Hum Reprod.* 1995;**10**(5):1123–9.

10. Palermo G, Joris H, Derde MP *et al.* Sperm characteristics and outcome of human assisted fertilization by subzonal insemination and intracytoplasmic sperm injection. *Fertil Steril.* 1993;**59**(4):826–35.

11. Palermo GD, Cohen J, Alikani M *et al.* Development and implementation of intracytoplasmic sperm injection (ICSI). *Reprod Fertil Develop.* 1995;**7**(2):211–17; discussion 217–8.

12. Palermo GD, Cohen J, Alikani M *et al.* Intracytoplasmic sperm injection: a novel treatment for all forms of male factor infertility. *Fertil Steril.* 1995;**63**(6):1231–40.

13. Tournaye H, Devroey P, Liu J *et al.* Microsurgical epididymal sperm aspiration and intracytoplasmic sperm injection: a new effective approach to infertility as a result of congenital bilateral absence of the vas deferens. *Fertil Steril.* 1994;**61**(6):1045–51.

14. Ludwig M, al-Hasani S, Kupker W *et al.* A new indication for an intracytoplasmic sperm injection procedure outside the cases of severe male factor infertility. *Eur J Obstet Gynecol Reprod Biol.* 1997;**75**(2):207–10.

15. Porcu E, Fabbri R, Seracchioli R *et al.* Birth of a healthy female after intracytoplasmic sperm injection of cryopreserved human oocytes. *Fertil Steril.* 1997;**68**(4):724–6.

16. Johnson L. Evaluation of the human testis and its age-related dysfunction. *Progr Clin Biol Res.* 1989;**302**:35–60; discussion 61–7.

17. Schalkoff ME, Oskowitz SP, Powers RD. Ultrastructural observations of human and mouse oocytes treated with cryopreservatives. *Biol Reprod.* 1989;**40**(2):379–93.

18. Van Blerkom J, Davis PW, Merriam J. The developmental ability of human oocytes penetrated at the germinal vesicle stage after insemination in vitro. *Hum Reprod.* 1994;**9**(4):697–708.

19. Vincent C, Pickering SJ, Johnson MH. The hardening effect of dimethylsulphoxide on the mouse zona pellucida requires the presence of an oocyte and is associated with a reduction in the number of cortical granules present. *J Reprod Fertil.* 1990;**89**(1):253–9.

20. Handyside AH, Kontogianni EH, Hardy K *et al.* Pregnancies from biopsied human preimplantation embryos sexed by Y-specific DNA amplification. *Nature.* 1990;**344**(6268):768–70.

21. Verlinsky Y, Kuliev A. Preimplantation polar body diagnosis. *Biochem Mol Med.* 1996;**58**(1):13–17.

22. Wilton L. Preimplantation genetic diagnosis for aneuploidy screening in early human embryos: a review. *Prenat Diagn.* 2002;**22**(6):512–18.

23. Bendikson KA, Neri QV, Takeuchi T *et al.* The outcome of intracytoplasmic sperm injection using occasional spermatozoa in the ejaculate of men with spermatogenic failure. *J Urol.* 2008;**180**(3):1060–4.

24. Edwards RG, Tarin JJ, Dean N *et al.* Are spermatid injections into human oocytes now mandatory? *Hum Reprod.* 1994;**9**(12):2217–19.

25. Fishel S, Green S, Bishop M *et al.* Pregnancy after intracytoplasmic injection of spermatid. *Lancet.* 1995;**345**(8965):1641–2.

26. Tesarik J, Mendoza C, Testart J. Viable embryos from injection of round spermatids into oocytes. *New Engl J Med.* 1995;**333**(8):525.

27. Tsai MC, Takeuchi T, Bedford JM *et al.* Alternative sources of gametes: reality or science fiction? *Hum Reprod.* 2000;**15**(5):988–98.

28. Osmanagaoglu K, Tournaye H, Kolibianakis E *et al.* Cumulative delivery rates after ICSI in women aged >37 years. *Hum Reprod.* 2002;**17**(4):940–4.

29. Sunderam S, Chang J, Flowers L *et al.* Assisted reproductive technology surveillance – United States, 2006. *MMWR Surveill Summ.* 2009;**58**(5):1–25.

30. Aboulghar MA, Mansour RT, Serour GI *et al.* Intracytoplasmic sperm injection and conventional in vitro fertilization for sibling oocytes in cases of unexplained infertility and borderline semen. *J Assist Reprod Genet.* 1996;**13**(1):38–42.

31. Fishel S, Aslam I, Lisi F *et al.* Should ICSI be the treatment of choice for all cases of in-vitro conception? *Hum Reprod.* 2000;**15**(6):1278–83.

32. Nyboe Andersen A, Carlsen E, Loft A. Trends in the use of intracytoplasmatic sperm injection marked variability between countries. *Hum Reprod Update.* 2008;**14**(6):593–604.

33. de Mouzon J, Lancaster P, Nygren KG *et al.* World Collaborative Report on Assisted Reproductive Technology, 2002. *Hum Reprod.* 2009;**24**(9):2310–2320.

34. Wright VC, Chang J, Jeng G *et al.* Assisted Reproductive Technology Surveillance – United States, 2005. *MMWR Surveill Summaries /CDC.* 2008;**57**(5):1–23.

35. Wang YA, Dean J, Badgery-Parker T *et al. Assisted Reproduction Technology in Australia and New Zealand*

2006. Assisted Reproduction Technology Series Number 12. Sydney: Australian Institute of Health and Welfare, National Perinatal Statistics Unit and Fertility Society of Australia; 2008.

36. World Health Organization. *WHO Laboratory Manual for the Examination and Processing of Human Semen and Sperm–Cervical Mucus Interaction.* 3rd edn. Geneva, WHO: 1992.

37. World Health Organization. *WHO Laboratory Manual for the Examination and Processing of Human Semen and Sperm–Cervical Mucus Interaction.* 4th edn. Geneva, WHO: 1999

38. World Health Organization. *WHO Laboratory Manual for the Examination and Processing of Human Semen and Sperm–Cervical Mucus Interaction.* 5th edn. Geneva, WHO: 2010.

39. Mallidis C, Howard EJ, Baker HW. Variation of semen quality in normal men. *Int J Androl.* 1991;**14**(2):99–107.

40. Schwartz D, Laplanche A, Jouannet P *et al.* Within-subject variability of human semen in regard to sperm count, volume, total number of spermatozoa and length of abstinence. *J Reprod Fertil.* 1979;**57**(2):391–5.

41. Cooper TG, Neuwinger J, Bahrs S *et al.* Internal quality control of semen analysis. *Fertil Steril.* 1992;**58**(1):172–8.

42. Matson PL. External quality assessment for semen analysis and sperm antibody detection: results of a pilot scheme. *Hum Reprod.* 1995;**10**(3):620–5.

43. Neuwinger J, Behre HM, Nieschlag E. External quality control in the andrology laboratory: an experimental multicenter trial. *Fertil Steril.* 1990;**54**(2):308–14.

44. Glazener CM, Coulson C, Lambert PA *et al.* The value of artificial insemination with husband's semen in infertility due to failure of postcoital sperm-mucus penetration – controlled trial of treatment. *Br J Obstet Gynaecol.* 1987;**94**(8):774–8.

45. Irvine DS, Aitken RJ, Lees MM *et al.* Failure of high intrauterine insemination of husband's semen. *Lancet.* 1986;**2**(8513):972–3.

46. Joffe M, Li Z. Association of time to pregnancy and the outcome of pregnancy. *Fertil Steril.* 1994;**62**(1):71–5.

47. Vine MF. Smoking and male reproduction: a review. *Int J Androl.* 1996;**19**(6):323–37.

48. Vine MF, Margolin BH, Morrison HI *et al.* Cigarette smoking and sperm density: a meta-analysis. *Fertil Steril.* 1994;**61**(1):35–43.

49. Kent-First MG, Kol S, Muallem A *et al.* The incidence and possible relevance of Y-linked microdeletions in babies born after intracytoplasmic sperm injection and their infertile fathers. *Mol Hum Reprod.* 1996;**2**(12):943–50.

50. McLachlan RI, Mallidis C, Ma K *et al.* Genetic disorders and spermatogenesis. *Reprod Fertil Develop.* 1998;**10**(1):97–104.

51. Reijo R, Lee TY, Salo P *et al.* Diverse spermatogenic defects in humans caused by Y chromosome deletions encompassing a novel RNA-binding protein gene. *Nat Genet.* 1995;**10**(4):383–93.

52. Simoni M, Gromoll J, Dworniczak B *et al.* Screening for deletions of the Y chromosome involving the DAZ (deleted in azoospermia) gene in azoospermia and severe oligozoospermia. *Fertil Steril.* 1997;**67**(3):542–7.

53. Vogt HJ. [sperm intolerance as a possible cause for infertility?]. *Der Hautarzt; Zeitschrift fur Dermatologie, Venerologie, und verwandte Gebiete.* 1996;**47**(4):312–13.

54. Repping S, Skaletsky H, Lange J *et al.* Recombination between palindromes p5 and p1 on the human Y chromosome causes massive deletions and spermatogenic failure. *Am J Hum Genet.* 2002;**71**(4):906–22.

55. Tal J, Ziskind G, Paltieli Y *et al.* ICSI outcome in patients with transient azoospermia with initially motile or immotile sperm in the ejaculate. *Hum Reprod.* 2005;**20**(9):2584–9.

56. Bonduelle M, Van Assche E, Joris H *et al.* Prenatal testing in ICSI pregnancies: incidence of chromosomal anomalies in 1586 karyotypes and relation to sperm parameters. *Hum Reprod.* 2002;**17**(10):2600–14.

57. Sutcliffe AG, Ludwig M. Outcome of assisted reproduction. *Lancet.* 2007;**370**(9584):351–9.

58. Palermo G, Neri QV, Takeuchi T *et al.* Genetic and epigenetic characteristics of ICSI children. *Reprod Biomed Online.* 2008;**17**(6):820–33.

59. Yanagimachi R, Bhattacharyya A. Acrosome-reacted guinea pig spermatozoa become fusion competent in the presence of extracellular potassium ions. *J Exp Zool.* 1988;**248**(3):354–60.

60. Barros C, Bedford JM, Franklin LE *et al.* Membrane vesiculation as a feature of the mammalian acrosome reaction. *J Cell Biol.* 1967;**34**(3):C1–5.

61. Bleil JD, Wassarman PM. Sperm–egg interactions in the mouse: sequence of events and induction of the acrosome reaction by a zona pellucida glycoprotein. *Develop Biol.* 1983;**95**(2):317–24.

62. Wassarman PM. Sperm receptors and fertilization in mammals. *Mount Sinai J Med NY.* 2002;**69**(3):148–55.

63. Palermo G, Joris H, Devroey P *et al.* Pregnancies after intracytoplasmic injection of single spermatozoon into an oocyte. *Lancet.* 1992;**340**(8810):17–18.

64. Vanderzwalmen P, Bertin G, Lejeune B *et al.* Two essential steps for a successful intracytoplasmic sperm

injection: injection of immobilized spermatozoa after rupture of the oolema. *Hum Reprod.* 1996;**11**(3):540–7.

65. Fishel S, Lisi F, Rinaldi L *et al.* Systematic examination of immobilizing spermatozoa before intracytoplasmic sperm injection in the human. *Hum Reprod.* 1995;**10**(3):497–500.

66. Gerris J, Mangelschots K, Van Royen E *et al.* ICSI and severe male-factor infertility: breaking the sperm tail prior to injection. *Hum Reprod.* 1995;**10**(3):484–6.

67. Palermo GD, Schlegel PN, Colombero LT *et al.* Aggressive sperm immobilization prior to intracytoplasmic sperm injection with immature spermatozoa improves fertilization and pregnancy rates. *Hum Reprod.* 1996;**11**(5):1023–9.

68. Van den Bergh M, Bertrand E, Biramane J *et al.* Importance of breaking a spermatozoon's tail before intracytoplasmic injection: a prospective randomized trial. *Hum Reprod.* 1995;**10**(11):2819–20.

69. Takeuchi T, Colombero LT, Neri QV *et al.* Does ICSI require acrosomal disruption? An ultrastructural study. *Hum Reprod.* 2004;**19**(1):114–17.

70. Dozortsev D, Rybouchkin A, De Sutter P *et al.* Sperm plasma membrane damage prior to intracytoplasmic sperm injection: a necessary condition for sperm nucleus decondensation. *Hum Reprod.* 1995;**10**(11):2960–4.

71. Christova Y, James P, Mackie A *et al.* Molecular diffusion in sperm plasma membranes during epididymal maturation. *Mol Cell Endocrinol.* 2004;**216**(1–2):41–6.

72. Palermo GD, Alikani M, Bertoli M *et al.* Oolemma characteristics in relation to survival and fertilization patterns of oocytes treated by intracytoplasmic sperm injection. *Hum Reprod.* 1996;**11**(1):172–6.

73. Palermo GD, Neri QV, Monahan D *et al.* Development and current applications of assisted fertilization. *Fertil Steril.* 2012;**97**(2):248–59.

74. Stricker SA. Comparative biology of calcium signaling during fertilization and egg activation in animals. *Develop Biol.* 1999;**211**(2):157–76.

75. Runft LL, Jaffe LA, Mehlmann LM. Egg activation at fertilization: where it all begins. *Develop Biol.* 2002;**245**(2):237–54.

76. Stice SL, Robl JM. Activation of mammalian oocytes by a factor obtained from rabbit sperm. *Mol Reprod Develop.* 1990;**25**(3):272–80.

77. Swann K. A cytosolic sperm factor stimulates repetitive calcium increases and mimics fertilization in hamster eggs. *Development.* 1990;**110**(4):1295–302.

78. Parrington J, Swann K, Shevchenko VI *et al.* Calcium oscillations in mammalian eggs triggered by a soluble sperm protein. *Nature.* 1996;**379**(6563):364–8.

79. Wolny YM, Fissore RA, Wu H *et al.* Human glucosamine-6-phosphate isomerase, a homologue of hamster oscillin, does not appear to be involved in Ca2+ release in mammalian oocytes. *Mol Reprod Develop.* 1999;**52**(3):277–87.

80. Dale B, Marino M, Wilding M. Sperm-induced calcium oscillations. Soluble factor, factors or receptors? *Mol Hum Reprod.* 1999;**5**(1):1–4.

81. Jones KT, Cruttwell C, Parrington J *et al.* A mammalian sperm cytosolic phospholipase c activity generates inositol trisphosphate and causes Ca2+ release in sea urchin egg homogenates. *FEBS Lett.* 1998;**437**(3):297–300.

82. Rice A, Parrington J, Jones KT *et al.* Mammalian sperm contain a Ca(2+)-sensitive phospholipase c activity that can generate INSP(3) from PIP(2) associated with intracellular organelles. *Develop Biol.* 2000;**228**(1):125–35.

83. Wu C, Stojanov T, Chami O *et al.* Evidence for the autocrine induction of capacitation of mammalian spermatozoa. *J Biol Chem.* 2001;**276**(29):26,962–8.

84. Parrington J, Jones ML, Tunwell R *et al.* Phospholipase c isoforms in mammalian spermatozoa: potential components of the sperm factor that causes Ca2+ release in eggs. *Reproduction.* 2002;**123**(1):31–9.

85. Saunders CM, Larman MG, Parrington J *et al.* PLC zeta: a sperm-specific trigger of Ca(2+) oscillations in eggs and embryo development. *Development.* 2002;**129**(15):3533–44.

86. Cox LJ, Larman MG, Saunders CM *et al.* Sperm phospholipase Czeta from humans and cynomolgus monkeys triggers Ca2+ oscillations, activation and development of mouse oocytes. *Reproduction.* 2002;**124**(5):611–23.

87. Palermo GD, Neri QV, Takeuchi T *et al.* ICSI: where we have been and where we are going. *Semin Reprod Med.* 2009;**27**(2):191–201.

88. Kashir J, Heindryckx B, Jones C *et al.* Oocyte activation, phospholipase C zeta and human infertility. *Hum Reprod Update.* 2010;**16**(6):690–703.

89. Yanagida K, Fujikura Y, Katayose H. The present status of artificial oocyte activation in assisted reproductive technology. *Reprod Med Biol.* 2008;**7**(3):133–42.

90. Vanden Meerschaut F, Nikiforaki D, De Gheselle S *et al.* Assisted oocyte activation is not beneficial for all patients with a suspected oocyte-related activation deficiency. *Hum Reprod.* 2012;**27**(7):1977–84.

91. Heytens E, Parrington J, Coward K *et al.* Reduced amounts and abnormal forms of phospholipase C zeta (PLCzeta) in spermatozoa from infertile men. *Hum Reprod.* 2009;**24**(10):2417–28.

92. Nasr-Esfahani MH, Deemeh MR, Tavalaee M. Artificial oocyte activation and intracytoplasmic sperm injection. *Fertil Steril.* 2010;**94**(2):520–6.

93. Yoon SY, Jellerette T, Salicioni AM *et al.* Human sperm devoid of PLC, zeta 1 fail to induce Ca(2+) release and are unable to initiate the first step of embryo development. *J Clin Invest.* 2008;**118**(11):3671–81.

94. Rogers NT, Hobson E, Pickering S *et al.* Phospholipase Czeta causes Ca2+ oscillations and parthenogenetic activation of human oocytes. *Reproduction.* 2004;**128**(6):697–702.

95. Spadafora C. Endogenous reverse transcriptase: a mediator of cell proliferation and differentiation. *Cytogenet Genome Res.* 2004;**105**(2–4):346–50.

96. Fields T, Neri QV, Hu JCY *et al.* A qualitative assay for sperm fertilization competence. Poster viewing session, ESHRE, July, Stockholm. *Hum. Reprod.* 2011;**26**(Suppl. 1):i349–53.

97. Aitken RJ, De Iuliis GN, McLachlan RI. Biological and clinical significance of DNA damage in the male germ line. *Int J Androl.* 2009;**32**(1):46–56.

98. Feliciano M, Neri QV, Kent-First M *et al.* Assays of sperm nuclear status do not correlate with ICSI success. *Hum Reprod.* 2004;**19**(Suppl. 1):i52.

99. Neri QV, Evenson D, Wehbe AS *et al.* Does DNA fragmentation in spermatozoa affect ICSI offspring development? *Hum Reprod.* 2004;**19**(Suppl. 1):i107.

100. Aitken RJ, De Iuliis GN. Origins and consequences of DNA damage in male germ cells. *Reprod Biomed Online.* 2007;**14**(6):727–33.

101. Bungum M, Humaidan P, Spano M *et al.* The predictive value of sperm chromatin structure assay (SCSA) parameters for the outcome of intrauterine insemination, IVF and ICSI. *Hum Reprod.* 2004;**19**(6):1401–8.

102. Chen C, Hu JCY, Neri QV *et al.* Kinetic characteristics and DNA integrity of human spermatozoa. *Hum Reprod.* 2011;**19**(Suppl. 1):i30.

103. Virro MR, Larson-Cook KL, Evenson DP. Sperm chromatin structure assay (SCSA) parameters are related to fertilization, blastocyst development, and ongoing pregnancy in in vitro fertilization and intracytoplasmic sperm injection cycles. *Fert and Steril.* 2004;**81**(5):1289–95.

104. Aitken RJ, De Iuliis GN. On the possible origins of DNA damage in human spermatozoa. *Mol Hum Reprod.* 2010;**16**(1):3–13.

105. Calvin HI, Bedford JM. Formation of disulphide bonds in the nucleus and accessory structures of mammalian spermatozoa during maturation in the epididymis. *J Reprod Fertil Suppl.* 1971;**13** (Suppl. 13): 65–75.

106. Brewer L, Corzett M, Balhorn R. Condensation of DNA by spermatid basic nuclear proteins. *J Biol Chem.* 2002;**277**(41):38,895–900.

107. Dadoune JP. Expression of mammalian spermatozoal nucleoproteins. *Microsc Res Techniq.* 2003;**61**(1):56–75.

108. Brewer L, Corzett M, Lau EY *et al.* Dynamics of protamine 1 binding to single DNA molecules. *J Biol Chem.* 2003;**278**(43):42,403–8.

109. Carrell DT. Epigenetics of the male gamete. *Fertil Steril.* 2012;**97**(2):267–74.

110. Hud NV, Allen MJ, Downing KH *et al.* Identification of the elemental packing unit of DNA in mammalian sperm cells by atomic force microscopy. *Biochem Biophys Res Comm.* 1993;**193**(3):1347–54.

111. Ward WS. Regulating DNA supercoiling: sperm points the way. *Biol Reprod.* 2011;**84**(5):841–3.

112. Vilfan ID, Conwell CC, Hud NV. Formation of native-like mammalian sperm cell chromatin with folded bull protamine. *J Biol Chem.* 2004;**279**(19):20,088–95.

113. Evenson D, Jost L. Sperm chromatin structure assay is useful for fertility assessment. *Methods Cell Sci Official J Soc In Vitro Biol.* 2000;**22**(2–3):169–89.

114. Evenson DP, Larson KL, Jost LK. Sperm chromatin structure assay: Its clinical use for detecting sperm DNA fragmentation in male infertility and comparisons with other techniques. *J Androl.* 2002;**23**(1):25–43.

115. Morris ID, Ilott S, Dixon L *et al.* The spectrum of DNA damage in human sperm assessed by single cell gel electrophoresis (Comet assay) and its relationship to fertilization and embryo development. *Hum Reprod.* 2002;**17**(4):990–8.

116. Sakkas D, Manicardi GC, Bizzaro D. Sperm nuclear DNA damage in the human. *Adv Exp Med Biol.* 2003;**518**:73–84.

117. van der Heijden GW, Ramos L, Baart EB *et al.* Sperm-derived histones contribute to zygotic chromatin in humans. *BMC Develop Biol.* 2008;**8**:34.

118. Zini A, Sigman M. Are tests of sperm DNA damage clinically useful? Pros and cons. *J Androl.* 2009;**30**(3):219–29.

119. Spano M, Bonde JP, Hjollund HI *et al.* Sperm chromatin damage impairs human fertility. The Danish first pregnancy planner study team. *Fertil Steril.* 2000;**73**(1):43–50.

120. Zini A, Bielecki R, Phang D *et al.* Correlations between two markers of sperm DNA integrity, DNA denaturation and DNA fragmentation, in fertile and infertile men. *Fertil Steril.* 2001;**75**(4):674–7.

121. Henkel R, Maass G, Hajimohammad M *et al.* Urogenital inflammation: changes of leucocytes and ROS. *Andrologia.* 2003;**35**(5):309–13.

122. Carrell DT, Liu L. Altered protamine 2 expression is uncommon in donors of known fertility, but common among men with poor fertilizing capacity, and may reflect other abnormalities of spermiogenesis. *J Androl.* 2001;**22**(4):604–10.

123. Moskovtsev SI, Willis J, Mullen JB. Age-related decline in sperm deoxyribonucleic acid integrity in patients evaluated for male infertility. *Fertil Steril.* 2006;**85** (2):496–9.

124. Moskovtsev SI, Willis J, White J *et al.* Sperm survival: relationship to age-related sperm DNA integrity in infertile men. *Archiv Androl.* 2007;**53**(1):29–32.

125. Plastira K, Msaouel P, Angelopoulou R *et al.* The effects of age on DNA fragmentation, chromatin packaging and conventional semen parameters in spermatozoa of oligoasthenoteratozoospermic patients. *J Assist Reprod Genet.* 2007;**24**(10):437–43.

126. Singh NP, Muller CH, Berger RE. Effects of age on DNA double-strand breaks and apoptosis in human sperm. *Fertil Steril.* 2003;**80**(6):1420–30.

127. Tamburrino L, Marchiani S, Montoya M *et al.* Mechanisms and clinical correlates of sperm DNA damage. *Asian J Androl.* 2012;**14**(1):24–31.

128. Griffin DK, Hyland P, Tempest HG *et al.* Safety issues in assisted reproduction technology: should men undergoing ICSI be screened for chromosome abnormalities in their sperm? *Hum Reprod.* 2003;**18**(2):229–35.

129. Hassold T, Hunt PA, Sherman S. Trisomy in humans: incidence, origin and etiology. *Curr Opin Genet Dev.* 1993;**3**(3):398–403.

130. Bonduelle M, Legein J, Buysse A *et al.* Prospective follow-up study of 423 children born after intracytoplasmic sperm injection. *Hum Reprod.* 1996;**11**(7):1558–64.

131. Ludwig M, Katalinic A. Malformation rate in fetuses and children conceived after ICSI: results of a prospective cohort study. *Reprod Biomed Online.* 2002;**5**(2):171–8.

132. Martin RH, Greene C, Rademaker AW. Sperm chromosome aneuploidy analysis in a man with globozoospermia. *Fertil Steril.* 2003;**79**(Suppl. 3):1662–4.

133. Colombero LT, Moomjy M, Sills ES *et al.* The role of structural integrity of the fertilising spermatozoon in early human embryogenesis. *Zygote.* 1999;**7**(2):157–63.

134. Palermo GD, Colombero LT, Hariprashad JJ *et al.* Chromosome analysis of epididymal and testicular sperm in azoospermic patients undergoing ICSI. *Hum Reprod.* 2002;**17**(3):570–5.

135. Rubio C, Simon C, Blanco J *et al.* Implications of sperm chromosome abnormalities in recurrent miscarriage. *J Assist Reprod Genet.* 1999;**16**(5):253–8.

136. Carrell DT, Wilcox AL, Lowy L *et al.* Elevated sperm chromosome aneuploidy and apoptosis in patients with unexplained recurrent pregnancy loss. *Obstet Gynecol.* 2003;**101**(6):1229–35.

137. Takeuchi T, Neri QV, Toschi M *et al.* The value of the sperm aneuploidy assay in men undergoing assisted reproductive technology. *Fertil Steril.* 2006;**86**(3, Suppl.):S513.

138. Hu JCY, Monahan D, Neri QV *et al.* The role of sperm aneuploidy assay. *Fertil Steril.* 2011;**96**(3S):S24–5.

139. Palermo G, Munne S, Cohen J. The human zygote inherits its mitotic potential from the male gamete. *Hum Reprod.* 1994;**9**(7):1220–5.

140. Palermo GD, Colombero LT, Rosenwaks Z. The human sperm centrosome is responsible for normal syngamy and early embryonic development. *Rev Reprod.* 1997;**2**(1):19–27.

141. Neri QV, Scala V, Rosenwaks Z *et al.* Assessment of the sperm centrosome. *Fertil Steril.* 2011;**96**(3, Suppl.): S235–S6.

142. Bartoov B, Berkovitz A, Eltes F. Selection of spermatozoa with normal nuclei to improve the pregnancy rate with intracytoplasmic sperm injection. *New Engl J Med.* 2001;**345**(14):1067–8.

143. Bartoov B, Berkovitz A, Eltes F *et al.* Real-time fine morphology of motile human sperm cells is associated with IVF-ICSI outcome. *J Androl.* 2002;**23**(1):1–8.

144. Antinori M, Licata E, Dani G *et al.* Intracytoplasmic morphologically selected sperm injection: a prospective randomized trial. *Reprod Biomed Online.* 2008;**16**(6):835–41.

145. Bartoov B, Berkovitz A, Eltes F *et al.* Pregnancy rates are higher with intracytoplasmic morphologically selected sperm injection than with conventional intracytoplasmic injection. *Fertil Steril.* 2003;**80**(6):1413–19.

146. Berkovitz A, Eltes F, Yaari S *et al.* The morphological normalcy of the sperm nucleus and pregnancy rate of intracytoplasmic injection with morphologically selected sperm. *Hum Reprod.* 2005;**20**(1):185–90.

147. Hazout A, Dumont-Hassan M, Junca AM *et al.* High-magnification ICSI overcomes paternal effect resistant to conventional ICSI. *Reprod Biomed Online.* 2006;**12**(1):19–25.

148. Zamboni L. The ultrastructural pathology of the spermatozoon as a cause of infertility: the role of electron microscopy in the evaluation of semen quality. *Fertil Steril.* 1987;**48**(5):711–34.

163

149. Fawcett DW, Ito S. Observations on the cytoplasmic membranes of testicular cells, examined by phase contrast and electron microscopy. *J Biophysic Biochem Cytol*. 1958;**4**(2):135–42.

150. Tanaka A, Nagayoshi M, Awata S *et al*. Are crater defects in human sperm heads physiological changes during spermiogenesis? *Fertil Steril*. 2009;**92**(3):S165.

151. Watanabe S, Tanaka A, Fujii S *et al*. No relationship between chromosome aberrations and vacuole-like structures on human sperm head. *Hum Reprod*. 2009;**24**(Suppl. 1):i94–6.

152. Baccetti B, Burrini AG, Collodel G *et al*. Crater defect in human spermatozoa. *Gamete Res*. 1989;**22**(3):249–55.

153. Kacem O, Sifer C, Barraud-Lange V *et al*. Sperm nuclear vacuoles, as assessed by motile sperm organellar morphological examination, are mostly of acrosomal origin. *Reprod Biomed Online*. 2010;**20**(1):132–7.

154. Peer S, Eltes F, Berkovitz A *et al*. Is fine morphology of the human sperm nuclei affected by in vitro incubation at 37 degrees C? *Fertil Steril*. 2007;**88**(6):1589–94.

155. Palermo GD, Hu JCY, Rienzi L *et al*. Thoughts on IMSI. In Racowsky C, Schlegel PN, Fauser BC *et al*., editors. *Biennial Review of Infertility*, Vol. **2**. New York, NY: Springer, 2011; 277–90.

156. Huszar G, Ozenci CC, Cayli S *et al*. Hyaluronic acid binding by human sperm indicates cellular maturity, viability, and unreacted acrosomal status. *Fertil Steril*. 2003;**79**(Suppl. 3):1616–24.

157. Jakab A, Sakkas D, Delpiano E *et al*. Intracytoplasmic sperm injection: a novel selection method for sperm with normal frequency of chromosomal aneuploidies. *Fertil Steril*. 2005;**84**(6):1665–73.

158. Yagci A, Murk W, Stronk J *et al*. Spermatozoa bound to solid state hyaluronic acid show chromatin structure with high DNA chain integrity: an acridine orange fluorescence study. *J Androl*. 2010;**31**(6):566–72.

159. Hu JCY. The role of HA selection on spermatozoon competence. *Hum Reprod*. 2012;**27**(Suppl. 2):73.

160. World Health Organization. *WHO Laboratory Manual for the Examination and Processing of Human Semen*. 5th edn. Cambridge: Cambridge University Press; 2010.

161. Schlegel PN, Girardi SK. Clinical review 87: in vitro fertilization for male factor infertility. *J Clin Endocrinol Metab*. 1997;**82**(3):709–16.

162. Palermo GD, Schlegel PN, Sills ES *et al*. Births after intracytoplasmic injection of sperm obtained by testicular extraction from men with nonmosaic Klinefelter's syndrome. *New Engl J Med*. 1998;**338**(9):588–90.

163. Monahan D, Neri QV, Schlegel P *et al*. The time spent in searching for testicular spermatozoa influences ICSI outcome. *Hum Reprod*. 2011;**26**(Suppl. 1):i73–5.

Sperm selection and ART outcome: a means to overcome the effects of aging and abnormal spermatogenesis?

Denny Sakkas

Introduction

In 1978, the culmination of knowledge in the technologies associated with in vitro fertilization (IVF) led to the first IVF birth in the world [1]. Subsequent pioneering work resulted in further improvements in the early 1980s, leading to births after drug-induced superovulation in the mother, the world's first "frozen embryo baby" and the first "donor egg baby." In 1986, the IVF technologies were adapted to assisting infertile males by achieving the world's first pregnancy and birth from a sperm retrieval operation performed on a patient with vasectomy [2]. Subsequently, breakthroughs in the use of micromanipulation allowed the treatment of males with more severe problems, especially low sperm counts, by using techniques such as partial zona dissection and sub-zonal sperm insemination. In 1992, the report of a successful pregnancy using intracytoplasmic sperm injection (ICSI) [3] revolutionized the ability to treat the male and opened up new avenues to treat the majority of males regardless of their etiology. In particular, both obstructive and non-obstructive azoospermic men could now be treated easily with excellent pregnancy outcomes.

These impressive advances have, however, led to the question of what type of paternal genome we are introducing into the egg when treating these males. In addition to the bioethical challenges these IVF technological improvements have raised, the trend in society to create a family later has also led to the treatment of couples in which the male is older.

Sperm quality in the aging male and the ICSI patient

Maternal age plays a significant role in any infertility treatment. The mean age of women that fail to achieve a pregnancy is higher than those that succeed. In fact the most recent SART results indicate that the percentage of IVF cycles resulting in live birth for a women aged < 35 is over 40% and this declines to less than 15% in women over the age of 40. Given the success of donor oocytes in older women and the knowledge about higher miscarriage rates it is evident that the high aneuploidy rates in eggs of older women are a major reason for this decline in pregnancy rates.

The aging male definitely has a less dramatic and obvious effect on reproductive success. Several years ago Wyrobek et al. [4] showed that advancing paternal age has differential effects on nuclear DNA damage, chromatin integrity, gene mutations, and aneuploidies in sperm. They found that after adjusting for potential confounders, male aging was significantly associated with increases in sperm DNA fragmentation and the achondroplasia mutation but not with sperm sex ratio, Apert syndrome mutations, sperm diploidies, or sperm aneuploidies involving chromosomes X, Y, or 21 within their cohort.

Clinical effects related to male age have been reported in numerous epidemiological studies. In 2006, Reichenberg et al. [5] reported a significant monotonic association between advancing paternal age and risk of autism spectrum disorder (ASD). They found that offspring of men 40 years or older were 5.75 times (95% confidence interval (CI) 2.65–12.46; $P < 0.001$) more likely to have ASD compared with offspring of men younger than 30 years. Other studies have also found an association with schizophrenia, however some recent studies indicate that there are combined effects related to maternal factors [6, 7]. The most intriguing studies investigating male age are those that examine the role of the aged male during natural fertility or when a couple is treated by either insemination or donor oocytes. When

Paternal Influences on Human Reproductive Success, ed. Douglas T. Carrell. Published by Cambridge University Press.
© Cambridge University Press 2013.

controlling for age of the woman, natural fertility was significantly reduced for men aged > 35 years [7]. Hassan and Killick [8] also found that increasing male age was associated with a significantly increased time to pregnancy, whereby males > 45 years were 4.6-fold and 12.5-fold more likely to have had a time to pregnancy of > 1 or > 2 years, respectively, compared with men < 25 years old. In women aged 35–39 years, when paternal age was > 40 years the adjusted odds ratio was 2.21 (95% CI 1.13–4.33) for delay in pregnancy onset [9]. In another French study [10] researchers studied the records of more than 17,000 couples treated by intrauterine insemination and found that women whose partners were 35 or older had more miscarriages than those who were with younger men, regardless of their own age. The men's ages also affected pregnancy rates, which were lower in the over-40s. Paternal age led to a decrease in the pregnancy rate from 12.3% before 30 years of age to 9.3% after 45 years of age ($P < 0.001$) and an increase in the miscarriage rate that more than doubled, from 13.7% before 30 years of age, to 32.4% after 45 years of age.

A number of studies have also examined the role of male age on outcomes of donor oocyte cycles. Girsh et al. [11] found a significant decline in pregnancy rates as the male partner became > 45 of age. Frattarelli et al. [12] also investigated outcomes in relation to oocyte donation and reported a significant increase in pregnancy loss, decrease in live birth rate, and decrease in blastocyst formation rate in cases where the male was > 50 years of age. There was no significant difference in implantation rate, pregnancy rate, or early embryo development through the cleavage stage (demonstrated by fertilization rate, embryo cleavage rate, percentage of non-fertilized or polyspermic embryos, rate of embryo arrest, or seven or more cell embryo development on day 3).

What are the underlying mechanisms affecting aging sperm? Unlike the dramatic rise in aneuploidy rates seen in the aging oocyte it is suspected that sperm undergo more subtle changes as the male gets older. Indeed, it may be that the aging effects and those seen in males with a variety of semen disorders (low sperm count, poor motility and morphology) are the same. The study of Wyrobek et al. [4] cited above showed that aging is related to increased sperm nuclear DNA damage. Increased sperm nuclear DNA damage is also more likely to occur in males diagnosed with low sperm numbers, poor motility, and/or poor morphology [13]. This

has now been confirmed in numerous publications. Recently, we found that the aging male also showed traits in spermatogenesis similar to those observed in males with azoospermia and varicocele [14]. Briefly, there was a universal increase in the expression of the Base Excision DNA repair enzyme PARP during the spermatocyte stage and this was a common trait in males aged over 50 and males with varicocele and azoospermia.

Identifying abnormal spermatogenesis

It is clear that ejaculated sperm can contain a heterogeneous population of spermatozoa that may possess abnormalities at various levels (Figure 16.1). This includes the membrane, mitochondria, centrioles, nuclear chromatin, nuclear DNA, and chromosome number. One area of sperm structure that has generated increasing interest in relation to both aging and male sperm assessment is that of the sperm nuclear DNA/chromatin structure.

In 1980, a paper in *Science* entitled "Relation of mammalian sperm chromatin heterogeneity to fertility" was published [15] which used flow cytometry measurements of heated sperm nuclei to reveal a significant decrease in resistance to *in situ* denaturation of spermatozoal DNA in samples from bulls, mice, and humans of low or questionable fertility when compared with others of high fertility. The authors proposed that there were changes in sperm chromatin conformation that were related to the diminished fertility. They then went on to suggest that flow cytometry of heated sperm nuclei could provide a new and independent determinant of male fertility.

In addition to this original methodology we have now become more skillful at measuring the abnormalities in the sperm nucleus. Numerous tests have been introduced for the analysis of sperm and in particular sperm nuclear DNA fragmentation (see review by Sakkas and Alvarez [16]). These tests include terminal deoxynucleotidyl transferase-mediated dUDP nick-end labeling (TUNEL) [17], Comet [18, 19], CMA_3 [19], *in situ* nick translation (ISNT) [13, 20], DNA breakage detection fluorescence *in situ* hybridization (DBD-FISH) [21], sperm chromatin dispersion test (SCD) [22], and the sperm chromatin structure assay (SCSA) [23, 24].

Sperm DNA fragmentation tests sometimes require an initial step of denaturation in order to detect DNA breaks: such as the SCSA, SCD, or Comet at acid or

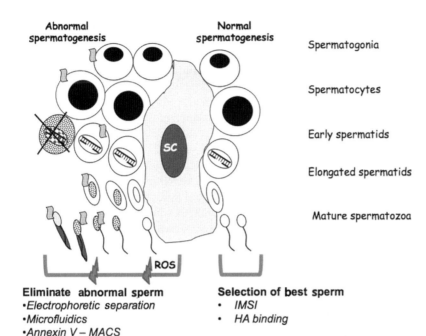

Spermatogonia

Spermatocytes

Early spermatids

Elongated spermatids

Mature spermatozoa

ROS

Eliminate abnormal sperm
- *Electrophoretic separation*
- *Microfluidics*
- *Annexin V – MACS*

Selection of best sperm
- IMSI
- HA binding

Figure 16.1. Spermatogenesis can lead to the production of spermatozoa (left side) with persistence of apoptotic marker proteins on the membrane (green flags) , retention of cytoplasm and membrane abnormalities (purple shading), and possession of nuclear DNA damage (black shading) . Both the normal and abnormal spermatozoa can then be damaged by Reactive Oxygen Species (ROS). These sperm can be eliminated from a sperm preparation using techniques that are designed to eliminate them from the final preparation. Normal spermatogenesis (right side) produces sperm carrying none of these traits. Individual normal sperm can be selected using high magnification intracytoplasmic morphologically selected sperm injection (IMSI) or by selecting sperm whose membranes possess the Hyaluronan receptor (HA binding). This figure is presented in color in the color plate section.

alkaline pH. When DNA damage is observed under acid or alkaline conditions and not under neutral pH conditions they are examining acid/alkali labile DNA sites [4]. Other tests such as TUNEL [17], ISNT [20] and Comet at neutral pH do not require an initial denaturation step and, therefore, measure single-stranded (ISNT, TUNEL, and Comet) or double-stranded (TUNEL and Comet) DNA breaks directly.

Controversy remains as to which tests give the best information and their overall utility. A recent meta-analysis [25] concluded that sperm DNA damage is associated with a significantly increased risk of pregnancy loss after IVF and ICSI. The protocol of analysis may actually prove to be more important however as Borini *et al.* [26] showed that sperm DNA fragmentation values in aliquots of the same spermatozoa used for IVF, measured by TUNEL, were significantly correlated with pregnancy outcome. This is in sharp contrast to the results reported by Bungum *et al.* [27] where no correlation was found between sperm DNA fragmentation values in the samples used for IVF, as measured by the SCSA test, and pregnancy outcome. Overall some controversy still remains about the utility of these tests [28].

In general the clinical results point to a greater utility of sperm DNA tests in relation to natural conception and intrauterine insemination rather than assisted reproduction fertility treatments such as

normal IVF and ICSI [25, 29]. It is important to note that the only final determinant is the quality of the sperm DNA in the fertilizing sperm. In techniques such as IVF or ICSI, where a lot of the natural selection and sperm competition is bypassed, it becomes more important to remove or isolate DNA-damaged sperm for treatment.

To date no sperm test can gauge the degree of sperm DNA damage in a single sperm. Only in animal studies is there a strict correlation between increasing amounts of DNA damage inducers, heat and radiation, and reproductive outcome [30, 31]. One such study by Ahmadi and Ng [31] showed that fertilization rates of around 60% were achieved when sperm were subjected to between 0 and 100 GY of radiation. Blastocyst development decreased from 49.8% in the control group to 2.3% with sperm exposed to doses of 100 GY, respectively. Of the transferred blastocyst in the control group, 33.9% developed into live fetuses while these rates were 20 and 0% when sperm were exposed to doses of 5 and 10 GY, respectively. The authors concluded that embryonic and fetal development are very much related to the degree of DNA damage.

Regardless of the test and the perceived effects these abnormalities have on reproductive outcome, it is clear that there is a higher penetration of patients likely to exhibit sperm DNA damage into the treatment pool via assisted reproduction treatment technologies. In contrast to creating tests to diagnose these patients the data have created a renewed interest in trying to select or deselect particular sperm so that their "abnormal" paternal effects are either limited or completely avoided.

Selecting the best sperm

The strategy to select the best sperm or to eliminate those that are abnormal from the population can be performed using various approaches. The population of sperm as a whole can be prepared or individual sperm can be isolated. The strategies to select or de-select sperm can be based on abnormalities representing different defects acquired during spermatogenesis or during sperm transport (Figure 16.1).

Sperm population preparation

In 1988 a paper by Aitken and Clarkson [32] demonstrated that centrifugal pelleting of unselected sperm populations from human ejaculates caused the production of reactive oxygen species (ROS) (superoxide and hydroxyl radicals) within the pellet which induced irreversible damage to the spermatozoa, and impairment of their fertilizing ability. Mortimer [33] therefore proposed that certain iatrogenic failures of IVF could be associated with sperm preparation techniques. Preparation of sperm with media containing antioxidants has been shown to improve the overall functional parameters of spermatozoa by reducing the ROS level [34].

The simple routine use of density gradient centrifugation has been shown to improve the quality of the sperm population. We have previously shown that when sperm samples from different men were prepared using density gradient techniques for ART and then stained using the chromomycin A3 (CMA3) fluorochrome, which indirectly demonstrates a decreased presence of protamine, and ISNT which examines for the presence of endogenous DNA nicks, a significant ($P < 0.001$) decrease in both CMA3 positivity and DNA strand breakage was observed. The mean difference of the percentage of DNA-damaged sperm prior to preparation and after density gradient centrifugation in over 100 men was 10.5% to 4.6% respectively. In effect the chance of selecting a damaged sperm was reduced by more than half [13, 35]. Spano et al. [36] also measured DFI and HDS on both the raw and prepared semen aliquots. They found that enriched cell suspensions contained sperm with better motility, morphology, HDS, and DFI.

A seemingly milder technique that prepares a sperm population has been reported by Aitken and colleagues. Briefly, this separation system consists of a cassette comprising two 400 µl chambers separated by a polycarbonate filter containing five micromol/l pores and bounded by a 15 kDa polyacrylamide membrane to allow the free circulation of buffer. Semen is introduced into one chamber, current applied (75 mA at variable voltage) and within seconds a purified suspension of spermatozoa is collected from the adjacent chamber. The spermatozoa collected in the adjacent chamber all show good count, viability, motility, and improvement in morphology and DNA integrity.

Some pregnancies have been reported using this system and a clinical trial showed that membrane-based electrophoresis was as effective as density gradient centrifugation in preparing sperm for IVF and ICSI, although it had the added benefit of being significantly faster [37]. Optimized modifications have recently been described that indicated more benefits when compared with conventional density gradient centrifugation technologies [38].

Another technology that could aid in the preparation of sperm populations is microfluidics. Microfluidic technology has been utilized in numerous biological applications specifically for miniaturization and simplification of laboratory techniques. Initial studies have sought to apply microfluidic technology to sperm preparation and showed promising results. They reported that the use of a microfluidic device, designed with two parallel laminar flow channels which preferentially separate motile spermatozoa into a separate outlet increased sperm motility in a sample from 44% to 98% and morphology from 10% to 22% [39]. Similar to the electrophoretic separation technology the removal of centrifugation has the potential to limit some of the iatrogenic preparation problems described earlier. These technologies may also prove useful in isolating motile spermatozoa from oligozoospermic samples, even with high amounts of non-motile gamete and/or non-gamete cell contamination.

De-selection of apoptotic spermatozoa

Although we still do not understand why some ejaculated sperm exhibit apoptotic marker proteins [40] we do know that it is not a trait exhibited by normal sperm. The presence of any apoptotic marker protein on the membrane of a spermatozoon is more likely to be associated with increased DNA damage, poor morphology, cytoplasmic retention, and numerous other abnormal traits. The presence of apoptotic-like ejaculated sperm, or more correctly, ejaculated sperm retaining apoptotic marker proteins on their membranes was shown in the late 1990s [40] and has since been verified by many independent studies [41–44]. Fas, phosphatidylserine, Bcl-X_L, p53, etc., could all be utilized to de-select spermatozoa from semen samples. A novel and promising technique of annexin V-conjugated microbeads (ANMB) – magnetic-activated cell sorting (MACS) has been shown to remove spermatozoa with phosphatidylserine externalization (marker of apoptosis) and produce a higher quality non-apoptotic sperm fraction. Furthermore these "negative-apoptotic marker" cells display higher fertilization rates when used for animal model IVF and ICSI. Magnetic-activated cell sorting is considered as a flexible, fast and simple cell sorting system for separation of large numbers of cells according to specific cell surface markers [45]. This technique has now been reported in several small clinical trials with some success [46, 47].

Selection of single spermatozoon for ICSI

Intracytoplasmic morphologically selected sperm injection

The use of morphological characteristics has been a mainstay for embryologists selecting embryos. Morphology has also been a key characteristic in assessing spermatozoa during semen analysis. Although the WHO and Kruger strict criteria have been used for many years in routine sperm assessment, in 2001 Bartoov and colleagues [48] reported a high magnification technique for selecting normal spermatozoa prior to ICSI. The selection of spermatozoa with normal nuclei was shown to improve the pregnancy rate with ICSI. They went on to verify this technique by performing ICSI using morphologically normal sperm, selected at > 6000 times magnification, in couples with repeated ICSI failures. Sixty-two couples, with at least two previous consequent pregnancy failures after ICSI, underwent a single ICSI trial preceded by morphological selection of spermatozoa with normal nuclei. Fifty of these couples were matched with couples who underwent a routine ICSI procedure at the same IVF center and exhibited the same number of previous ICSI failures. The matching study revealed that the pregnancy rate after modified ICSI was significantly higher than that of the routine ICSI procedure (66% vs 30%). Antinori et al. [49] conducted a prospective randomized study to assess the advantages of intracytoplasmic morphologically

selected sperm injection (IMSI) over the conventional ICSI procedure in the treatment of patients with severe oligoasthenoteratozoospermia. As reported above, IMSI was based on a preliminary motile sperm organellar morphology examination under ×6600 high magnification. A total of 446 couples with at least two previous diagnoses of severe oligoasthenoteratozoospermia, three years of primary infertility, the woman aged 35 years or younger, and an undetected female factor were randomized to IVF microinsemination treatments: ICSI ($n = 219$; group 1) and IMSI ($n = 227$; group 2). A comparison between the two different techniques was made in terms of pregnancy, miscarriage, and implantation rates. The data showed that IMSI resulted in a higher clinical pregnancy rate (39.2% vs 26.5%; $P = 0.004$) than ICSI when applied to severe male infertility cases. Despite their initial poor reproductive prognosis, patients with two or more previous failed attempts benefited the most from IMSI in terms of pregnancy (29.8% vs 12.9%; $P = 0.017$) and miscarriage rates (17.4% vs 37.5%). A recent meta-analysis demonstrated no significant difference in fertilization rate between ICSI and IMSI groups. However, a significantly improved implantation (odds ratio (OR) 2.72; 95% CI 1.50–4.95) and pregnancy rate (OR 3.12; 95% CI 1.55–6.26) was observed in IMSI cycles. Moreover, the results showed a significantly decreased miscarriage rate (OR 0.42; 95% CI 0.23–0.78) in IMSI cycles as compared with ICSI cycles [50].

The traits of the morphologically selected sperm have also been investigated and Wilding et al. [51] found a positive association between high-magnification selection of sperm cells with normal nuclear shape and sperm DNA integrity (by TUNEL assay). A noticeable improvement in clinical outcomes (implantation and birth rates) was also observed in patients with previously failed ICSI cycles when treated with IMSI.

The use of IMSI appears promising (see review by Nadalini et al. [52]). Some drawbacks are however present, in particular the belief that it is a complicated technique that cannot be routinely performed and it can take a long time to identify the sperm under high magnification.

Another microscope-based technology that is showing promise is one that analyzes birefringence in the sperm head. Gianaroli et al. [53] recently performed a prospective randomization including 71 couples with severe male factor infertility and performed ICSI using polarized light for sperm selection which permitted analysis of the pattern of birefringence in the sperm head. Twenty-three patients had their oocytes injected with acrosome-reacted spermatozoa, 26 patients' oocytes were injected with non-acrosome-reacted spermatozoa, and in 22 patients both reacted and non-reacted spermatozoa were injected. They found no effect on the fertilizing capacity and embryo development of either type of sperm, whereas the implantation rate was higher in oocytes injected with reacted spermatozoa (39.0%) vs those injected with non-reacted spermatozoa (8.6%). The implantation rate was 24.4% in the group injected with both reacted and non-reacted spermatozoa. They concluded that spermatozoa that have undergone the acrosome reaction seem to be more prone to supporting the development of viable ICSI embryos.

Sperm binding to hyaluronic acid (HA)

Another technique that utilizes the concept of selecting spermatozoa that have undergone normal spermatogenesis is the HA binding assay. During human spermiogenesis, the elongated spermatids undergo a plasma membrane remodeling step which facilitates formation of the zona pellucida and HA-binding sites. Human sperm that bind to HA exhibit attributes similar to that of zona pellucida-bound sperm, including minimal DNA fragmentation, normal shape, and low frequency of chromosomal aneuploidies [54]. In 2005 Jakab et al. [55] reported that selection of HA-bound spermatozoa significantly decreased the percentage of sperm showing both apoptotic marker proteins and aneuploidies. It was suggested that clinical use of HA-mediated sperm selection could ultimately solve the pertinent problem of aneuploidies and DNA fragmentation when ICSI is performed with immature sperm samples.

A number of studies have now indicated that HA-bound sperm selected for the ICSI procedure may lead to increased implantation rates. In one such study, Parmegiani et al. [56] showed that in 293 couples treated with HA-ICSI vs 86 couples treated with conventional ICSI (historical control group) that all outcome measures i.e. fertilization, embryo quality, implantation, and pregnancy were the same or improved in the HA-bound sperm group. The implantation rate was increased from 10.3% in conventional ICSI to 17.1% in the HA group. A clinical trial assessing the same technology by Worrilow et al. [57] has also shown that clinical pregnancy rates are improved when using HA-selected sperm compared with conventional ICSI. Furthermore, HA binding can be used as a diagnostic semen analysis platform prior to treatment. In preliminary results from a multi-center clinical trial Worrilow et al. [57] has shown that when patients with less than 65% binding efficiency are prescreened and selected prior to ICSI their success rates are improved by using this technology.

Overcoming reactive oxygen species exposure

It could be argued however that whatever the preparation technique used or the protection offered to the spermatozoa it may still be too late. Post-testicular sperm DNA damage can also be induced by reactive oxygen species (ROS) or after exposure to ionizing radiation is associated with nucleotide damage of the 8-OHdG type.

A radical approach to circumvent this type of damage occurring in the epididymis is using testicular sperm. A number of reports have now shown that sperm DNA damage is significantly lower in the seminiferous tubules compared with the cauda epididymis [58] or ejaculated sperm [59]. These reports indicate that the use of testicular sperm in couples with repeated pregnancy failure in ART and high sperm DNA fragmentation in semen result in a significant increase in pregnancy rates in these couples [59, 60]. Moreover, a recent report shows that pregnancy rates in first cycles of TESA–ICSI in these couples are relatively high [16]. The use of testicular sperm may however not always solve the problem since sperm DNA damage may also occur in the seminiferous tubule epithelium by apoptosis or be due to defects in chromatin remodeling during the process of spermiogenesis.

Future approaches to sperm selection

A number of novel new technologies are being developed which may also serve the purpose of allowing better sperm selection prior to classical IVF or ICSI. These include the use of Raman spectroscopy to non-invasively distinguish the DNA packaging and protamine content between normal and abnormal cells [61]. In this study it was shown that the relative protein content per cell and DNA packaging efficiencies are distributed over a relatively wide range for sperm cells with both normal and abnormal shape. Their findings indicate that single cell Raman spectroscopy could be a valuable tool in assessing the quality of sperm cells.

Other molecular techniques may allow the analysis of sperm populations in the future. For example, DNA methylation patterns of key developmental genes have been shown to differ in spermatozoa and this may impact embryo development [62]. Interesting results are also being generated from proteomic [63] and RNA [64] analysis of sperm which will create a database for identifying key factors implicated in defective sperm function and aid in both diagnosis and treatment.

Conclusions

The noted decline in live birth rates and miscarriages in relation to increasing age and sperm containing nuclear DNA damage is putting a greater onus on the need to improve our knowledge of the molecular basis of male infertility. The effect of the paternal genome on reproductive outcome is definitely coming under more scrutiny. New tools to more accurately diagnose and select individual sperm will subsequently allow us to counsel and treat couples with greater confidence and efficiency.

References

1. Steptoe PC, Edwards RG. Birth after the reimplantation of a human embryo. *Lancet.* 1978;**2** (8085):366.

2. Temple-Smith PD, Southwick GJ, Yates CA *et al.* Human pregnancy by in vitro fertilization (IVF) using sperm aspirated from the epididymis. *J In Vitro Fert Embryo Transf.* 1985;**2**(3):119–22.

3. Palermo G, Joris H, Devroey P *et al.* Pregnancies after intracytoplasmic injection of single spermatozoon into an oocyte. *Lancet.* 1992;**340** (8810):17–18.

4. Wyrobek AJ, Eskenazi B, Young S *et al.* Advancing age has differential effects on DNA damage, chromatin integrity, gene mutations, and aneuploidies in sperm. *Proc Natl Acad Sci USA.* 2006;**103**(25):9601–6.

5. Reichenberg A, Gross R, Weiser M *et al.* Advancing paternal age and autism. *Arch Gen Psychiatry.* 2006;**63**(9):1026–32.

6. Malaspina D, Harlap S, Fennig S *et al.* Advancing paternal age and the risk of schizophrenia. *Arch Gen Psychiatry.* 2001;**58**(4):361–7.

7. Dunson DB, Colombo B, Baird DD. Changes with age in the level and duration of fertility in the menstrual cycle. *Hum Reprod.* 2002;**17**(5):1399–403.

8. Hassan MA, Killick SR. Effect of male age on fertility: evidence for the decline in male fertility with increasing age. *Fertil Steril.* 2003;**79**(Suppl. 3):1520–7.

9. de La Rochebrochard E, Thonneau P. Paternal age > or = 40 years: an important risk factor for infertility. *Am J Obstet Gynecol.* 2003;**189**(4):901–5.

10. Belloc S, Cohen-Bacrie P, Benkhalifa M *et al.* Effect of maternal and paternal age on pregnancy and

11. Girsh E, Katz N, Genkin L *et al.* Male age influences oocyte-donor program results. *J Assist Reprod Genet.* 2008;**25**(4):137–43.

12. Frattarelli JL, Miller KA, Miller BT *et al.* Male age negatively impacts embryo development and reproductive outcome in donor oocyte assisted reproductive technology cycles. *Fertil Steril.* 2008;**90**(1):97–103.

13. Tomlinson MJ, Moffatt O, Manicardi GC *et al.* Interrelationships between seminal parameters and sperm nuclear DNA damage before and after density gradient centrifugation: implications for assisted conception. *Hum Reprod.* 2001;**16**(10):2160–5.

14. El-Domyati MM, Al-Din AB, Barakat MT *et al.* Deoxyribonucleic acid repair and apoptosis in testicular germ cells of aging fertile men: the role of the poly (adenosine diphosphate-ribosyl)ation pathway. *Fertil Steril.* 2009;**91**(5 Suppl.):2221–9.

15. Evenson DP, Darzynkiewicz Z, Melamed MR. Relation of mammalian sperm chromatin heterogeneity to fertility. *Science.* 1980;**210**(4474):1131–3.

16. Sakkas D, Alvarez JG. Sperm DNA fragmentation: mechanisms of origin, impact on reproductive outcome, and analysis. *Fertil Steril.* 2010;**93**(4):1027–36.

17. Gorczyca W, Traganos F, Jesionowska H *et al.* Presence of DNA strand breaks and increased sensitivity of DNA in situ to denaturation in abnormal human sperm cells: analogy to apoptosis of somatic cells. *Exp Cell Res.* 1993;**207**(1):202–5.

18. Hughes CM, Lewis SE, McKelvey-Martin VJ *et al.* A comparison of baseline and induced DNA damage in human spermatozoa from fertile and infertile men, using a modified Comet assay. *Mol Hum Reprod.* 1996;**2**(8):613–19.

19. Manicardi GC, Bianchi PG, Pantano S *et al.* Presence of endogenous nicks in DNA of ejaculated human spermatozoa and its relationship to chromomycin a3 accessibility. *Biol Reprod.* 1995;**52**(4):864–7.

20. Bianchi PG, Manicardi GC, Bizzaro D *et al.* Effect of deoxyribonucleic acid protamination on fluorochrome staining and in situ nick-translation of murine and human mature spermatozoa. *Biol Reprod.* 1993;**49** (5):1083–8.

21. Fernandez JL, Vazquez-Gundin F, Delgado A *et al.* DNA breakage detection-FISH (DBD-FISH) in human spermatozoa: technical variants evidence different structural features. *Mutat Res.* 2000;**453**(1):77–82.

22. Fernandez JL, Muriel L, Rivero MT *et al.* The sperm chromatin dispersion test: a simple method for the determination of sperm DNA fragmentation. *J Androl.* 2003;**24**(1):59–66.

23. Larson KL, DeJonge CJ, Barnes AM *et al.* Sperm chromatin structure assay parameters as predictors of failed pregnancy following assisted reproductive techniques. *Hum Reprod.* 2000;**15**(8):1717–22.

24. Evenson DP, Larson KL, Jost LK. Sperm chromatin structure assay: its clinical use for detecting sperm DNA fragmentation in male infertility and comparisons with other techniques. *J Androl.* 2002;**23**(1):25–43.

25. Zini A, Boman JM, Belzile E *et al.* Sperm DNA damage is associated with an increased risk of pregnancy loss after IVF and ICSI: systematic review and meta-analysis. *Hum Reprod.* 2008;**23**(12):2663–8.

26. Borini A, Tarozzi N, Bizzaro D *et al.* Sperm DNA fragmentation: paternal effect on early post-implantation embryo development in Art. *Hum Reprod.* 2006;**21**(11):2876–81.

27. Bungum M, Humaidan P, Axmon A *et al.* Sperm DNA integrity assessment in prediction of assisted reproduction technology outcome. *Hum Reprod.* 2007;**22**(1):174–9.

28. Collins JA, Barnhart KT, Schlegel PN. Do sperm DNA integrity tests predict pregnancy with in vitro fertilization? *Fertil Steril.* 2008;**89**(4):823–31.

29. Evenson DP, Wixon R. Data analysis of two in vivo fertility studies using sperm chromatin structure assay-derived DNA fragmentation index vs. Pregnancy outcome. *Fertil Steril.* 2008;**90**(4):1229–31.

30. Setchell BP, Ekpe G, Zupp JL *et al.* Transient retardation in embryo growth in normal female mice made pregnant by males whose testes had been heated. *Hum Reprod.* 1998;**13**(2):342–7.

31. Ahmadi A, Ng SC. Fertilizing ability of DNA-damaged spermatozoa. *J Exp Zool.* 1999;**284**(6):696–704.

32. Aitken RJ, Clarkson JS. Significance of reactive oxygen species and antioxidants in defining the efficacy of sperm preparation techniques. *J Androl.* 1988;**9** (6):367–76.

33. Mortimer D. Sperm preparation techniques and iatrogenic failures of in-vitro fertilization. *Hum Reprod.* 1991;**6**(2):173–6.

34. Donnelly ET, McClure N, Lewis SE. Glutathione and hypotaurine in vitro: effects on human sperm motility, DNA integrity and production of reactive oxygen species. *Mutagenesis.* 2000;**15**(1):61–8.

35. Sakkas D, Manicardi GC, Tomlinson M *et al.* The use of two density gradient centrifugation techniques and the swim-up method to separate spermatozoa with chromatin and nuclear DNA anomalies. *Hum Reprod.* 2000;**15**(5):1112–16.

36. Spano M, Cordelli E, Leter G *et al.* Nuclear chromatin variations in human spermatozoa undergoing swim-up and cryopreservation evaluated by the flow cytometric

sperm chromatin structure assay. *Mol Hum Reprod.* 1999;**5**(1):29–37.

37. Fleming SD, Ilad RS, Griffin AM *et al.* Prospective controlled trial of an electrophoretic method of sperm preparation for assisted reproduction: comparison with density gradient centrifugation. *Hum Reprod.* 2008;**23** (12):2646–51.

38. Aitken RJ, Hanson AR, Kuczera L. Electrophoretic sperm isolation: optimization of electrophoresis conditions and impact on oxidative stress. *Hum Reprod.* 2011;**26**(8):1955–64.

39. Schuster TG, Cho B, Keller LM *et al.* Isolation of motile spermatozoa from semen samples using microfluidics. *Reprod Biomed Online.* 2003;**7**(1):75–81.

40. Sakkas D, Mariethoz E, St John JC. Abnormal sperm parameters in humans are indicative of an abortive apoptotic mechanism linked to the FAS-mediated pathway. *Exp Cell Res.* 1999;**251**(2):350–5.

41. Sakkas D, Moffatt O, Manicardi GC *et al.* Nature of DNA damage in ejaculated human spermatozoa and the possible involvement of apoptosis. *Biol Reprod.* 2002;**66**(4):1061–7.

42. Cayli S, Sakkas D, Vigue L *et al.* Cellular maturity and apoptosis in human sperm: creatine kinase, caspase-3 and Bcl-XL levels in mature and diminished maturity sperm. *Mol Hum Reprod.* 2004;**10**(5):365–72.

43. Mahfouz RZ, Sharma RK, Poenicke K *et al.* Evaluation of poly(ADP-ribose) polymerase cleavage (cPARP) in ejaculated human sperm fractions after induction of apoptosis. *Fertil Steril.* 2009;**91**(5 Suppl.):2210–20.

44. Oehninger S, Morshedi M, Weng SL *et al.* Presence and significance of somatic cell apoptosis markers in human ejaculated spermatozoa. *Reprod Biomed Online.* 2003;**7**(4):469–76.

45. Said TM, Agarwal A, Zborowski M *et al.* Utility of magnetic cell separation as a molecular sperm preparation technique. *J Androl.* 2008;**29**(2):134–42.

46. Polak de Fried E, Denaday F. Single and twin ongoing pregnancies in two cases of previous ART failure after ICSI performed with sperm sorted using annexin V microbeads. *Fertil Steril.* 2010;**94**(1):351 e15–18.

47. Rawe VY, Boudri HU, Alvarez Sedo C *et al.* Healthy baby born after reduction of sperm DNA fragmentation using cell sorting before ICSI. *Reprod Biomed Online.* 2010;**20**(3):320–3.

48. Bartoov B, Berkovitz A, Eltes F. Selection of spermatozoa with normal nuclei to improve the pregnancy rate with intracytoplasmic sperm injection. *N Engl J Med.* 2001;**345**(14):1067–8.

49. Antinori M, Licata E, Dani G *et al.* Intracytoplasmic morphologically selected sperm injection: a prospective

randomized trial. *Reprod Biomed Online*. 2008;**16**(6):835–41.

50. Souza Setti A, Ferreira RC, Paes de Almeida Ferreira Braga D *et al.* Intracytoplasmic sperm injection outcome versus intracytoplasmic morphologically selected sperm injection outcome: a meta-analysis. *Reprod Biomed Online*. 2010;**21**(4):450–5.

51. Wilding M, Coppola G, di Matteo L *et al.* Intracytoplasmic injection of morphologically selected spermatozoa (IMSI) improves outcome after assisted reproduction by deselecting physiologically poor quality spermatozoa. *J Assist Reprod Genet*. 2011;**28**(3):253–62.

52. Nadalini M, Tarozzi N, Distratis V *et al.* Impact of intracytoplasmic morphologically selected sperm injection on assisted reproduction outcome: a review. *Reprod Biomed Online*. 2009;**19**(Suppl. 3):45–55.

53. Gianaroli L, Magli MC, Ferraretti AP *et al.* Birefringence characteristics in sperm heads allow for the selection of reacted spermatozoa for intracytoplasmic sperm injection. *Fertil Steril*. 2010;**93**(3):807–13.

54. Huszar G, Jakab A, Sakkas D *et al.* Fertility testing and ICSI sperm selection by hyaluronic acid binding: clinical and genetic aspects. *Reprod Biomed Online*. 2007;**14**(5):650–63.

55. Jakab A, Sakkas D, Delpiano E *et al.* Intracytoplasmic sperm injection: a novel selection method for sperm with normal frequency of chromosomal aneuploidies. *Fertil Steril*. 2005;**84**(6):1665–73.

56. Parmegiani L, Cognigni GE, Ciampaglia W *et al.* Efficiency of hyaluronic acid (HA) sperm selection. *J Assist Reprod Genet*. 2010;**27**(1):13–16.

57. Worrilow K, Huynh H, Bowers J *et al.* The clinical impact associated with the use of pICSI derived embryos. *Fertil Steril*. 2009;**92**(3):O146.

58. Steele EK, McClure N, Maxwell RJ *et al.* A comparison of DNA damage in testicular and proximal epididymal spermatozoa in obstructive azoospermia. *Mol Hum Reprod*. 1999;**5**(9):831–5.

59. Greco E, Scarselli F, Iacobelli M *et al.* Efficient treatment of infertility due to sperm DNA damage by ICSI with testicular spermatozoa. *Hum Reprod*. 2005;**20**(1):226–30.

60. Alvarez JG. Aplicaciones clinicas del estudio de fragmentacion del DNA espermatico. *Revista Argentina de Andrologia*. 2008;5.

61. Huser T, Orme CA, Hollars CW *et al.* Raman spectroscopy of DNA packaging in individual human sperm cells distinguishes normal from abnormal cells. *J Biophotonics*. 2009;**2**(5):322–32.

62. Hammoud SS, Nix DA, Zhang H *et al.* Distinctive chromatin in human sperm packages genes for embryo development. *Nature*. 2009;**460**(7254):473–8.

63. Aitken RJ, Baker MA. The role of proteomics in understanding sperm cell biology. *Int J Androl*. 2008;**31**(3):295–302.

64. Ostermeier GC, Goodrich RJ, Diamond MP *et al.* Toward using stable spermatozoal RNAs for prognostic assessment of male factor fertility. *Fertil Steril*. 2005;**83**(6):1687–94.

Variability of human semen quality: caution in interpreting semen analysis data

Kenneth I. Aston

Introduction

The standard semen analysis is a fundamental tool in the evaluation of male fertility potential. Although it is a staple of the Andrology laboratory and the best first-line tool currently available to estimate male fertility potential, it is critical that clinicians be aware of the limitations of the assay and that interpretation of results and clinical decisions be made within the context of those limitations. This chapter will provide a brief overview of the parameters evaluated by the standard semen analysis and will review the data available that illustrate the limitations of this tool in the diagnosis of male-factor infertility. In addition, currently available adjunctive sperm tests as well as future directions for the development of improved male fertility diagnostic tools will be briefly discussed.

Semen analysis

The World Health Organization's *Laboratory Manual for the Examination, and Processing of Human Semen*, 5th edition (WHO 5) recommends that semen analyses be performed after 2–7 days of sexual abstinence [1]. Following semen collection by masturbation or with the use of a sterile, non-spermicidal condom, the sample is maintained at 37 °C and allowed to liquefy for 15–60 minutes, after which the semen analysis is performed.

After liquefaction, the sample is assessed for abnormal viscosity and general appearance (opacity, color, etc.), and the total ejaculate volume and pH are measured. Initial microscopic evaluation of the sample at low power allows the identification of sperm aggregation, agglutination, round cells, and gross abnormalities.

Subsequently, the sample is observed at 200× or 400× magnification for the evaluation of sperm motility and concentration. Sperm motility, generally based on the

evaluation of 200 cells, is classified according to the motility category: progressive motility, non-progressive motility, and immotility. Increased sperm motility correlates with natural pregnancy rates as well as conception rates following intrauterine insemination [2–5].

Concentration determination is performed on the thoroughly mixed semen sample using a hemocytometer or similar counting chamber. Sperm are typically immobilized and diluted using a solution of sodium bicarbonate and formalin in water, then counted. Sperm concentration and total sperm count (measures of the sperm production capacity of the testes) correlate with time to pregnancy and pregnancy rates [5–7].

In addition to sperm motility and count, sperm vitality is another important metric assessed during the semen analysis. Sperm vitality is indirectly ascertained using two primary tests of membrane integrity, dye exclusion and hypo-osmotic swelling (HOS) tests. Vitality testing is performed as soon as possible after liquefaction of the sample.

The dye exclusion test employs the use of the membrane-impermeant stain eosin followed by counter-staining with nigrosin, which facilitates sperm identification. In viable sperm with intact plasma membranes, eosin will not penetrate the cell, whereas non-viable sperm with damaged membranes will stain readily. Evaluation of vitality following eosin-nigrosin staining simply involves determining the percentages of eosin-stained (red or pink) and unstained (white) sperm heads on a dry smear of the stained preparation using brightfield optics at 1000× magnification with oil immersion [8]. Typically 200 sperm are evaluated for this test.

The HOS test is performed by mixing a semen sample with hypo-osmotic medium composed of sodium citrate and D-fructose in water. In the hypo-osmotic solution,

Paternal Influences on Human Reproductive Success, ed. Douglas T. Carrell. Published by Cambridge University Press.
© Cambridge University Press 2013.

sperm membranes of membrane-intact sperm will swell, while non-viable sperm will not respond to hypo-osmotic conditions [9]. Sperm are evaluated following an exposure of at least 30 minutes to hypo-osmotic medium. Membrane swelling is ascertained using phase contrast microscopy at 200× or 400×. Sperm cells exhibiting a coiled tail or various degrees of tail swelling are counted as reacted (viable), and unreacted sperm are considered non-viable. As with the eosin-nigrosin test, 200 sperm are counted for the HOS test.

In addition to the above, the assessment of sperm morphology is another important element of the semen analysis. The proportion of morphologically normal sperm is related to time to pregnancy and both in vivo and in vitro pregnancy rates [10–13]. Early studies observed an enrichment of morphologically normal sperm in the potentially fertilizing fraction of sperm, those recovered from endocervical mucus and from the surface of the zona pellucida post-coitus [14, 15]. Sperm morphology evaluation involves preparing a semen smear on a slide followed by air-drying, fixing, staining, and cover-slipping the slide, and finally examining the slide under brightfield conditions at 1000× magnification with oil immersion. The percentage of normal forms is optimally determined after assessing approximately 200 sperm. A morphologically normal sperm based on WHO 5 criteria displays a smooth, regularly contoured, oval-shaped head with a well-defined acrosomal region, minimal vacuoles, a slender midpiece about the same length as, and aligned with, the sperm head, minimal residual cytoplasm, and a uniform principal piece approximately 10 times the length of the head without any sharp bends [1].

Considerations in the interpretation of semen analysis results

While the standard semen analysis provides potentially valuable information in evaluating a man's fertility potential, a clear understanding of several factors is important in interpreting semen analysis results and using those results for clinical decision making. These factors can essentially be summarized by two primary assessments: (1) the reliability of semen analysis results (i.e. how closely the reported semen analysis results reflect the actual semen parameters of an individual), and (2) the clinical significance or prognostic value of the semen parameters evaluated by a standard semen analysis. The reliability of semen analysis results is limited by human error and a myriad

of extrinsic factors that can result in significant intra-individual variability in semen parameters across multiple ejaculates. These limitations, while not insignificant, can be largely controlled by the faithful implementation of quality control measures and consistent adherence to proper laboratory protocols. Probably the more significant limitation of semen analysis data is inherent in the assay itself. The standard semen analysis provides a very superficial assessment of the reproductive capacity of an individual. While incontrovertible clinical correlates have been reported, and reference ranges have been established for each of the semen parameters analyzed based on the best data available, there are many aspects of sperm function that are not captured by the standard semen analysis. Nevertheless, in spite of its shortcomings, the semen analysis remains the cornerstone for fertility assessment in the male.

Reliability of semen analysis results

In interpreting the results of a semen analysis, it is important to be aware of limitations in the reliability of the assay. The limitations of assay reliability are derived from two main sources: technician variability/human error and normal fluctuations in semen parameters within an individual based on natural biological processes or extrinsic factors that affect spermatogenic efficiency or sperm function [16].

Random and systematic errors in semen analyses

As semen analyses are performed manually, and most of the tests performed are somewhat objective, there will naturally be some margin of error associated with each result. The magnitude of error depends upon the test, as some are more subjective or prone to error than others.

Semen analysis errors can be random or systematic in nature. Random errors are simply the result of statistical probabilities – errors that arise by chance as a result of sampling errors, due to the random distribution of sperm displaying a particular parameter [16]. This type of error can easily be assessed by evaluation of repeat assays performed by the same technician on the same sample using the same equipment. Systematic errors, or biases, are errors that arise due to procedural factors, so errors are consistently altered in a single direction and are thus more difficult to assess and control.

Several groups have evaluated inter- and intra-technician variability of semen analysis measures. While variability varies greatly between studies, coefficients of variation (CV) for sperm concentration, motility, and morphology are almost universally > 10%, and often in the range of 20–30% or higher. For example, evaluation of the performance of sperm concentration determination for 10 andrology laboratories by Neuwinger *et al.* demonstrated CVs of 23–73% with higher concentrations yielding the lowest CVs. In the same study, CVs for morphology between labs were 25% for normal heads and 87% for normal midpieces, and the CV for sperm motility was 21%. This study also demonstrated the apparent systematic differences between laboratories, as the CVs for internal quality control (QC) were significantly lower at 10%, 8%, and 8% for concentration, normal head morphology, and motility respectively [17]. A more recent study of 20 laboratories found CVs for sperm concentration, morphology, and progressive motility ranged from 29–52%, 17–26%, and 39–71% respectively [18]. Another study evaluated semen analysis variability among technicians from different laboratories who were all trained at a central laboratory. This model resulted in improved consistency between technicians with CVs of 12.6–15.2% for concentration and 10.5% for motility. Further, intra-technician CVs were 10.3–12.5% for concentration and 5.2% for motility [19].

Given the demonstrated variability in semen analysis results between and within laboratories, clearly internal and external QC as part of a quality assurance (QA) program is critical in ensuring that accuracy and precision for the various semen analysis parameters are maximized [20, 21]. These measures serve to detect and control for systematic errors. The regular assessment of technician competency using QC samples prepared in the laboratory or purchased from a commercial source allows for the routine monitoring of technician performance to ensure values for each test by each technician consistently fall within acceptable limits.

In addition to the use of appropriate QC programs to minimize systematic errors, increasing sampling size can minimize random or sampling errors. The WHO recommends the assessment of 200 sperm in duplicate for each test in the standard semen analysis [1]. As more sperm are assessed for a particular test, the confidence interval (CI) narrows. However, the statistical advantage of increasing sample size diminishes rapidly as greater than 200 sperm are assessed [16], so 200 has been determined to be the optimal balance between effort and diminishing returns. In addition, there is a balance between the resulting decrease in statistical sampling error and the increased time required and potential decreased accuracy on the part of the technician with increased workload.

Also important in minimizing random and systematic errors is the establishment of written standard operating procedures (SOPs). These documents serve as a reference for training and re-training and become the foundation for careful and consistent procedures. These SOPs should be followed strictly by all technicians regardless of experience level to ensure that all assays are performed according to protocol, thus minimizing the potential for errors due to slight modifications to procedures.

With proper training, careful adherence to laboratory SOPs, and consistent monitoring of technician performance with a faithfully implemented QA program, random and systematic errors can be minimized such that they will fall within acceptable and predictable limits [22]. While errors will not be eliminated, with the proper controls in place and an understanding of the potential for controlled errors, these factors should not have a significant negative impact on clinical decisions.

Intra-individual variability in semen parameters

While systematic and random errors can clearly impact semen analysis results, another important source for variability in semen parameters is intra-individual biological variability. Numerous intrinsic and extrinsic factors can affect semen parameters in an individual. Due to the inherent variation, which can be significant in some cases, the WHO recommends that at least two semen analyses be performed for each individual prior to clinical decision making [1].

Variations in semen parameters within an individual are the result of a variety of factors, some of which are predictable and can be controlled for, and others that are more stochastic or unpredictable. Factors that have been demonstrated to impact semen parameters include abstinence time, collection method, collection time, and the presence of bacteriospermia and elevated leukocytes in semen, as well as numerous environmental and therapeutic exposures. Some of these factors affect semen parameters only slightly, while others can have a profound impact. In addition, significant intra-individual variation in semen parameters is observed in the absence of known contributory factors, likely due to seemingly inconsequential day-to-day exposures to heat, pollutants, radiation, and other factors, or other uncharacterized factors that affect spermatogenic efficiency either directly or indirectly.

Numerous studies have evaluated the effect of abstinence time on sperm concentration, total count, and motility. The WHO recommends that semen analyses be performed following 2–7 days of sexual abstinence [1]. Even within that window, it has been demonstrated that increased periods of abstinence generally result in increased semen volume, increased total sperm count, and decreased motility [23–28]. An early study of 36 normal subjects reported sperm concentration, volume, and total count increased on average 13×10^6/mL, 0.4 mL, and 87×10^6 respectively for each day of increased abstinence time [26]. Recently, a large study evaluating the semen parameters of 5,240 men for which two semen analyses had been performed reported CVs of 28% for semen volume, 29% for sperm concentration, 34% for motility, 29% for morphology, and 30% for total motile sperm count. In this study abstinence time had a significant effect on all of these parameters except morphology [28].

While abstinence time has the best studied and generally the most profound effect on semen parameters, other factors have also been demonstrated to affect semen analysis results. Modest, but significant diurnal and seasonal effects have been reported to affect sperm concentration, motility, and morphology [29–32]. In addition, history of fever or other exposures that increase scrotal temperature can have a negative impact on sperm concentration, morphology, and motility [33, 34], and increased seminal leukocytes are associated with significantly reduced sperm concentration, motility, and normal morphology [35].

These and numerous other factors can significantly affect semen parameters. It is impossible to account for or isolate all of these factors when evaluating the results of a semen analysis. This intra-individual variability is the primary reason that it is helpful to obtain more than one semen analysis from each patient [1]. Figure 17.1 illustrates the variation in sperm concentration and total sperm number in five healthy young men assigned to a male hormone contraception study. The study involved multiple collections spanning a 1.5-year period [1]. Similar magnitudes in intra-individual variation have been described for many of the other semen parameters.

Strict adherence to abstinence times, care in identifying other factors that might influence semen quality, and the performance of at least two semen analyses from each patient are all important in overcoming the inherent variability in semen parameters and obtaining reliable semen analysis results.

Prognostic limitations of the semen analysis

Semen analyses are generally performed with the primary goal of assessing the fertility potential of an individual and using that information to determine if, and/or what, clinical interventions might be appropriate to help an infertile couple to successfully conceive. In some regards, the semen analysis is appropriate and sufficient for this task, but often semen analyses fall short of accomplishing this goal, particularly in the diagnosis of subfertility. The semen analysis in its current form offers a relatively superficial view of male fertility potential. The prognostic limitations and the need for a more informative semen analysis has been the subject of much discussion in the andrology community [36–39].

The parameters assessed by a semen analysis, including sperm concentration and total count, total motility and progressive motility, viability, morphology and observations such as increased round cells, etc., have important prognostic value. However semen analysis results often give an inconclusive or incomplete picture of the fertility status or the best treatment option for a patient. Indeed male-factor infertility can be, and likely often is, the culprit for a couple's infertility even when the semen parameters evaluated by a semen analysis fall within normal ranges.

Conditions such as azoospermia, severe oligozoospermia, asthenozoospermia, and complete globozoospermia can be diagnosed by the semen analysis and explain the cause of infertility. However it is often important to perform additional testing to characterize the underlying cause for these conditions. For example, in the case of azoospermia, testing to rule out obstruction or absence of vas deferens is necessary [40]. In cases of non-obstructive azoospermia or severe oligozoospermia, Y chromosome microdeletion testing and karyotype analysis can be valuable in identifying the underlying genetic cause for spermatogenic impairment [40]. The results of these tests can offer valuable insight for the patient and clinician in determining the best treatment strategies. For example, for patients with complete globozoospermia, fertilization is likely only possible with ICSI and may

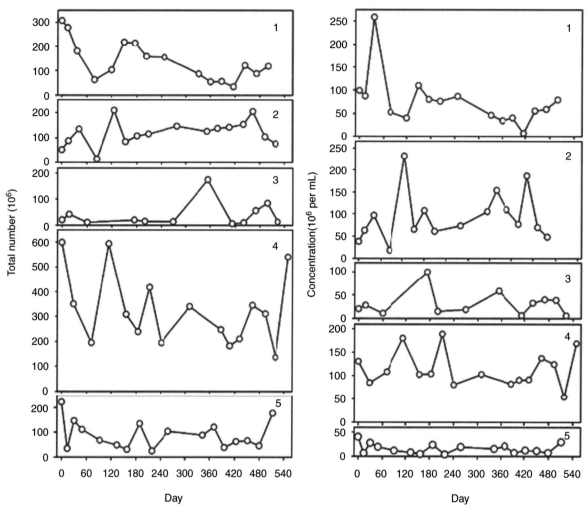

Figure 17.1. Variation in total sperm number and sperm concentration in five young healthy men over a 1.5-year period [1].

necessitate artificial oocyte activation using a calcium ionophore [41]. Similarly, in cases where no motile sperm are identified, selection of viable sperm using strategies such as pentoxifylline (PTX) incubation or the hypo-osmotic swelling test followed by ICSI is generally indicated [42].

The WHO 5 manual offers the best data to date to objectively evaluate and interpret semen analysis results. Reference limits for this edition of the manual were generated by computing the 5th percentiles of the various semen parameters from almost 2,000 men from 14 countries whose partners conceived within 12 months of ceasing the use of contraception (Table 17.1) [43]. Importantly, these values do not represent cut-offs to define infertility. By definition,

in a random population of fertile men, 95% would be expected to display semen parameters above the lower reference limit. The corollary to this is that any given semen parameter would fall below the lower reference limit in 5% of fertile men. Conversely, many infertile and subfertile men have semen parameters that exceed these limits. The reference limits are established to guide clinical diagnosis, not to define infertility or subfertility.

Advanced sperm testing

A significant deficiency in the current semen analysis is that current methods fail in large measure to assess the functional parameters of sperm. The semen analysis does a fine job at assessing spermatogenic efficiency

Table 17.1 Lower reference limits (5th centiles and their 95% confidence intervals) for semen parameters [1].

Parameter	Lower reference limit
Semen volume (mL)	1.5 (1.4–1.7)
Total sperm number (10^6/ejaculate)	39 (33–46)
Sperm concentration (10^6/mL)	15 (12–16)
Total motility, PR+NP (%)	40 (38–42)
Progressive motility, PR (%)	32 (31–34)
Vitality, live spermatozoa (%)	58 (55–63)
Sperm morphology, normal forms (%)	4 (3.0–4.0)

NP, non-progressive motility; PR, progressive motility.

by determining the number and viability of sperm produced. Unfortunately the only functional parameter assessed by the semen analysis is the motility of sperm. While a sufficient number of motile sperm is an important requirement for successful fertilization and normal embryo development, there are numerous other factors, some known and others unknown that are required for proper sperm function. This is due to the complex process of fertilization and early development.

In order for successful fertilization to occur in vivo, sperm have to traverse the harsh environment of the female reproductive tract, reach the cumulus oocyte complex in the fallopian tube, penetrate the cumulus mass and the zona pellucida by mechanical and enzymatic means, bind to and fuse with the oolemma, trigger the resumption of meiosis in the oocyte, introduce an intact haploid chromosome complement to the ooplasm which must then successfully de-condense to form the male pronucleus and subsequently fuse with the female pronucleus to undergo mitotic cell divisions. In addition, emerging data indicate other sperm factors such as various RNA species carried by the sperm, and the epigenetic architecture of the sperm nucleus impact embryo development [44–48]. The semen analysis does little to assess the capacity of the sperm to successfully complete all of the processes required for successful fertilization and embryo development.

Numerous additional tests designed to augment semen analysis results have been employed in male infertility testing [36, 38]. Some of the available diagnostic tests include tests for sperm DNA damage (Comet,

TUNEL, SCSA) [49], aneuploidy testing [50], and tests of chromatin composition [51]. While clinical correlates between infertility and sperm DNA damage, aneuploidy rates, and chromatin structure have been demonstrated, these tests are not routinely used for a variety of reasons.

In the case of DNA damage assessment, each of the available methods has advantages and disadvantages [52]. General limitations of DNA damage tests are that they can be labor intensive and require significant experience to master, and in some cases can require significant initial investment. While data are accumulating as to their clinical utility, routine clinical adoption of these tests will require additional assay standardization and significantly more prospective clinical data.

Sperm aneuploidy screening likewise can be a technically difficult and relatively costly test, and is not indicated in most cases of male-factor infertility. It may be indicated in cases of oligozoospermia, particularly when accompanied by recurrent, unexplained pregnancy loss or IVF failure [50].

Tests of sperm chromatin composition including acridine orange staining, aniline blue staining, chromomycin A3 staining, protamine ratio assessment by acid gel electrophoresis, among others have all been demonstrated to correlate to some degree with clinical data, but significantly more research will be required before any of these tests can be adopted for routine clinical use [51].

In addition to these advanced tests, a number of functional tests have been devised to better assess the capacity of sperm to successfully fertilize an oocyte. These tests include the hemizona assay [53], the sperm penetration assay [54], and the acrosome reaction test [55]. These tests likewise offer important information regarding different facets of sperm function not assessed by the standard semen analysis, however the tests are generally quite technical with significant inter-laboratory variability. They are used routinely in some clinical laboratories, but have not reached the status of mainstream due to the technical limitations as well as a general lack of prospective clinical studies.

Conclusions

It is only in the past few years that we have begun to appreciate the epigenetic complexity of sperm as well as the apparent importance of the correct epigenetic architecture of sperm for fertility [44–46, 56]. In addition, incremental progress is being made to characterize novel genetic causes of male infertility [57–59]. Likewise changes in the transcriptomes and proteomes of sperm and semen in infertile compared with fertile men are currently being elucidated [47, 60]. Increased understanding in these arenas will be critical in advancing diagnostic capabilities in infertile men.

The standard semen analysis will continue to be an important fundamental assessment of male fertility potential, however it is likely that the assay will evolve with the advent of new technologies and with the increased understanding of the etiologies of male-factor infertility that is sure to come in the years and decades ahead. As characterization of the molecular signatures (DNA sequence, epigenetic state, and RNA and protein expression) of fertile and infertile sperm increases, new tools for the precise assessment of fertility status will likely become available. As genomic tools become increasingly accessible and affordable, and clinically relevant tests are developed and validated, these tools will likely be widely applied as a supplement to the limited data generated by the current semen analysis. These advances will serve to improve diagnosis and treatment in the infertile male.

References

1. World Health Organization. *WHO Laboratory Manual for the Examination and Processing of Human Semen.* 5th edn. Geneva: World Health Organization; 2010.

2. Dong F, Sun Y, Su Y *et al.* Relationship between processed total motile sperm count of husband or donor semen and pregnancy outcome following intrauterine insemination. *Syst Biol Reprod Med.* 2011;**57**(5):251–5.

3. Demir B, Dilbaz B, Cinar O *et al.* Factors affecting pregnancy outcome of intrauterine insemination cycles in couples with favourable female characteristics. *J Obstet Gynaecol.* 2011;**31**(5):420–3.

4. Larsen L, Scheike T, Jensen TK *et al.* Computer-assisted semen analysis parameters as predictors for fertility of men from the general population. The Danish first pregnancy planner study team. *Hum Reprod.* 2000;**15**(7):1562–7.

5. Zinaman MJ, Brown CC, Selevan SG *et al.* Semen quality and human fertility: a prospective study with healthy couples. *J Androl.* 2000;**21**(1):145–53.

6. Merviel P, Heraud MH, Grenier N *et al.* Predictive factors for pregnancy after intrauterine insemination (IUI): an analysis of 1038 cycles and a review of the literature. *Fertil Steril.* 2010;**93**(1):79–88.

7. Slama R, Eustache F, Ducot B *et al.* Time to pregnancy and semen parameters: a cross-sectional study among fertile couples from four European cities. *Hum Reprod.* 2002;**17**(2):503–15.

8. Bjorndahl L, Soderlund I, Kvist U. Evaluation of the one-step eosin-nigrosin staining technique for human sperm vitality assessment. *Hum Reprod.* 2003;**18**(4):813–16.

9. Jeyendran RS, Van der Ven HH, Perez-Pelaez M *et al.* Development of an assay to assess the functional integrity of the human sperm membrane and its relationship to other semen characteristics. *J Reprod Fertil.* 1984;**70**(1):219–28.

10. Chan SY, Wang C, Chan ST *et al.* Predictive value of sperm morphology and movement characteristics in the outcome of in vitro fertilization of human oocytes. *J In Vitro Fert Embryo Transf.* 1989;**6**(3):142–8.

11. Coetzee K, Kruge TF, Lombard CJ. Predictive value of normal sperm morphology: a structured literature review. *Hum Reprod Update.* 1998;**4**(1):73–82.

12. Ombelet W, Menkveld R, Kruger TF *et al.* Sperm morphology assessment: historical review in relation to fertility. *Hum Reprod Update.* 1995;**1**(6):543–57.

13. Menkveld R, Wong WY, Lombard CJ *et al.* Semen parameters, including WHO and strict criteria morphology, in a fertile and subfertile population: an effort towards standardization of in-vivo thresholds. *Hum Reprod.* 2001;**16**(6):1165–71.

14. Fredricsson B, Bjork G. Morphology of postcoital spermatozoa in the cervical secretion and its clinical significance. *Fertil Steril.* 1977;**28**(8):841–5.

15. Menkveld R, Franken DR, Kruger TF *et al.* Sperm selection capacity of the human zona pellucida. *Mol Reprod Dev.* 1991;**30**(4):346–52.

16. Bjorndahl L. What is normal semen quality? On the use and abuse of reference limits for the interpretation of semen analysis results. *Hum Fertil (Camb).* 2011;**14**(3):179–86.

17. Neuwinger J, Behre HM, Nieschlag E. External quality control in the andrology laboratory: an experimental multicenter trial. *Fertil Steril.* 1990;**54**(2):308–14.

18. Gandini L, Menditto A, Chiodo F *et al.* From the European Academy of Andrology. Italian pilot study for an external quality control scheme in semen analysis and antisperm antibiotics detection. *Int J Androl.* 2000;**23**(1):1–3.

19. Brazil C, Swan SH, Tollner CR *et al.* Quality control of laboratory methods for semen evaluation in a multicenter research study. *J Androl.* 2004;**25**(4):645–56.

20. Dunphy BC, Kay R, Barratt CL *et al.* Quality control during the conventional analysis of semen, an essential exercise. *J Androl.* 1989;**10**(5):378–85.

21. Palacios ER, Clavero A, Gonzalvo MC *et al.* Acceptable variability in external quality assessment programmes for basic semen analysis. *Hum Reprod.* 2012;**27**(2):314–22.

22. Mortimer D, Shu MA, Tan R. Standardization and quality control of sperm concentration and sperm motility counts in semen analysis. *Hum Reprod.* 1986;**1**(5):299–303.

23. Levitas E, Lunenfeld E, Weiss N *et al.* Relationship between the duration of sexual abstinence and semen quality: analysis of 9,489 semen samples. *Fertil Steril.* 2005;**83**(6):1680–6.

24. De Jonge C, LaFromboise M, Bosmans E *et al.* Influence of the abstinence period on human sperm quality. *Fertil Steril.* 2004;**82**(1):57–65.

25. Blackwell JM, Zaneveld LJ. Effect of abstinence on sperm acrosin, hypoosmotic swelling, and other semen variables. *Fertil Steril.* 1992;**58**(4):798–802.

26. Schwartz D, Laplanche A, Jouannet P *et al.* Within-subject variability of human semen in regard to sperm count, volume, total number of spermatozoa and length of abstinence. *J Reprod Fertil.* 1979;**57**(2):391–5.

27. Mortimer D, Templeton AA, Lenton EA *et al.* Influence of abstinence and ejaculation-to-analysis delay on semen analysis parameters of suspected infertile men. *Arch Androl.* 1982;**8**(4):251–6.

28. Leushuis E, van der Steeg JW, Steures P *et al.* Reproducibility and reliability of repeated semen analyses in male partners of subfertile couples. *Fertil Steril.* 2010;**94**(7):2631–5.

29. Carlsen E, Petersen JH, Andersson AM *et al.* Effects of ejaculatory frequency and season on variations in semen quality. *Fertil Steril.* 2004;**82**(2):358–66.

30. Cagnacci A, Maxia N, Volpe A. Diurnal variation of semen quality in human males. *Hum Reprod.* 1999;**14**(1):106–9.

31. Yogev L, Kleiman S, Shabtai E *et al.* Seasonal variations in pre- and post-thaw donor sperm quality. *Hum Reprod.* 2004;**19**(4):880–5.

32. Centola GM, Eberly S. Seasonal variations and age-related changes in human sperm count, motility, motion parameters, morphology, and white blood cell concentration. *Fertil Steril.* 1999;**72**(5):803–8.

33. Carlsen E, Andersson AM, Petersen JH *et al.* History of febrile illness and variation in semen quality. *Hum Reprod.* 2003;**18**(10):2089–92.

34. Jung A, Schuppe HC. Influence of genital heat stress on semen quality in humans. *Andrologia.* 2007;**39**(6):203–15.

35. Domes T, Lo KC, Grober ED *et al.* The incidence and effect of bacteriospermia and elevated seminal leukocytes on semen parameters. *Fertil Steril.* 2012;**97**(5):1050–5.

36. Lamb DJ. Semen analysis in 21st century medicine: the need for sperm function testing. *Asian J Androl.* 2010;**12**(1):64–70.

37. Liu DY, Baker HW. Evaluation and assessment of semen for IVF/ICSI. *Asian J Androl.* 2002;**4**(4):281–5.

38. Natali A, Turek PJ. An assessment of new sperm tests for male infertility. *Urology.* 2011;**77**(5):1027–34.

39. De Jonge C. Semen analysis: looking for an upgrade in class. *Fertil Steril.* 2012;**97**(2):260–6.

40. Oates RD. Clinical evaluation of the infertile male with respect to genetic etiologies. *Syst Biol Reprod Med.* 2011;**57**(1–2):72–7.

41. Taylor SL, Yoon SY, Morshedi MS *et al.* Complete globozoospermia associated with PLCzeta deficiency treated with calcium ionophore and ICSI results in pregnancy. *Reprod Biomed Online.* 2010;**20**(4):559–64.

42. Mangoli V, Mangoli R, Dandekar S *et al.* Selection of viable spermatozoa from testicular biopsies: a comparative study between pentoxifylline and hypoosmotic swelling test. *Fertil Steril.* 2011;**95**(2):631–4.

43. Cooper TG, Noonan E, von Eckardstein S *et al.* World Health Organization reference values for human semen characteristics. *Hum Reprod Update.* 2010;**16**(3):231–45.

44. Hammoud SS, Nix DA, Hammoud AO *et al.* Genome-wide analysis identifies changes in histone retention and epigenetic modifications at developmental and imprinted gene loci in the sperm of infertile men. *Hum Reprod.* 2011;**26**(9):2558–69.

45. Hammoud SS, Nix DA, Zhang H *et al.* Distinctive chromatin in human sperm packages genes for embryo development. *Nature.* 2009;**460**(7254):473–8.

46. Carrell DT, Hammoud SS. The human sperm epigenome and its potential role in embryonic development. *Mol Hum Reprod.* 2010;**16**(1):37–47.

47. Hamatani T. Human spermatozoal RNAs. *Fertil Steril.* 2012;**97**(2):275–81.

48. Krawetz SA, Kruger A, Lalancette C *et al.* A survey of small RNAs in human sperm. *Hum Reprod.* 2011;**26**(12):3401–12.

49. Schulte RT, Ohl DA, Sigman M *et al.* Sperm DNA damage in male infertility: etiologies, assays, and outcomes. *J Assist Reprod Genet.* 2010;**27**(1):3–12.

50. Templado C, Vidal F, Estop A. Aneuploidy in human spermatozoa. *Cytogenet Genome Res.* 2011;**133**(2–4):91–9.

51. Kazerooni T, Asadi N, Jadid L *et al.* Evaluation of sperm's chromatin quality with acridine orange test, chromomycin a3 and aniline blue staining in couples with unexplained recurrent abortion. *J Assist Reprod Genet.* 2009;**26**(11–12):591–6.

52. Shamsi MB, Imam SN, Dada R. Sperm DNA integrity assays: diagnostic and prognostic challenges and implications in management of infertility. *J Assist Reprod Genet.* 2011;**28**(11):1073–85.

53. Burkman LJ, Coddington CC, Franken DR *et al.* The hemizona assay (HZA): development of a diagnostic test for the binding of human spermatozoa to the human hemizona pellucida to predict fertilization potential. *Fertil Steril.* 1988;**49**(4):688–97.

54. Yanagimachi R, Yanagimachi H, Rogers BJ. The use of zona-free animal ova as a test-system for the assessment of the fertilizing capacity of human spermatozoa. *Biol Reprod.* 1976;**15**(4):471–6.

55. Sanchez R, Toepfer-Petersen E, Aitken RJ *et al.* A new method for evaluation of the acrosome reaction in viable human spermatozoa. *Andrologia.* 1991;**23**(3):197–203.

56. Miller D, Brinkworth M, Iles D. Paternal DNA packaging in spermatozoa: more than the sum of its parts? DNA, histones, protamines and epigenetics. *Reproduction.* 2010;**139**(2):287–301.

57. Aston KI, Carrell DT. Genome-wide study of single-nucleotide polymorphisms associated with azoospermia and severe oligozoospermia. *J Androl.* 2009;**30**(6):711–25.

58. Tuttelmann F, Simoni M, Kliesch S *et al.* Copy number variants in patients with severe oligozoospermia and Sertoli-cell-only syndrome. *PLoS One.* 2011;**6**(4):e19426.

59. Hu Z, Xia Y, Guo X *et al.* A genome-wide association study in Chinese men identifies three risk loci for non-obstructive azoospermia. *Nat Genet.* 2012;**44**(2):183–6.

60. du Plessis SS , Kashou AH, Benjamin DJ *et al.* Proteomics: a subcellular look at spermatozoa. *Reprod Biol Endocrinol.* 2011;**9**:36.

Semen characteristics and aging: technical considerations regarding variability

Lars Björndahl

Introduction

A general consideration in medicine is the expected changes in organ functions with increasing age. Therefore many scientists have attempted the challenge to determine possible age-dependent changes in semen characteristics. There are, however, a number of hurdles that can cause bias and lead to wrong conclusions.

In this review, only classical semen analysis characteristics have been addressed. In recent years, studies attempting to measure the integrity of sperm DNA have become increasingly common, although the exact nature of what the different methods actually measure is not known in detail [1]. Sperm DNA investigations are covered more extensively in Chapters 2 and 9.

Biological and physiological sources of variation

It is well known that in a healthy, fertile man semen sample characteristics can vary a lot from one sample to another. The main cause for this is the variability of the different organ functions necessary to produce an ejaculate. For a certain man, it is likely that one of the most stable factors is the testicular output of spermatozoa. The hypothalamic–pituitary control of sperm production is based on LH and FSH stimulation leading to maintained androgen production in the testis and in general sustained peripheral androgen levels in the body in healthy aging men [2] – contrary to the disappearance of hormonal stimulation occurring in women at menopause. Although hypogonadism may not be a very common problem, it is still important to consider the possibility of hypogonadism in men with signs of poor sperm production and offer a full clinical investigation.

An element in ejaculate formation that is likely to have a non-pathological variability is the transport of spermatozoa from the storage in the tail of the epididymis to the urethra. This function is primarily dependent on the activity of the autonomic nervous system, the vas deferens consisting of smooth musculature with one of the densest autonomic innervations in the body [3]. Besides considerable non-pathological variation this also means that early autonomic neuropathology in, for example, diabetes mellitus is, at least theoretically, likely to affect the function of the vas deferens and sperm transport to the urethra.

Another part of ejaculation that is under autonomic nerve control is the activation and emptying of the accessory sex glands, the prostate, and the seminal vesicles. Unlike for instance urine production, as far as it is known, accessory sex gland secretion is not a continuous phenomenon but almost completely dependent on the duration and intensity of sexual stimulation [4]. It is not known how the sequential emptying of the prostate and seminal vesicles is controlled, but judging from studies on the sequence of ejaculation [5] and on the urological diagnosis of ejaculatory duct obstruction [6, 7], it appears that pathological obstructions for the normal transport of spermatozoa to the urethra can cause abnormal sequence of ejaculation and abnormal contact between seminal vesicular fluid and spermatozoa, causing impairment of sperm motility, survival, and DNA protection [5].

Thus, variability in semen characteristics is significant even without any disorders involved. This makes it difficult to detect if there are any small, age-dependent changes occurring with increasing age.

Paternal Influences on Human Reproductive Success, ed. Douglas T. Carrell. Published by Cambridge University Press.
© Cambridge University Press 2013.

Variation due to bias in the selection of study participants

Ideally, an age-dependent variation in semen characteristics should be investigated in the "general population." This is not easy to achieve; not every man can be expected to volunteer providing at least one semen sample for such a research purpose. Contrary to laboratory investigations involving other body fluids, collection of semen samples is connected to sexuality. Therefore one cannot be sure to what extent volunteers from the general population are truly representative for this group [8].

If the representativeness can be questioned for recruitments from the general population, it is even more questionable to use patient groups to make conclusions regarding general trends related to increasing age. Patients referred for semen analysis are usually already selected because of infertility problems. It is not unlikely that disorders causing subfertility or infertility among older men in this population are more severe compared with younger men in the population – the older men probably have tried for far longer before seeking help or suffer from a secondary infertility (while older men without problems to conceive will not be included in the study group).

A third problem related to study participants is that the individuals in the population that is investigated have very different backgrounds. A younger man has not experienced the same environment as older men – they were not fetuses, children, and adolescents during the same time periods. For instance the incidence of testis cancer has been shown to be very different in different birth cohorts [9]. Thus, it may be that effects attributed to "age" are more an effect of the year of birth [10]. To address this issue, it is essential to investigate semen characteristics of the same population at different time points, where each man can be his own control.

Variability due to choice of laboratory methods

When evaluating the strength of evidence in studies on a possible relation between age and semen characteristics the choice of methods can be of great significance. If methods are not robust and low numbers of participants have been included, then the uncertainty inherent to the procedures can actually prevent true relations from being discovered. To a certain degree an increased number of participants may at least partially compensate for

technical inadequacy, but it is less demanding in terms of workload to follow international recommendations on standardized and robust laboratory techniques, as described elsewhere [2, 11, 12].

A review of the literature regarding aging and semen quality

There is no unanimous conclusion regarding relations between age and semen characteristics. If there are true changes with increasing age, the problems with lack of standardization of methods and bias in selection of study participants obscure the results and conceal the differences. In the condensed summary of the results here, a huge variety of characteristics have been aggregated into a few common entities like "concentration," "motility," "morphology" etc. Many studies have come to the conclusion based on group differences between different age cohorts, while a few have done correlation analyses between age and different semen parameters and also presented "R" or "R^2" values from which it can be concluded that although the relation can be considered statistically significant, increased age typically causes less than 1% of the variability in the semen characteristic investigated. Since most studies have not included this element of analysis, the "level of influence" has not been useful to include in this review.

Only one study involved investigations on the same individual at different ages – and this study only comprised one individual at 40 and 50 years of age, respectively. The significance of the data is therefore very limited until more individuals are included at younger and older ages.

Studies on non-patients

Among studies of individuals not primarily investigated for subfertility (Table 18.1) 8/14 studies did not find a difference in sperm concentration. Among those that found a difference, one discovered increased sperm concentration and five a decrease with increasing age. When total sperm number was studied 5/9 did not find any difference and four revealed a decrease. For motility 3/12 saw no change and 9/12 found a decrease. For sperm morphology one study reported both a decrease ("WHO criteria") and no difference ("strict criteria"), although these criteria were supposed to be the same [13, 14], thus disclosing the general problem of poor global standardization. Among the other studies reporting on sperm morphology, two found a decrease by

Table 18.1 Summary of findings in studies involving participants which had not been primarily referred for infertility investigation. When results are reported for a combined population, all groups contributing are given as "participants." Computer-assisted sperm analysis (CASA): HTM, Hamilton Thorne; VP50, CP50 Semen analyzer; SM, Strömberg Mika.

Reference	Study type	Participants	N	Age	Methods	Abstinence	Volume	pH	Concentration	Total number	Motility	CASA	Morphology	% Live
Zhu et al., 2011 [16]	P	General population	998	20–60	WHO 92		=		=	=	↓		↓	
Brahem et al., 2011 [17]	P	Fertile donors	50	25–65	WHO 99		=		=	=	=		=[1]	=
Colin et al., 2010 [18]	P	Fertile donors	25	20–68	WHO 10				↓[2]					
Winkle et al., 2009 [19]	P	Donor	84	?-?	WHO 99				=[3]		=		=	
Sergerie et al., 2006 [20]	?	Fertile donors	1	40, 50	WHO 99				=	=	=		=	=
Sloter et al., 2006 [21]	P	Employees	90	22–80	CASA HTM				=	=		=[4],↓[5]		
Hellstrom et al., 2006 [22]	R	Erectile dysfunction	1174	45–80	Overstreet et al., 1997 [23]		↓		=	↓			↓	
Pasqualotto et al., 2005 [24]	R	Prevasectomy men	889	24–67	WHO 99/ CASA VP50		↓		↓[6]		↓	=	=[7],↓[8]	
Henkel et al., 2005 [25]	P	Patients and donors	157	21–57	WHO ?/ CASA SM				↓		↓	↓[9]		
Singh et al., 2003 [26]	R	Patients, donors, prevasectomy men	66	20–57	WHO 99/ CASA HTM	↑			↓	=	↓		=	

Table 18.1 (cont.)

Reference	Study type	Participants	N	Age	Methods	Abstinence	Volume	pH	Concentration	Total number	Motility	CASA	Morphology	% Live
Eskenazi et al., 2003 [27]	R	Employees	97	22–80	WHO 92/ CASA HTM		↓		=	↓	↓			
Luetjens et al., 2002 [28]	P	General population	27	22–29 60–71	WHO 99		=		=		↓		=	
Bonde et al., 1998 [10]	P	Occupational exposure	1196	20–56	WHO 80	↑			↓[10]	↓				
Haidl et al., 1996 [29]	P	Secondary infertile patients Fertile donors	29 35	45–63 26–35	WHO 92	=			↓		↓		=	
Mladenovic et al., 1994 [30]	R	Fathers Grandfathers	24 15	25–36 60–84	WHO 80	↑	=		↑	↑	↓		=	
Sartorelli et al., 2001 [31]	P	Donors	7 5	59–74 23–39	WHO 92		↓		↓	↓	↓		=	↓

[1] David system.
[2] Makler counting chamber.
[3] Makler counting chamber.
[4] Motile, rapid, progressive.
[5] LIN, VSL, VAP.
[6] Makler counting chamber.
[7] Tygerberg strict criteria.
[8] WHO criteria.
[9] VAP, VSL, VCL, LIN, ALH.
[10] Makler counting chamber.

Table 18.2 Summary of findings in studies involving primarily patients referred for infertility investigation. Study type: P, Prospective, R, Retrospective. Participants: when selected from treatment groups: IUI, intrauterine insemination; IVF, in vitro fertilization; ICSI, intracytoplasmic sperm injection; OD, oocyte donation; VE, prevasectomy men. Computer-assisted sperm analysis (CASA): HTM, Hamilton Thorne; SM, Strömberg Mika; MC, Mika Cell.

Reference	Study Type	Participants	N	Age	Methods	Abstinence	Volume	pH	Concentration	Total number	Motility	CASA	Morphology	% Live
Rybar et al., 2011 [32]	P	IVF	153	20–61	WHO 99		=		=		=		=	
Nijs et al., 2011 [33]	P	IVF-ICSI	278	25–56	WHO 99		=		=		=		=	
Brahem et al., 2011 [17]	P	Infertility	140	24–76	WHO 99		↓		↑	=	=		=[1]	↓
Paasch et al., 2010 [34]	P?	Infertility	2157	17–67	WHO 99 / CASA MC					↓	↓	↓	↓	
Mukhopadhyay et al., 2010 [35]	R	Infertility	3729		WHO 80–99		=		↑[2]		↓		↓	
Molina et al., 2010 [36]	R	Infertility	9168	20–77	WHO 92		↓			↓[3]	↓		↑	↓
Cardona Maya et al., 2009 [37]	R	Infertility	1364	17–59	WHO 92		↓		↓[4]	↓	↓		↓	
Winkle et al., 2009 [19]	P	Infertility	320	24–56	WHO 99		=		=[5]	↓	=		=[6]	
Girsh et al., 2008 [38]	R	Infertility	484	25–60	WHO 92		↓		↓[7]	↓	↓		↓[8]	
Henkel et al., 2007 [39]	R	Infertility	1942	17–66	WHO 99		↓	↑	↑	↓	↓		↓	
Levitas et al., 2007 [40]	R	IUI	6022	<25->55	WHO 99	↑	↓		↑[9]	↓	↓		↓	
Plastira et al., 2007 [41]	P	ICSi	25	20–50	WHO 99		=		=		=		↓	
Siddighi et al., 2007 [42]	P	Infertility	186	<30->45	?				=		↓		=	↓
Zavos et al., 2006 [43]	P	IVF IUI	792	20–60	WHO 99		↓		↓	↓	↓		↓	↓

Table 18.2 (cont.)

Reference	Study Type	Participants	N	Age	Methods	Abstinence	Volume	pH	Concentration	Total number	Motility	CASA	Morphology	% Live
Henkel et al., 2005 [25]	R	Infertility	2111	17–66	WHO ? / CASA SM		↓		↑		↓		=[10]	
Henkel et al., 2005 [25]	P	Infertility + donors	157	21–57	WHO ?				↓		↓	↓		
Singh et al., 2003 [26]	R	Infertility +donors+VE	66	20–57	WHO 99 / CASA HTM	↑				=	↓		=	
Eskenazi et al., 2003 [27]	R	Infertility	904	20–66	WHO 99 / CASA ?		↓	=	↓	↓	↓		↓	
Paulson et al., 2001 [44]	R	IVF	441	22–64	?		=	=	=	↑	=		=	
Centola and Eberly, 1999 [45]	R	Infertility	1434	19–67	WHO 92 / CASA HTM		=		↓		↓	=		
Bellver et al., 2008 [46]	R	IUI, IVF, OD	3669	19–71	?		↓		↓		↓			

[1] David system.
[2] Makler counting chamber.
[3] Makler counting chamber.
[4] Makler counting chamber.
[5] Makler counting chamber.
[6] Not WHO.
[7] Makler counting chamber.
[8] SperMac staining, not WHO.
[9] Makler counting chamber.
[10] Düsseldorf system.

increasing age and eight could not reveal a change. Only three studies reported vitality results – two saw no change and one reported a decrease.

Studies on patients in subfertile couples

Studies based on patients referred for infertility investigations (Table 18.2) showed a very varied picture of sperm concentration variability: 6/18 showed no difference, 5/18 had an increase and 7/18 a decrease. For total sperm number the results were more consistent: 7/10 showed a decrease, 2/10 found no change and 1/10 revealed an increase. For motility 6/20 found no change and 7/20 revealed a decrease. For morphology 8/14 studies found no difference and 6/14 showed a decrease. All four studies reporting live or dead spermatozoa showed a decrease in proportion of live spermatozoa by increasing age.

Conclusion

Most studies on reproductive functions face unique problems that are not otherwise common in modern medical science in that fertility is a matter involving two individuals and not only one person. Another aspect is that recruitment of "controls" is influenced by social and cultural problems – is it at random which men volunteer to participate as healthy (and fertile) sperm donors? Furthermore, it is not simple to define what often is called "male factor" from a scientific point of view. On top of this (and partially due to difficulties to define, recruit, and study men other than those who are part of a subfertile couple) comes lack of standardization and in general quite poor technical standards in semen laboratories.

Therefore it is difficult to come to a unanimous conclusion of the literature in this field. The most consistent change by increased age was a decrease in sperm motility. This may be at least partially due to longer abstinence time, but cannot be taken as evidence for a loss of fertility potential, not least since observed differences are small and there are no sharp limits between fertile and infertile [15].

References

1. Barratt CL, Aitken RJ, Bjorndahl L et al. Sperm DNA: organization, protection and vulnerability: from basic science to clinical applications – a position report. *Hum Reprod.* 2010;**25**(4):824–38.

2. Barratt CL, Bjorndahl L, Menkveld R et al. ESHRE special interest group for andrology basic semen analysis course: a continued focus on accuracy, quality, efficiency and clinical relevance. *Hum Reprod.* 2011;**26**(12):3207–12.

3. Wagner G, Sjösten NO. Autonomic pharmacology and sexual function. In Sjösten A, editor. *The Pharmacology and Endocrinology of Sexual Function.* Amsterdam: Elsevier Science Publishers; 1988.

4. Yamamoto Y, Sofikitis N, Mio Y et al. Influence of sexual stimulation on sperm parameters in semen samples collected via masturbation from normozoospermic men or cryptozoospermic men participating in an assisted reproduction programme. *Andrologia.* 2000;**32**(3):131–8.

5. Björndahl L, Kvist U. Sequence of ejaculation affects the spermatozoon as a carrier and its message. *Reprod Biomed Online.* 2003;**7**(4):440–8.

6. Dohle GR. Inflammatory-associated obstructions of the male reproductive tract. *Andrologia.* 2003;**35**(5):321–4.

7. Fisch H, Lambert SM, Goluboff ET. Management of ejaculatory duct obstruction: etiology, diagnosis, and treatment. *World J Urol.* 2006;**24**(6):604–10.

8. Gandini L, Lombardo F, Culasso F et al. Myth and reality of the decline in semen quality: an example of the relativity of data interpretation. *J Endocrinol Invest.* 2000;**23**(6):402–11.

9. Richiardi L, Bellocco R, Adami HO et al. Testicular cancer incidence in eight northern European countries: secular and recent trends. *Cancer Epidemiol Biomarkers Prevent.* 2004;**13**(12):2157–66.

10. Bonde JP, Kold Jensen T, Brixen Larsen S et al. Year of birth and sperm count in 10 Danish occupational studies. *Scand J Work, Environ Health.* 1998;**24**(5):407–13.

11. World Health Organization. *WHO Laboratory Manual for the Examination and Processing of Human Semen.* 5th edn. Geneva: WHO; 2010.

12. Björndahl L, Mortimer D, Barratt CLR et al. *A Practical Guide to Basic Laboratory Andrology.* 1st edn. Cambridge: Cambridge University Press; 2010.

13. World Health Organization. *WHO Laboratory Manual for the Examination of Human Semen and Sperm-Cervical Mucus Interactions.* 4th edn. Cambridge: Cambridge University Press; 1999.

14. Mortimer D, Menkveld R. Sperm morphology assessment – historical perspectives and current opinions. *J Androl.* 2001;**22**(2):192–205.

15. Björndahl L. What is normal semen quality? On the use and abuse of reference limits for the interpretation of semen analysis results. *Hum Fertil (Camb).* 2011;**14**(3):179–86.

16. Zhu QX, Meads C, Lu ML et al. Turning point of age for semen quality: A population-based study in Chinese men. *Fertil Steril.* 2011 Sep;**96**(3):572–6.

17. Brahem S, Mehdi M, Elghezal H *et al.* The effects of male aging on semen quality, sperm DNA fragmentation and chromosomal abnormalities in an infertile population. *J Assist Reprod Genet.* 2011;**28**(5):425–32.

18. Colin A, Barroso G, Gomez-Lopez N *et al.* The effect of age on the expression of apoptosis biomarkers in human spermatozoa. *Fertil Steril.* 2010;**94**(7):2609–14.

19. Winkle T, Rosenbusch B, Gagsteiger F *et al.* The correlation between male age, sperm quality and sperm DNA fragmentation in 320 men attending a fertility center. *J Assist Reprod Genet.* 2009;**26**(1):41–6.

20. Sergerie M, Mieusset R, Daudin M *et al.* Ten-year variation in semen parameters and sperm deoxyribonucleic acid integrity in a healthy fertile man. *Fertil Steril.* 2006;**86**(5):1513 e11–18.

21. Sloter E, Schmid TE, Marchetti F *et al.* Quantitative effects of male age on sperm motion. *Hum Reprod (Oxford).* 2006;**21**(11):2868–75.

22. Hellstrom WJ, Overstreet JW, Sikka SC *et al.* Semen and sperm reference ranges for men 45 years of age and older. *J Androl.* 2006;**27**(3):421–8.

23. Overstreet JW, Brazil C. Semen analysis. In Lipschulz LI, Howards SS, editors. *Infertility in the Male.* 3rd edn. St Louis, MO: Mosby Year Book, Inc; 1997, pp. 487–90.

24. Pasqualotto FF, Sobreiro BP, Hallak J *et al.* Sperm concentration and normal sperm morphology decrease and follicle-stimulating hormone level increases with age. *BJU Int.* 2005;**96**(7):1087–91.

25. Henkel R, Maass G, Schuppe HC *et al.* Molecular aspects of declining sperm motility in older men. *Fertil Steril.* 2005;**84**(5):1430–7.

26. Singh NP, Muller CH, Berger RE. Effects of age on DNA double-strand breaks and apoptosis in human sperm. *Fertil Steril.* 2003;**80**(6):1420–30.

27. Eskenazi B, Wyrobek AJ, Sloter E *et al.* The association of age and semen quality in healthy men. *Hum Reprod (Oxford).* 2003;**18**(2):447–54.

28. Luetjens CM, Rolf C, Gassner P *et al.* Sperm aneuploidy rates in younger and older men. *Hum Reprod (Oxford).* 2002;**17**(7):1826–32.

29. Haidl G, Jung A, Schill WB. Ageing and sperm function. *Hum Reprod (Oxford).* 1996;**11**(3):558–60.

30. Mladenovic I, Micic S, Papic N *et al.* Sperm morphology and motility in different age populations. *Archiv Androl.* 1994;**32**(3):197–205.

31. Sartorelli EM, Mazzucatto LF, de Pina-Neto JM. Effect of paternal age on human sperm chromosomes. *Fertil Steril.* 2001;**76**(6):1119–23.

32. Rybar R, Kopecka V, Prinosilova P *et al.* Male obesity and age in relationship to semen parameters and sperm chromatin integrity. *Andrologia.* 2011;**43**(4):286–91.

33. Nijs M, De Jonge C, Cox A *et al.* Correlation between male age, WHO sperm parameters, DNA fragmentation, chromatin packaging and outcome in assisted reproduction technology. *Andrologia.* 2011;**43**(3):174–9.

34. Paasch U, Grunewald S, Kratzsch J *et al.* Obesity and age affect male fertility potential. *Fertil Steril.* 2010;**94**(7):2898–901.

35. Mukhopadhyay D, Varghese AC, Pal M *et al.* Semen quality and age-specific changes: a study between two decades on 3,729 male partners of couples with normal sperm count and attending an andrology laboratory for infertility-related problems in an Indian city. *Fertil Steril.* 2010;**93**(7):2247–54.

36. Molina RI, Martini AC, Tissera A *et al.* Semen quality and aging: analysis of 9,168 samples in Cordoba, Argentina. *Arch Esp Urol.* 2010;**63**(3):214–22.

37. Cardona Maya W, Berdugo J, Cadavid Jaramillo A. The effects of male age on semen parameters: analysis of 1364 men attending an andrology center. *Aging Male: Official J Int Soc Study Aging Male.* 2009;**12**(4):100–3.

38. Girsh E, Katz N, Genkin L *et al.* Male age influences oocyte-donor program results. *J Assist Reprod Genet.* 2008;**25**(4):137–43.

39. Henkel R, Maass G, Jung A *et al.* Age-related changes in seminal polymorphonuclear elastase in men with asymptomatic inflammation of the genital tract. *Asian J Androl.* 2007;**9**(3):299–304.

40. Levitas E, Lunenfeld E, Weisz N *et al.* Relationship between age and semen parameters in men with normal sperm concentration: analysis of 6022 semen samples. *Andrologia.* 2007;**39**(2):45–50.

41. Plastira K, Angelopoulou R, Mantas D *et al.* The effects of age on the incidence of aneuploidy rates in spermatozoa of oligoasthenozoospermic patients and its relationship with ICSI outcome. *Int J Androl.* 2007;**30**(2):65–72.

42. Siddighi S, Chan CA, Patton WC *et al.* Male age and sperm necrosis in assisted reproductive technologies. *Urol Int.* 2007;**79**(3):231–4.

43. Zavos PM, Kaskar K, Correa JR *et al.* Seminal characteristics and sexual behavior in men of different age groups: is there an aging effect? *Asian J Androl.* 2006;**8**(3):337–41.

44. Paulson RJ, Milligan RC, Sokol RZ. The lack of influence of age on male fertility. *Am J Obstet Gynecol.* 2001;**184**(5):818–22; discussion 822–4.

45. Centola GM, Eberly S. Seasonal variations and age-related changes in human sperm count, motility, motion parameters, morphology, and white blood cell concentration. *Fertil Steril.* 1999;**72**(5):803–8.

46. Bellver J, Garrido N, Remohi J *et al.* Influence of paternal age on assisted reproduction outcome. *Reprod Biomed Online.* 2008;**17**(5):595–604.

Index